REGULATING
romance

Main Points

① Youth Sexuality
② Marriage and HIV
③ Gender & Antiretrovirals
④ Mobility, Extractive Economies
   and Sex Trade

→ Analyzes the dynamics of morality, desire, aspiration
→ 300 love letters written by Ugandan youth

REGULATING *romance*

YOUTH LOVE LETTERS, MORAL ANXIETY, AND INTERVENTION IN UGANDA'S TIME OF AIDS

shanti parikh

Vanderbilt University Press
Nashville

This book is printed on acid-free paper.
Manufactured in the United States of America

Library of Congress Cataloging-in-Publication Data on file
LC control number 2015003150
LC classification number RA643.86.U33P37 2015
Dewey class number 362.19697'920096761—dc23

ISBN 978-0-8265-1777-7 (hardcover)
ISBN 978-0-8265-1778-4 (paperback)
ISBN 978-0-8265-1779-1 (ebook)

I dedicate this book
to the memory of my parents:

Arvind Mukundrai Parikh
Eleanor Vernice Joyner Parikh

Contents

Illustrations

Figures

All photos were taken by the author unless otherwise stated.

Acknowledgments

This book is dedicated to people who have worked to alleviate the impact of the HIV epidemic and of inequality in Uganda and elsewhere in the world for the past thirty-plus years. Although what follows is a critique of interventions and their unintended consequences, the epidemic would likely be far worse without these workers' tireless efforts.

My greatest debt is to the residents of the Iganga region in eastern central Uganda who graciously allowed me into their lives from 1996 to 2015. I am especially grateful to the region's young people for sharing their love letters and the private stories from which these missives emerge. I have tried to represent the richness of their lives and their desires, but no doubt my accounts are partial and biased.

The companionship and dedication of a group of research assistants sustained me during each field research period and kept me connected to Iganga while in the United States. To Janet Kagoda and Gerald Isabirye Kigenyi—thank you for your years of diligent research assistance and keeping me intellectually accountable and engaged. We were joined by an equally steadfast group of assistants: Salim Wantati, Steven Waiswa, Ronald Ojambo, Ruth Nakaima, and Robert Butwala during my initial project on the history of coming of age and premarital romance, and Moses Mwesigwa, Harriet Mugulusi, John Ibemba, Francis Kyakulaga, and Charles Ojambo on subsequent projects. Many evenings of laughing, dancing, and singing as we organized research data and tasks are fondly remembered. I extend my deepest gratitude to my hosts in Bulubandi village, Mrs. Agaati Ojambo and her family, who welcomed me into their home and their lives despite my endless questions.

I had the honor of many insightful conversations with elders in the Iganga region. Thank you to my initial teachers, Mr. and Mrs. Peter Kigenyi; the wisemen of Bulubandi, the late Imam Kassan Wantati and the late Marichi Maiso; Mirembe Proscovia and the late Margaret Nakidodo, community women's leaders; the late Christopher Isabirye; Florence Kumunu, hero to many; the courageous Reverend Jackson and Nurse Catherine Njuba from IDAAC (Integrated Development Activities and AIDS Concern); the dedicated Nurse Rose and other staff at Iganga District Hospital; Bulubandi Literacy Group; the Iganga health officer, Mr. David Muwanguzi; and members of various cultural groups and HIV support groups spread throughout the region. Numerous teachers, staff, and students in Iganga invested time in this project even though youth romance was not a topic that most schools wanted to discuss openly. I wish to express special appreciation to David Balaba of Kings Secondary School, Father Damien Grimes of Namasagali Secondary School College, and the headmasters and staff at Nakigo Secondary School, Kasokoso Primary School, and Iganga Parents Secondary School, for allowing me the opportunity to spend time in their schools. And to all the young people in Iganga—my heartfelt thanks for teaching me about youth romance, hopes, and fears; I am inspired by your optimism, your enjoyment of laughter, and your care for your peers.

This project benefited from my having access to materials and perspectives on gender, sexuality, and regulation from a variety of people working at agencies in Iganga, including the Probate (Domestic Affairs) Office, the Family Planning Agency, the District Hospital and Ministry of Health, the Iganga Magistrate and Busoga High Courts, and the Iganga branch of the Uganda Taxi Operators and Drivers Association (UTODA). Many media outlets, sexual health and HIV organizations, women's and children's rights organizations, and government offices in Kampala also gave me access to their materials; I owe a special note of thanks to the newspaper *Straight Talk*, CBS and Simba radio stations, the publications *The Red Pepper* and *Chic*, Save the Children (Denmark), the Uganda AIDS Commission, and FIDA-Uganda (Federación Internacional de Abogadas, or International Federation of Women Lawyers).

Makerere Institute for Social Research (MISR) provided more than an academic affiliation. The faculty, researchers, and staff of MISR, together with Makerere University School of Public Health, provided an intellectual home to critical dialogue about this project. I received research clearance from Institutional Review Boards (IRBs) in the United States and the Uganda National Council of Science and Technology (UNCST). Funding for research and analysis was provided by a Henry Hart Rice fellowship, a Leadership Alliance fellowship, the Yale Center for International and Area Studies, a Fulbright New Century Scholar fellowship (Global Feminisms), American Recovery and Reinvestment Act (ARRA) NIH Grant 2933-66027, and National Institutes of Health (NIH) R01 Grant 41724-01A1.

More people have helped refine my analysis and read pieces of this book over the years than I can mention here. In addition to those in Uganda, mentioned above, I have been fortunate to receive input from faculty and students at Washington University in St. Louis and Yale University. I especially want to recognize my faculty advisors at Yale—Harold Scheffler, Linda-Anne Rebhun, and Kamari Clarke—for their guidance and insight during the early stages of this project. Thank you to my brilliant collaborators on the NIH project, especially Jennifer Hirsch, who commented on an earlier draft, and also Daniel Smith, Holly Wardlow, Harriet Phinney, and Constance Nathanson for many fun and intellectually stimulating meetings. Jennifer Cole provided useful organizational comments, as did her students in her course at the University of Chicago; Susan Whyte reminded me of value of the ethnographic story; and Richard Parker offered his insights on sexuality, desire, and structural violence. In addition, I would be remiss if I did not mention the engaging conversations that I had with faculty and students when I presented on various parts of this project, including Duke University's Sexualities Colloquium; St. Mary's College Women, Gender, and Sexuality Colloquium; University of Arizona's Women, Gender, and Sexuality Studies Mapping Insurgencies Conference; the Sex and Secrecy International Conference at the University of Witwatersrand; University of Illinois's African Studies Symposium; University of Michigan's African Development and Human Security Project (ADHSP); and Harvard University's African Studies Workshop.

Chapter 5 is based on material that appears in "From auntie to disco: The bifurcation of risk and pleasure in sex education in Uganda," in *Sex in Development*, edited by V. Adams and S. L. Pigg, 125–58. Durham, NC: Duke University Press; copyright 2005. Chapter 6 is an expansion of ideas considered in "'They arrested me for loving a schoolgirl': Ethnography, HIV, and a feminist assessment of the age of consent law as a gender-based structural intervention in Uganda," *Social Science & Medicine* 74 (11): 1774–82; copyright 2012.

Preparation of this manuscript has benefited from the reliable assistance of a number of students at Washington University: David Iffrig, Claire Chaney, Dan Bromberg, Rubabin Tooba, Heather Meiers, Scott Leif, Mattew Lee, and Tess Croner, as well as other students who assisted along the way. I am truly appreciative of the patience and the meticulous editorial eye of Michael Ames, director of Vanderbilt University Press, and the rest of the production and editing staff.

Finally, to my deliciously mischievous boys and endlessly supportive husband: my deepest gratitude and love. Thank you for bearing with me as I put this book to rest—my aspiring superhero, Julian Arvind; his always-in-motion big brother, Jason David; and my loving husband, Jason K. Wilson. Come, let's go play!

Introduction

On a hot day typical of the dry season in Iganga Town in the east-central part of Uganda, a lovesick Sam Mukungu penned these tender words to his beloved Birungi:

HEY!

LOVER,

It is with much preasure to have this chance of comminucating to you, How is life treating you all over that end Let me hope (wish) that you are "okay" on my side I am not okay due to much thought I have about you, In fact I don't know what I can (say) tell you about my life (thinking of you) or love because I have come to atime when I start thinking about you and I don't want to do anything even sleeping at time I start crying but lover why do you make me cry so I am requesting you by kindly to keep all the promise please be pacient and I am requesting by kindly try as much as you can to come as per the promise but remember all what I told you and what you told me?

In fact I have much to say but let me wait up to when we meet am sorry that I am missing you but let me pray up to when God allows us to meet so let me end here by wishing you the best in all what you do Good bye

I remain yours in

Love,

Sam[1]

Sam scribed the letter to his girlfriend, a nursing student in the nearby city of Jinja, as he sat in my research office-*cum*-makeshift living quarters in Iganga Town. Curious about what was keeping the typically jovial young man so focused and melancholy, I asked. He had not seen his dear Birungi for some time, he explained, because he lacked the money to arrange travel and her parents were discouraging her. Seeing my interest in the letter, Sam offered to give me a copy. He carefully wrote it out by hand, ensuring that the layout and penmanship resembled the original. Sam's letter became the catalyst for future conversations about his love for Birungi—his feelings, future dreams, and eventual heartbreak.

Sam and Birungi had been classmates in secondary school when they began their relationship. A year into their relationship, Sam's father died. Without the income from his father's prominent position with the local police department, Sam had to sit out of school periodically as his mother, Agnes, scrambled for school fees for his six younger siblings and two orphan relatives who lived with them. After performing poorly on the national standardized exam, Sam decided to drop out of school to pursue earning his

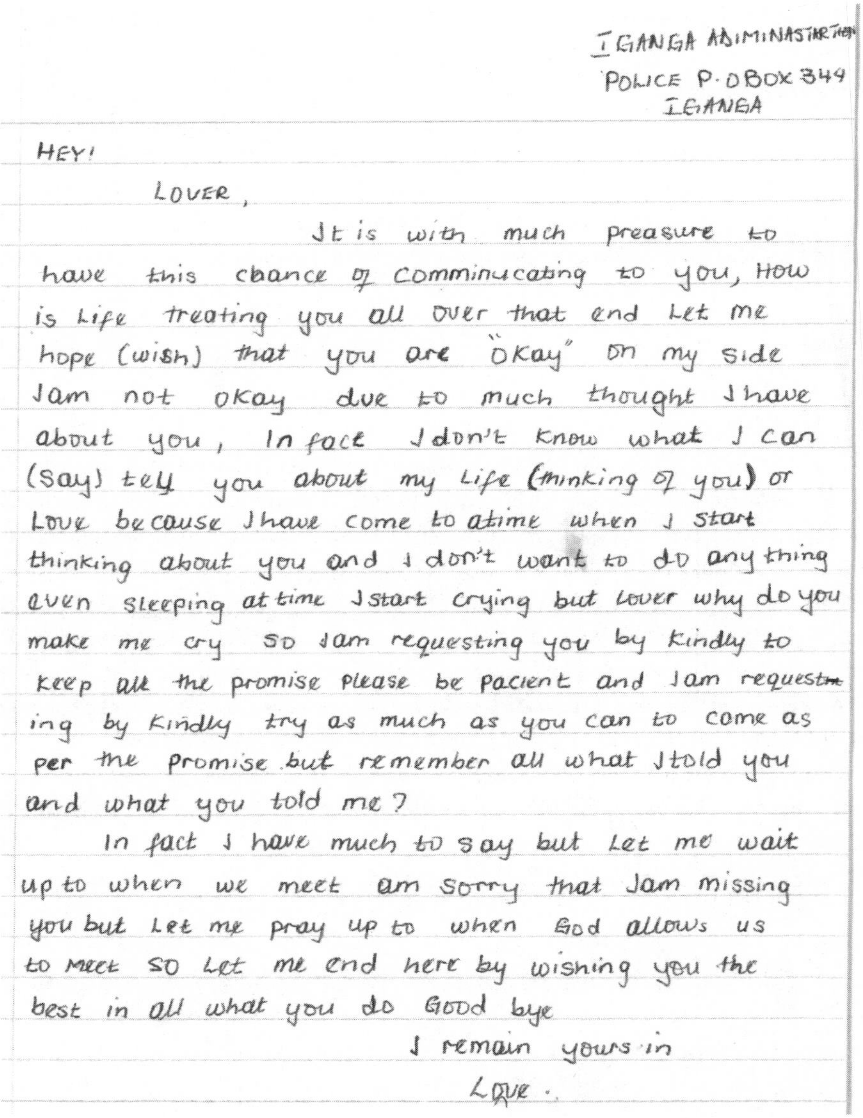

IGANGA ADIMINASTARTION
POLICE P.O BOX 349
IGANGA

HEY!

LOVER,

It is with much preasure to have this chance of comminucating to you, How is life treating you all over that end Let me hope (wish) that you are "Okay" on my side Jam not Okay due to much thought I have about you, In fact I don't know what I can (Say) tell you about my Life (minking of you) or Love because I have come to atime when I start thinking about you and i don't want to do anything even sleeping at time I start crying but Lover why do you make me cry so Jam requesting you by kindly to keep all the promise please be pacient and Jam requesting by kindly try as much as you can to come as per the promise but remember all what I told you and what you told me?

In fact I have much to say but Let me wait up to when we meet am sorry that Jam missing you but Let me pray up to when God allows us to meet So Let me end here by wishing you the best in all what you do Good bye

I remain yours in

LOVE.

FIGURE 1. Sam Mukungu's love letter to Birungi

own income. His late father's co-workers gave him an unsalaried position at the police department, which bestowed on him symbolic entrance and insight into the world of adult manhood. He hoped the position would turn into a formal appointment, but it never did and he was retained merely as an errand boy.

Birungi's family background and educational trajectory were markedly different from Sam's. She came from an educated, professional middle-class family in town, she easily finished secondary school, and she followed the health-care path of her older siblings, eventually settling in Jinja for her nursing practicum. When possible, Sam sent Birungi money, not only as a sign of his affection but also as a strategy to secure his place among her possible other suitors, though he was not able to send money and gifts as regularly as or in the amount that he would have liked.

Throughout their relationship, the young couple's privileging of romantic desire over the Basoga ideal of family involvement and approval gave both Sam's mother and Birungi's parents reason to disapprove of the relationship. There were economic issues at play as well. Agnes believed that her eldest son had no business chasing after the nursing student that "he couldn't afford," as she told me one day as we walked to town. Birungi's parents agreed about the economic mismatch: Sam's lower socioeconomic status and educational attainment did not fit their vision of their daughter's upwardly mobile future. Birungi's parents sent Sam several threatening messages about actions they would take if he continued to "fill their daughter's head with lofty dreams."

But neither Birungi's parents nor Agnes had reason to worry. The attractive and bright young woman had developed her own dreams about her future, and she and her classmates began socializing with a group of older professional men in Jinja town who treated them to day trips on the weekends and evenings out in bars and pool halls in neighboring towns. Her new cosmopolitan connections offered the pleasures and possibilities of a modern life, while Sam remained in his provincial rural setting, struggling to establish his post-secondary-school masculine identity and status. Several months after the letter-writing incident, a visibly distraught Sam informed me that Birungi had no desire to continue their relationship and had broken off all communication with him.

To medicate his broken heart and career frustrations, Sam became a regular patron of the outdoor drinking area of town, Kasokoso, where he socialized with an assortment of *nakyewombekeire* (single or "free" young women; literally "a woman who lives on her own"). His mother expressed concern and disappointment about her son's behavior as an "idle young man," but also empathized with him: his romantic aspirations had been squelched by the reality that his heartfelt hopes and feelings were no match for the economic stability and upward social mobility possibilities that employed men offered to his Birungi. While Sam was criticized for his life of debauchery, it is not unlikely that the wives of Birungi's older male companions cast her in the same socially threatening category as Iganga's *nakyewombekeire*, seeing her as a nubile paramour with insufficient supervision from her family to keep her from disrupting marriage. As Agnes worried about Sam's reputation and health, she received news that one of her adolescent daughters was six months pregnant by a young man. She had tried to discourage her daughter's entanglement with him, but without the threat of withholding financial support, her efforts were much less successful than those of Birungi's parents.

I fortuitously stumbled upon Sam's letter while conducting research on historical transformations of heterosexual premarital romantic relationships among youth in Iganga, a predominately Basoga ethnic region.[2] A year into the project, my research assistants and I had gathered colorful coming-of-age narratives from older Basoga about culturally ideal routes to marriage as well as their actual premarital lived experiences. Compared to the eagerness with which elders recounted their premarital romantic tales and mishaps, young people tended to be reserved and guarded as they did their best to politely evade my questions. They were certainly experiencing romance and desire in their feelings and actions, as demonstrated in Sam's letter and our subsequent conversations. However, uncovering this affective world was a methodologically tricky task, particularly in a context in which moral and social anxiety around youth sexuality had driven their sexual relationships further away from the historical surveilling eye of concerned adults.

Sam's letter and the over three hundred others I eventually collected offer a window into what Michelle Fine has called "the missing discourse of desire" that is often neglected in scholarship, development reports, and media stories on youth (1988; see also Tolman 1994). Letters and stories of youthful hopes of love and the structural obstacles that stubbornly take these dreams on a circuitous route motivate this ethnography on the politics of intervention and its consequences on youth sexuality in postcolonial Uganda. I had not expected that what began as a routine premarital and marital life history of Agnes in 1996 and the fortuitous encounter with Sam's love letter would evolve into this survey of an unpredictable series of events that reveal the complex interactions of youth as romantically desiring social actors, and that I would learn both about the wider conditions that turn their hopes into what Lauren Berlant (2011) called a "cruel optimism," and the anxieties that emerge when the (social and medical) risks of love and poverty are combined. I return to the story of Sam and Agnes throughout this book and particularly in the concluding chapter.

Regulating Romance: Protecting and Policing Youthful Sexuality

Regulating Romance is an ethnographic study of the unintended consequences of interventions around sexuality that emerge within a particular place and historical trajectory. At the center of this ethnography are the lives of residents of Iganga as they confront a historically nagging tension, with young people's romantic desires and dreams on the one hand, and anxieties surrounding possible negative social and medical outcomes of youthful love on the other.[3] Concern about the sexuality of premarital young people and particularly unmarried females has a long history in the region (as it does elsewhere in the world); however, this anxiety has been heightened since the onset of the epidemic and, ironically, as a consequence of the country's aggressive HIV efforts. As explored throughout this book, the country's bold HIV efforts have facilitated the rapid emergence of competing moralities about sexual propriety, debates what a modern sexuality should look like, and conflicts about how best to design interventions to shape sexual and moral landscapes. During numerous research visits to Iganga between 1996 and 2015, as well as through many e-mail exchanges and phone conversations with residents during and since that period, I have become intimately familiar with the politics of interventions around youthful sexuality and the female body, as well as the persistent economic precarities, social uncertainties, and kinship struggles that throw young people's romantic desires into disarray. I have witnessed youth relationships unfold in what resembles the classic interplay between wider phenomena and everyday actions of individuals (Bourdieu 1977; Giddens 1984). Anthropologists and others conducting ethnographic research use the concept "lived experience" to capture how individual actions are shaped by historical and wider forces. Erica C. James examines "routines of ruptures" that punctuate the lives of Haitians, arguing that the notion of lived experiences of insecurity (*ensekirite*) "incorporates not only the threats residing in material space but also the perception of unseen malevolent forces that covertly intervene in Haitian society—whether such forces are natural or supernatural, individual or collective, organized or arbitrary, or domestic or foreign" (2010:8).

My inquiries into interventions around sexuality benefit from several intellectual genealogies. One is the feminist challenge Carole Vance issues in the introduction to her edited volume *Pleasure and Danger: Exploring Female Sexuality*, which resulted from the seminal 1982 Barnard Conference on Sexuality. At the conference, which uniquely brought together feminist scholars and activists, Vance chided both groups for exploring only one aspect of women's experiences with sexuality—danger or pleasure. She urged participants to break from their ideological agendas and instead consider the complicated dialectic between the danger and pleasure that is ever present in the lives of women.[4] In *Pleasure and Danger*, she writes, "Sexuality is simultaneously a domain of restriction, repression, and danger as well as a domain of exploration, pleasure, and agency. . . . The hallmark of sexuality is its complexity: its multiple meanings, sensations, and connections. It is all too easy to cast sexual experiences as either wholly pleasurable or dangerous; our culture encourages us to do so" (1984a:1–5). The call for examining both pleasure and risk ignited controversy: some asked, for instance, how can pornography or prostitution ever be pleasurable for the women being exploited? Decades later, however, the assumption that women (and men) can and do exert individual agency in situations of desperation and inequality and create meaning and significance is now commonplace in sexuality studies.

My dedication to studying the subjectivity of local actors is also motivated by calls made in postcolonial studies from the 1970s onwards that drew attention to the ways in which the voices and subjectivities of brown-skinned, formerly colonized people in the global South are silenced in global North representations about lives and suffering in the global South. This group of scholars includes but is not limited to Frantz Fanon, Edward Said, Toni Morrison, Gayatri Spivak, Chandra T. Mohanty, bell hooks, Ann Ducille, and Homi Bhabha. For example, in her oft-cited article, "Can the Subaltern Speak?," Spivak argues that the practice of *sati* (widow-burning) in India became an important pretext for colonial intercessions, justifying the expansion of the empire for the moral and humanitarian purpose of "white men saving brown women from brown men" (1988:296). Racialized ideologies created the myth of brutal masculinity and female docility and an overarching hypersexualized blackness that emerged and proliferated during the colonial project throughout Asia, Africa, and Latin America through representations of local practices—such as polygyny, female circumcision, widow inheritance and sacrifice, or burqas—that were constructed as offensive to Western sensibilities (see Fanon 1967). Spivak and other postcolonial scholars theorize about the legacies of European colonialism, calling for a critical exploration that foregrounds subjectivities and voices of formerly colonized people but does so in ways that appreciate the contradictory and complex entanglements with global capitalism, inequalities, and knowledge production.

While explorations into local subjectivities and enactments of desire are now the standard in ethnographies on sexuality and race, such inquiries lag behind in the studies on sexual health that guide much policy and program development. Sexual health research remains focused on understanding risk, vulnerability, and access to protective techniques, with the ultimate aim of developing and evaluating interventions to abate negative outcomes of risk. I share this aim. But, as John Gagnon and Richard Parker (1994:16) pointed out early in the AIDS epidemic, by limiting our analytic focus to risk and defining risk in terms of health outcomes, we miss crucial aspects of what shapes people's quest for intimacy and ignore the reality that desire, prestige, personal significance, social obligations, and much else remain large components of people's pursuit of or entry into the sexual liaisons that may be putting them at risk, however "risk" is understood.[5]

Research into sentiment and romance has been particularly limited in the area of ethnographic studies among youth, mainly because they are still seen as passing through a liminal state during which most relationships end and hence are taken as ephemeral. However, for the youth with whom I interacted in Iganga, youthful desires are more than just juvenile fantasies. Imagining their futures is one of their main preoccupations as they simultaneously consider how to survive amid economic and social uncertainties. On a more cynical note, acknowledging that affection is the basis for intimate relationships in communities with poor sexual health outcomes would uncomfortably disrupt the bourgeois and Western-centric assumption that better behaviors and cultural practices such as companionate relationships would vaccinate the poor against negative sexual health outcomes. We know that this formula is not sufficient (e.g., Sobo 1995; Parikh 2007; Hirsch et al. 2010; Smith 2014). Love has never been a prophylaxis for bad outcomes. Context is key. I conceptualize this context in Iganga as the sexual economy, and not simply as an economy structured by the money-for-sex (or, transactional sex) exchanges so common in the literature on HIV and sexuality in Africa and among poor people elsewhere. Rather, I propose a framework of sexual economy that appreciates the network of interactions among the emotions, competing moral authorities, sexual possibilities, social obligations, kinship systems, and economic and gender inequalities that shape and give meaning to youth sexual liaisons—or, the interaction of symbolic, material, and affective significance.

Uganda and the Paradox of the HIV Success Story: Anxiety around the Sexuality of Young Females

Uganda offers a unique setting for a study on interventions, sexual culture, and moral anxiety. The resource-poor country is regularly touted as the first global HIV success story. Known as the global "epicenter of AIDS" in the late 1980s, with national prevalence reaching 18.5 percent (over 30 percent in urban sentinel sites), the country recorded an impressive 70 percent reduction in the following decades, with the national average falling to 6.4 percent by the time the 2004/2005 AIDS Indicator Survey was compiled (UAC 2012; Asiimwe-Okiror, Musinguzi, and Madraa 1996; Wawer, Sewankambo, et al. 1994).[6] Credit for this dramatic decline is often given to then-newly empowered president Yoweri Museveni and later to what became known as Uganda's magic bullet—the ABC (abstinence, be faithful, and condom use) model, a model that would be replicated around the world.[7] When the country's HIV prevalence crept back up to 7.3 percent by 2011, global attention from donors and researchers again followed (UAC 2014). Uganda has no doubt been at the center of global HIV discussions.

Extensive literature exists about the extent of and reasons for Uganda's impressive decline in and subsequent increase. However, virtually no analytic attention has been given to the *unintended* consequences that the country's aggressive and massive HIV efforts have had on how communities reconceptualize and deal with specific targeted populations. As Michel Foucault and others observe, the process of developing a surveillance system for tracking a social problem heightens the visibility and control of actors and acts deemed to be at higher risk or outside newly constructed norms (Foucault 1990). This codification of risk categories and acts by a cast of experts leads to what Berlant has called "the paradox of partial legibility," in which certain acts and aspects of identity are reified and recognized as problematic while others are simultaneously rendered invisible (1997:1). The naming and dissemination of information about a social problem can work to incite a moral panic, which, as Roger Lancaster points out, "often express[es], in an irrational, spectral, or misguided way, other social anxieties" (2011:23). The ironic outcome of awareness campaigns in Uganda and elsewhere has been the surfacing of "other social anxieties" that have been codified as "risk" groups. In local and popular speech, the risk group becomes *the cause* of other social problems instead of *the result* of existing problems, such that, for example, the freely floating young *nakyewombekeire*, idle young men, and more recently the queer black body in Uganda all become targets for critiques about moral decline, as opposed to being viewed as results of economic precarity and social uncertainties.

Even before the HIV epidemic, young females had received much attention from international agencies, for data had showed the impact of gender inequality on the outcome of women and girls. The United Nations made the 1980s the Decade for Women, proposing programs and strategies for empowering women—messages that were picked up in Uganda and in other developing countries. The Decade for Women was followed by the 1990s UN focus on children's rights, setting off new initiatives to address the plight of the girl child, making the brown- and black-skinned girl child in formerly colonized countries in the global South the international symbol for Western humanitarian efforts.

During the late 1980s, while the girl child was the center of UN efforts, HIV surveillance reports simultaneously began to show that adolescent girls in Uganda were disproportionately affected by HIV compared to their male counterparts. The alarming 5:1 ratio of girls to boys being infected with HIV in Uganda was a statistic frequently reproduced in the media and recited in local speeches and campaigns. Even after a reduction in the country's overall HIV rates and a significant decline among girls, adolescent females remained almost nine times more likely than adolescent males to test positive for HIV (MOH and ORC Macro 2006:101). At the height of Uganda's HIV epidemic, the country also had one of the highest teen pregnancy rates in the world. When I commenced my research on this topic, 43 percent of girls between the ages of 15 and 19 had given birth (UBOS 1996). Although the rate of teen pregnancy had decreased to 31 percent in 2001 and to 25 percent in 2011, Uganda's rate remained among the highest globally (UBOS and ICF International 2012; Neema, Musisi, and Kibombo 2004:15).

Although the HIV epidemic and teen pregnancy are important backdrops for this study, this is not an ethnography *about* the epidemic, sexual risk, or risk reduction practices. Nor is this book an evaluation of HIV control efforts. Rather, this book takes HIV as a "social fact" woven into lives and landscapes. Not only has the widespread knowledge of HIV shaped sexual and moral economies, but the bio-legitimacy of the epidemic has engendered an influx of economic, technical, and medical resources. From intimate experiences of caring for dying parents, siblings, aunts, uncles, and neighbors to the omnipresence of HIV in the public sphere, HIV is neither exotic nor extraordinary for youth in Iganga. Rather, it is another unfortunate and mundane fact of everyday life.

While this book is not directly about HIV, it does, however, intend to contribute methodologically and theoretically to the vast amount of literature about the epidemic and about sexual health more generally. Given that sub-Saharan Africa is home to an estimated 70 percent of the world's HIV cases and the site of around 72 percent of AIDS-related deaths as of 2011 (UNAIDS 2012), it is no surprise that an enormous amount of behavioral research exists on sexual risk. Much of this research can be classified into two types—sexual KABP (sexual knowledge, attitudes, behaviors, and practices) studies, and analyses of population-level health data, behavioral investigations, and serosurveys, such as ICF International's Demographic and Health Surveys (DHS). Remarkably, however, although there is a great body of research on sexual activities and networks, we know far less about the *effects* of HIV as a social phenomenon, and how over thirty years of interventions have shaped community understandings of sexuality.

The person-centered approach of ethnographic investigations has made important contributions to the vast body of literature about the epidemic and global health in general. The discipline's *methodological* foregrounding of lived experiences through devices such as Arthur Kleinman's illness narratives (1988) and its long-standing tradition of participant observation (Malinowski 1922) are suited for revealing the complexities and nuances behind quantitative data (see also Nichter 2008; Biehl and Petryna 2013; Hahn and Harris 1999). Analytically, I draw from Marxist-informed critical theory (often known in anthropology as "political economy"), which considers interactions among historical, regional, and global inequalities and processes and lived experiences (Roseberry 1988). With methodological and analytic tools attuned to toggling among various levels of analysis and between the recent past and contemporary events, anthropology has been at the forefront of demonstrating that the disproportionally high distribution of negative outcomes among poorer and marginalized groups is the product of structural forces such as global and regional inequalities and access, rather than of "individual moral failings or a breakdown in social rules" (J. S. Hirsch, Meneses, et al. 2007).[8]

This book advances a critical anthropology of interventions, and makes three arguments.[9] First, the Uganda case demonstrates that thrusting discussions of sexuality into the public sphere in ways not previously experienced—as was occasioned by the country's aggressive and bold HIV control efforts—brings to the surface local contestations over gender, sexuality, and morality that may reinforce existing hierarchies. Second, like other programs around identified "risk groups," interventions designed to protect young people from undesirable social and health outcomes and model them into proper moral adults also leads to the intensified policing of the adolescent and young adult body—particularly adolescent female sexuality—in ways that exacerbate tensions between generations and genders and leads to new avenues of social and medical risk. The imagined *nakyewombekeire* becomes the public moral object upon which residents in Iganga and the nation-state debate virtue, and a scientific project through which public health, development, and donor agencies monitor and assess the health and well-being of society and the success of their interventions. Third, against this backdrop of increased surveillance, youth love letters provide both a practical space for articulating and an analytic window into understanding how youth simultaneously resist and appropriate regulatory discourses that aim to mold or discipline their sexuality. Their letters reveal how these youthful subjects imagine and make sense of the place of their affection-seeking selves and practices within the context of heightened anxiety surrounding youth sexuality—an anxiety that most clearly has been played out in public health campaigns since the beginning of the epidemic.

Signs of the Times: Global Politics, Interventions, and Iatrogenic Effects

The year 1981 was a watershed moment for youth sexuality around the world. Researchers as well as casual followers of the HIV epidemic easily associate 1981 with the official beginning of the global infectious disease, with the June 5 publication of "Pneumocystis pneumonia—Los Angeles," an article in the Centers for Disease Control's *Morbidity and Mortality Weekly Report* (*MMWR*). It is doubtful that many of these same observers will also recall that only two months after the *MMWR* announcement, a channel named MTV (Music Television) was making another intervention into modern, youthful sexuality. On August 1, 1981, MTV broadcast the first music video, revolutionizing the way youthful bodies, desire, and sexual freedom could be packaged and circulated around the world (Williams 1991).[10] Even for those without access to cable television in their homes, this new electronic music genre rapidly accelerated the speed at which sexually explicit depictions of youthful bodies could stimulate the imaginations of audiences around the globe, in what David Harvey (1989) has called the "time-space" compression enabled by technology. The virus and the video both targeted youthful bodies. While the HIV epidemic motivated the circulation of messages about deadly risk, popular culture distributed images of delightful and, some would argue, hedonistic pleasures.[11] Religious fundamentalists intensified a moral crusade, attempting to redomesticate unrestrained sexuality and force it back behind the closed door of (mythical) heterosexual, monogamous marriage. Although this tension between new avenues of sexual freedom and intensified moral crusades is not new, HIV ushered in a new era in the global culture wars over sexuality. In this section, I turn to the recent past to situate shifts in Uganda's HIV messages within the wider global political landscape, with two aims. I want to draw the reader's attention to (1) how recent genealogies of

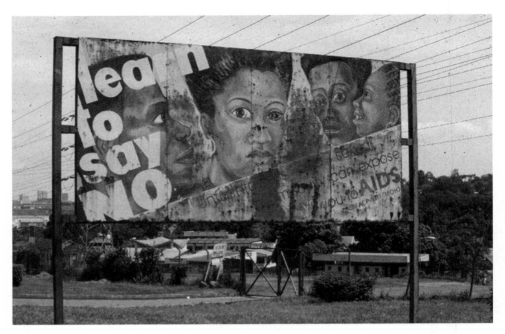

FIGURE 2. "Learn to say no," Africa's first HIV billboard, built in the mid-1980s

interventions into sexuality in Uganda are wrapped up in cultural wars within the country, and (2) how these internal wars are fueled by an international cast of powerful donors and policy makers, with Uganda's largest HIV funder, the United States, having a significant role in what has transpired.

In 1986, a year before US president Ronald Reagan mentioned HIV in a public speech, Africa's first AIDS billboard was unveiled outside of Kampala, along the Trans-Africa Highway. The historic billboard displayed the cartoon-like faces of two couples, each pair consisting of an innocent protagonist (one male, one female) and an alluring potential sexual partner. The sign warned its intergenerational audience, "Learn to say NO. Unfaithfulness and sexual promiscuity can expose you to AIDS" (Figure I.2). The international media, including the *New York Times* and the *International Herald Tribune*, later published photos of the billboard in stories about the courageous East African president who was tackling the AIDS epidemic. A public health official in Kampala whom I interviewed reflected on President Yoweri Museveni's bold response, arguing that at that point saving people was more important than not offending them. The language of the inaugural HIV billboard was clear and uniquely direct for the time. HIV was about sex, fear, and death.

A decade later, the famous billboard stood rusted and weather-beaten, the bottom of it peppered with tattered flyers announcing local concerts, religious revivals, and political candidates. The billboard loomed larger than other elements in the surrounding built environment, but a decade after its debut it had faded into the background and seemed virtually invisible to local residents and long-distance commuters who traveled on the highway. Compared to the doom and fear evoked in the inaugural "Say No"

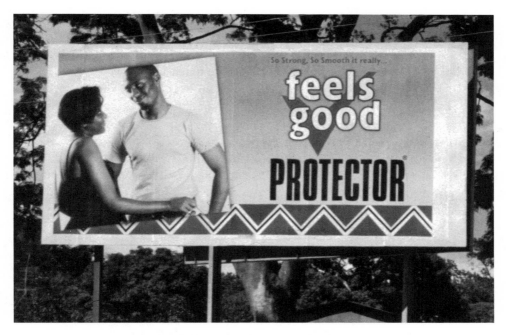

FIGURE 3. "Feels good" condom billboard, built in the mid-1990s

sign, a colorful 1998 billboard at the opposite end of the capital on the road to the airport appeared youthfully playful and hopeful, marking a new era in HIV messaging. The vibrant billboard resembled that of a Madison Avenue marketing firm, advertising the condom as chic, sexy, and modern risk-reduction technology. The ad featured an attractive young couple dressed in stylish urban wear, embracing each other. The young smiling woman was confidently reaching for a "Protector" (perhaps a play on "protect her") condom in the back jean pocket of her well-built lover (Figure I.3). Using effective social marketing strategies, the billboard attempted to sell the viewers a new trend—a modern relationship. The "price" of being in a modern relationship was using a condom, participating in open discussions of sexuality, and engaging with women with enough sexual agency to talk about safer sex. The visible urgency of the epidemic and the relatively liberal global climate of the mid-1990s allowed the taboo pairing of youth and sex to be publicly named and, as some argued, even encouraged with the suggestive phrase "Feels Good."

But the Madison Avenue–style condom billboard was not without its critics. Condom promotion campaigns that were more visibly featured galvanized social conservatives who were growing increasingly uncomfortable with the explicit messages that they maintained were based on foreign ideas and promoted Western immoral sensibilities. Opponents of public condom promotion joined the chorus with global critics of comprehensive sexual education, and claimed that safe-sex campaigns were akin to sexual abuse and aroused otherwise dormant sexual desires (Irvine 1999; Patton 1996).

By the early 2000s, the global climate around public health discussions about condoms and safer sex had dramatically shifted (Girard 2004). The highly influential evangelical movement, to which US president George W. Bush owed a political debt, played a major role in the global policy shift. The political arm of the evangelical movement spread its moral prescription to the global South through Bush's 2002 faith-based initiatives and then through his 2003 PEPFAR (President's Emergency Plan for AIDS Relief) program. PEPFAR guaranteed $15 billion for five years to combat global HIV, tuberculosis, and malaria primarily in fifteen hard-hit "focus countries."[12] The program consolidated US public funding for international HIV efforts into one program to be allocated according to specific guidelines established by US elected lawmakers and with virtually no input from key agencies in recipient countries.[13] A target of much criticism was PEPFAR's 2005 directive that "66 percent of resources dedicated to prevention of HIV from sexual transmission must be used for activities that encourage abstinence and fidelity" (Kohn 2005). This directive put constraints on condom promotion and comprehensive sexuality education for youth (IOM 2007). The new US law guaranteed that "safer sex" and condom campaigns would be replaced by evangelically inflected and now well-funded "no sex" slogans and programs.[14] The abstinence and "be faithful" messages that had always been part of what later became known as Uganda's famous ABC (abstinence, be faithful, use condoms) approach became the main public health message for countries receiving PEPFAR support (Figure I.4).

The shift away from what some observers called a "pragmatic approach" and the turn toward a moral approach resonated with Uganda's growing evangelical movement and its most visible and popular advocate, first lady Janet Museveni (see, for example, Kinsman 2010; Epstein 2005). Nonpartisan reports had found that "the abstinence-until-marriage budget allocation . . . hampers [prevention] efforts," is not based in evidence-based science, and "has greatly limited the ability of Country Teams to develop and implement comprehensive prevention programs that are well integrated with each other," but the global morality crusade grew more vigilant with funding and ideological backing from the United States (IOM 2007:113).[15] The initial PEPFAR decade saw an intensification of the neoliberal notion of individual responsibility and public health messages based on the premise of rational thought, which started with the assumption that "given enough information, people will act on rational decisions designed to maximize their well-being" (Paxson 2002:309). Uganda's epidemic proved that this was not the case. The virus continued to spread among people armed with both knowledge and moral ideologies but who either lacked the power or tools to negotiate less risky sex or were driven by something other than medical risk avoidance, such as the desire to reproduce, express affection, seek pleasure, confirm their commitment to a partner, or conform to group norms.

This conflict played itself out on the ground. As the moral crusade around sexuality as a way to fight HIV grew, something unexpected and embarrassing happen in Uganda—HIV prevalence and incidence began increasing (Shafer et al. 2008). Policy analysts and critics of PEPFAR's overly prescriptive guidelines who had warned of the consequences of relying heavily on an ideology- and morality-based health model had evidence to support their claims (CHANGE 2005; Evertz 2010; GAO 2006; Jamison and Padian 2006). The global debate as to whether PEPFAR policies were inimical to HIV efforts came to a head when critiques of PEPFAR observed that Uganda had

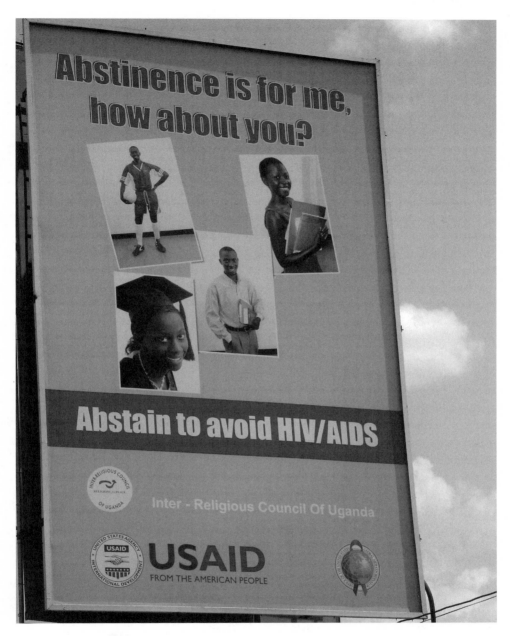

FIGURE 4. Abstinence billboard, PEPFAR-funded, built in the early 2000s

experienced a dangerously low level of condom supplies between late 2004 and early 2005 (Das 2005; ABC 2005; Ssejoba 2004; Bass 2005; Wakabi 2008). The condom shortage controversy exposed the clear global cleavage between the two ideologically opposed groups—Bush's PEPFAR and the multicountry opponents consolidated under the United Nations (Wakabi 2009; Altman 2005; BBC 2004b; Bass 2005; CHANGE 2005; Mogwanja 2005; Boseley 2005).

Alongside the "no sex" youth programs, a new set of campaigns focusing on sexually networking adults appeared. Some observers interpreted Uganda's uptick or a less significant decrease in prevalence among adult and married people as suggesting that HIV campaigns were not going far enough in condemning concurrent partnering (Halperin and Epstein 2004; Halperin, Steiner, et al. 2004; Mah and Halperin 2008). Others maintained that simply focusing on a cultural fix was not sufficient if underlying structural factors (such as labor-related migration, poverty, and gender inequality) facilitating concurrent multiple partnerships were not addressed (M. N. Lurie and Rosenthal 2010; see also Parker, Easton, and Klein 2000). Using the language of individual choice to target people's ability to change behavior and the phrase "side dish" to describe concurrent liaisons, the One Love sexual networking campaign further cemented HIV infection as an *individual* choice while successfully silencing any discussion of *contextual* factors (see Kasyate 2010; Namubiru 2013). The cultural fix model was promoted to the public through the "To live a good life, get off the sexual network!" campaign led by the Uganda Health Marketing Group and funded by USAID (Figure I.5).

The assumptions underlying the cultural fix messages were not without criticism from within Uganda. For instance, Sylvia Tamale, a feminist Ugandan legal scholar and activist, argued that the spread of the conservative HIV messages were further evidence that Ugandans "have uncritically bought into the 'risky cultural practices' frame, which is racist, moralistic and paternalistic. It has also become the main resource of public health advocates and policy makers, resulting in two decades of muddled approaches to HIV prevention in Africa with minimal success" (quoted in *PlusNews* 2010; see also Agot 2007, 2008). Uganda's cultural wars intensified and gained global attention during the events surrounding Uganda's proposed 2009 "Kill the Gays Bill," as it was called by global gay rights supporters. The vulnerable bodies of young people once again emerged as central to a moral debate, as a main public justification for the bill was to punish and ward off Western cultural intrusion, which the antigay movement argued was penetrating the country through an "underground 'gay' movement" that was recruiting in schools by offering students money (Lively 2009).[16] My brief chronicle of the shifts in HIV prevention messages is intended to show how interventions in Uganda in general are entangled with global cultural wars and changing notions of responsibility and respectability.

Entering Iganga: Histories of Sexual and Gender Anxiety among the Basoga

In *Law without Precedent: Legal Ideas in Action in the Courts of Colonial Busoga* (1969), anthropologist Lloyd Fallers quotes a subcounty chief: "You ask why the woman is never the accused in adultery cases. But if someone were to steal your shoes, would you accuse the shoes?" (101). The 1950s research of Fallers initially led me to Iganga in 1995 for exploratory research.[17] I was particularly drawn to Fallers's courtroom data in *Law without Precedent*, which had led him to conclude that "gender disputes were an integral part of Busoga life." As a feminist scholar, I was also intrigued by Fallers's analytic blinders about the workings of patriarchy and women's acts of refusal.

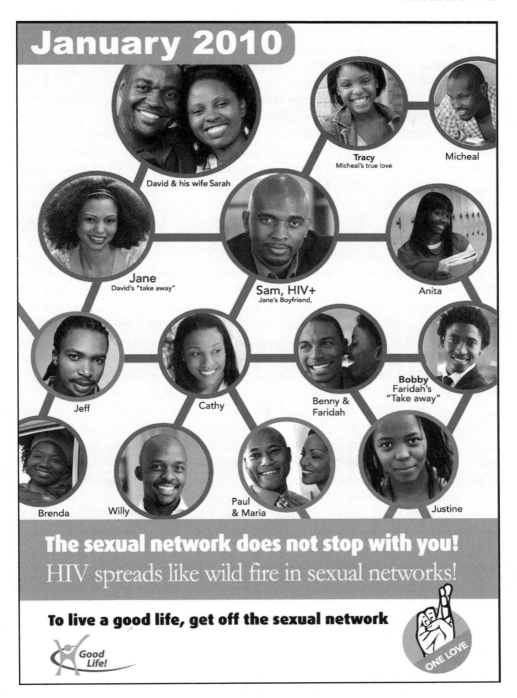

FIGURE 5. "Get off the sexual network" campaign poster, circa 2009

The "gender disputes" he details commonly concerned male conflicts over female sexuality—arguments about which man had legitimate rights over a woman (her father through his blood right or another man through the payment of bridewealth), or cases where compensation was demanded from men who had "seduced" another man's wife or daughter without consent from her male guardian. In the defining and addressing of local problems, colonial courts along with missionary agents engaged themselves in the creation of new types of morality (Peterson 2006). The project of morality-making was highly gendered. The exclusion of women from the colonial court system served to strengthen and bring new meanings to existing practices of patriarchy and male privilege. British colonial administrators' collaboration with male local leaders alienated women from centers of official power and decision making. This gender inequality in access to state resources played itself out in how problems of the time were conceptualized and interventions developed. For instance, a council investigating the decline of cash crops and hence tax revenue argued that "female weakness" was not only "the chief threat to stable marriage" but also to blame for the lack of adequate farm labor (Fallers 1969:105–8). As a solution, the council suggested establishing policies to reinforce husbands' authority over wives (105).[18] These patriarchal interventions, however, did not go without resistance from women, and some women sought ways to gain control over labor and sexuality despite social ostracization and demonization.[19] Here we see the historical antecedent of today's socially denounced *nakyewombekeire* and her role in moral decline (see also Hodgson and McCurdy 2001; P. J. Davis 2000; Dinan 1983; La Fontaine 1974; Summers 2000).

Fallers's detailed ethnographic work offered an ideal historical baseline from which to begin my research on transformations in premarital sexuality. I headed to villages around Iganga Town where Fallers had conducted his research. I spoke with the then-elderly son of one of his key informants and took a tour of the sub-county headquarters where Fallers observed many of the court proceedings contained in his book. Not surprisingly, since the time of his research much had changed in Iganga. The most notable change was the social geography of Basoga life. Black life in the 1940s and 1950s under British colonial rule was centered in the villages as colonial administrators regulated and restricted the movement and settlement of Africans to and within Iganga Town. While there were a couple of poor black residential areas to house urban laborers, public urban life was dominated by whites, with Indians present in the small business sector. Post-independence policies and developments have opened up towns to black Ugandans and transformed the once lively rural communities into quiet enclaves for the elderly, as well as small children and their mothers. Young and adult men, as well as an increasing number of women, typically leave the village during the day to work or, as is commonly said, "search for money," while other men and women out-migrate for longer periods in search of income and other resources. School-age children likewise leave to attend classes. Younger residents who have the ability and desire to move out of rural villages do so and relocate to town or peri-urban villages in hopes of accessing educational or work opportunities. Given the changes in the social geography and my project's focus on the localization of nationally and globally originated interventions, I instead selected a site closer to Iganga Town.

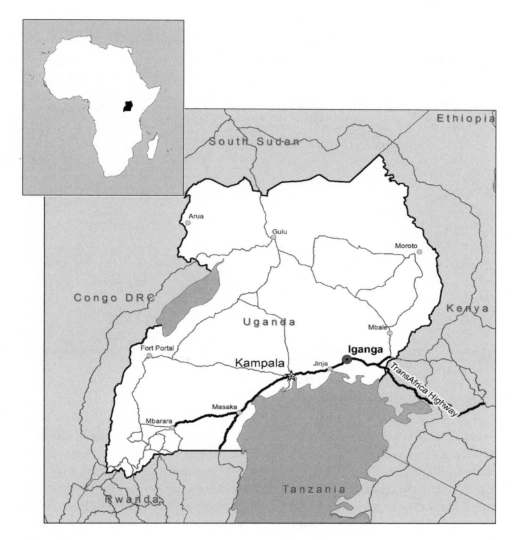

MAP 1. Uganda with Iganga Town and Trans-Africa Highway

Lying about seventy-five miles northeast of Uganda's capital city of Kampala and along the infamous international Trans-Africa Highway, which transported HIV throughout eastern and central Africa, Iganga Town is the social, administrative, and commercial hub of Iganga District (see Map 1). The town has a residential population with an average annual growth rate of between 5 to 7 percent, rising from 5,958 in 1969 to 39,472 in 2002 and to an estimated 53,870 in 2014 (UBOS 2010, 2014). The day and commuter population in the town is much greater than reflected in the national population census, increasing an estimated 60 percent during the day as people from outlying villages commute to the town to access jobs, services, goods, schools, social networks, and other opportunities (AMICAALL 2004).

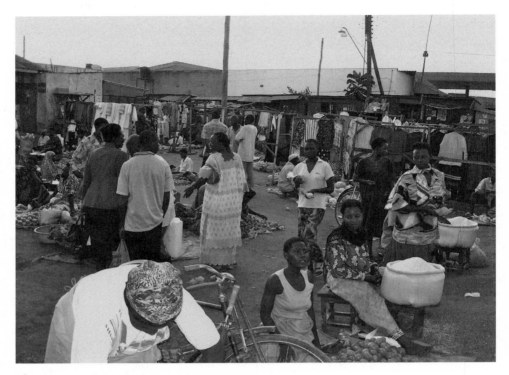

FIGURE 6. Evening kayola (bazaar) in Iganga Town

Iganga Town plays a major role in the romantic lives of young people. Whether they are passing through it on their way to and from school, or running errands for their parents, the town provides a space for young people to interact not only with other young people but also with ideas and goods from elsewhere. The early evening *kayola* (bazaar) is of particular importance. "Business is brisk," writes Obbo (1991) about the *kayola*. "Things are cheap and it attracts people from all socio-economic classes" (103). It is a vibrant scene, lasting from 3:30 p.m. until 9:30 p.m. or later. The *kayola* provides a uniquely coed and semi-anonymous space for youth romance, where young people can meet their sweethearts, exchange glances with potential lovers, or deliver messages for friends, and if need be, all discovered activities can be easily denied as coincidental (Figure I.6).

Though Iganga's poverty rate is 55 percent, there is a growing visible professional middle class in Iganga. Its members relocate to the area to work in one of the existing or newly opened branches of a company, development agency, government office, or re-tail venue (AMICAALL 2004).[20] The presence of young professionals has dramatically changed the availability of luxury goods and other aspects of the consumer market-place, as well as the demand for civic institutions to connect all residents (rich or poor, younger or older) to regional and global economies. These changes have enabled Iganga residents to forge and imagine identities and to gain access to resources based on non-kin relations. Today, Iganga residents draw from both kin networks and wider civic networks (such as schools, religious congregations, and occupations) for access to status and wealth, and young people draw on those networks to craft modern identities.

As evidence of how the shift from kin- to civic-identity is having a negative impact on Iganga, residents often point to the decline of and delay in the formal engagement or introduction ceremony (*kwandhula*) that marks the official solemnization of a marriage among the Basoga. Elders commonly say that young men today make what is frequently referred to as "crocodile requests," meaning that they ask for permission after they have already taken the daughter and before bridewealth has been exchanged, and that young women give themselves away too easily. Women's rights organizations and the government have attacked bridewealth as the brokering of a daughter's sexuality, but the policies they have designed to protect young women (such as the age of consent law) are appropriated locally to take care of anxieties stemming from the independence of young women and reinforce patriarchal control over young women and youth romance more generally.

Research Methods

Discretion is central to Basoga notions of respectability and maturity. The willful act of nondisclosure captures the essence of researching the intimate lives of people not only in Iganga but certainly in many locations in the world, posing endless methodological obstacles (see Lewontin 1995). Hence, building trust, remaining open-minded and being methodologically creative are central tenets to researchers studying sexuality. The use of multiple methods and an iterative research process enabled my research assistants and me to triangulate findings gained from different methods as well as to explore the multivalent meanings and significance behind people's actions and stories.

Interviews and Longitudinal Case Studies
Over the course of this project, I conducted approximately 250 interviews with younger and older people from different socioeconomic backgrounds and family situations about their experiences with premarital romance, relationships, and sexuality. Some of the interviews were formal, and others informal. Some were recorded, and others were unrecorded but documented. The breakdown of these interviews is as follows: In addition to informal interviews with young people, I also collected around seventy in-depth interviews with youth and approximately twenty-five longitudinal case studies of young people that spanned over several years and as they progressed into young adulthood and sometimes into marriage, childbearing, and even marital dissolution. Longitudinal case studies provide insight into the way a person's romantic desires and practices change over the course of adolescence and into adulthood, and how these changes take place because of educational trajectories and reproductive experiences (see Johnson-Hanks 2006). Since a major aim of this research was to examine youth sexuality as a historical process, I also collected sexual histories from older people about their premarital relationships. Between 1996 and 1998 I collected coming-of-age and sexual histories from forty men and women (twenty men and twenty women) between the ages of thirty-five and eighty-five years old, and about forty informal or unstructured life histories with

older people. I conducted follow-up interviews with about half of these older people in 2000, 2002, 2004, 2006, and 2015. I interviewed an additional seventy-two adults and older people in 2004 as part of a multicountry comparative ethnographic project on love, marriage, and HIV risk funded by the National Institutes of Health (see J. S. Hirsch, Wardlow, Smith, et al. 2010; Parikh 2007).[21]

In sampling for and writing about age categories I use a combination of people's age (or estimated age) and local perception of the person's age category. In this book, I define "youth" less by a person's biological age or the legal criteria of eighteen years or younger. Rather, following the social practice of residents of Iganga and scholarship on adolescence beginning with G. Stanley Hall's 1904 magnum opus, I take "youth" to be determined by an intersection of an individual's reproductive and marital histories, level of economic and social independence, school status, and community- and self-perception. For instance, Iganga residents might not generally consider a seventeen-year-old female who is married with two children a youth, although she would be considered a youth by development agencies and the law. However, another seventeen-year-old female, who may or may not have a child and is not married, who resides with her natal relatives, has aspirations of continuing with school, and does not work full time might very well be considered a youth in Iganga and this book. As the political economy of youth suggests, a family's socioeconomic status, access to resources, and ability to provide security for its young can prolong the life stage of youth but also create the socially problematic and promising category of adolescence.

Given that this is an ethnography about generational change, age-related categories are invoked in two ways throughout as a way of illuminating temporal transformations. First, I use two general categories—"older" people and "younger" people—when referring to the social cleavage and tensions between adults (such as parents, older relatives and residents, authority figures, and policy makers) and unmarried young people (who are semidependent on parents, relatives, and other older people). Second, I am also interested in illuminating the gradual social changes that have occurred in Iganga, so I further divide "older" people into three cohorts.[22] Although there is slippage and no definitive boundaries among these age groups, I roughly delineate the groups according to their marital and reproductive status and the historical period during which they came of age. "Young adults" are defined as either people who are married or people who are not currently married but are over the age of thirty during my study, many of whom would have come of age when HIV was already a reality. "Adults" refers to married people who are over the age of forty or who have adolescent children and who came of age sometime after Uganda gained independence from the British in 1962. Finally, "elders" are people over fifty or with grandchildren, who came of age during British colonialism. What follows thus engages in ethnographic theorizing about generational transformations occurring over four age-related categories as the country transitioned through specific social, political, and economic changes.

In my analysis of life histories of older people I pay attention to their version of the *ideal* Basoga custom and how this ideal relates to the narrators' own lived experiences. The use of oral histories to reconstruct the past has generated lively debate among historians of Africa since Jan Vansina's 1965 seminal text *Oral Tradition* (see also

Adenaike and Vansina 1996). And while, as Philip Setel observes, "the idea that 'once upon a time' there were clear and rigidly obeyed cultural rules and social institutions governing sexuality is not truer for Africa than it is for Europe" (1999:27), elders' historical narratives can nonetheless serve as important ideological moral commentary about present social problems, as well as illuminating the ways in which residents resisted and appropriated colonial and more recent sources of influence.[23] In addition to reflecting elders' life histories, the historical context of this book is informed by travelers' journals written by British missionaries and explorers (Ashe 1890; Roscoe 1915, 1922; Speke 1863) and earlier academic works by anthropologists and historians (D. W. Cohen 1977, 1986; Fallers 1964, 1965, 1969; Mudoola 1974; Nabwiso-Bulima 1967; Nayenga 1976; Tuma 1980; Larimore 1959).

I also conducted interviews with a number of key informants who have unique insight into particular areas of sexuality, sexual culture, youth, gender, or HIV. The AIDS industry is the largest, most visible, and best funded sector in Uganda directly addressing issues of adolescent sexuality; therefore, I interviewed individuals and gathered information from various testing, monitoring, counseling, education, funding, and advocacy agencies. In both Iganga and Kampala I interviewed policy makers, HIV and public health professionals, and women's rights activists. I also interacted with clinics and agencies in Iganga that worked with youth, including IDAAC (Integrated Development Activities and AIDS Concern), Family Planning International, and Marie Stopes International. Religion plays a major role in public ideas about propriety and morality; therefore, in addition to attending religious services, I also interviewed leaders of the main religious affiliations in Iganga, which included Catholicism, Islam, Pentecostalism, and various forms of Protestantism, about their perspectives on gender, premarital sexuality, and cultural change. Other key informants, I call "sexperts," provided information on local sex culture and sex education. Such people included sex education teachers, *ssengas* (paternal aunts, or the people designated to educate betrothed girls about sexual matters), and local healers who specialize in STIs, HIV, or matters of love.

Finally, I spoke with publishers and editorial staff working in various mass media and public culture outlets. My conversations with them were often about their general observations about the public's reaction to the content, intention, and overtly sexual images and messages circulated by the media, and at other times I specifically asked about a particular piece or show from their respective media platform that generated public attention. From the two daily newspapers, I clipped gossip columns and articles on AIDS, sexuality, and gender issues, as well as various sex and health advice columns. I collected back issues of *Straight Talk* (a monthly newspaper insert for youth on sexuality), which had been founded in 1993, and regularly bought copies of Uganda's popular tabloids, of which *Chic* and *Spice* magazines and *Bukedde* newspaper were the earliest. More recent publications include *The Red Pepper* and *Rolling Stone*; the latter was closed down after being sued for running pictures of people they accused of being gay (Rice 2011). These publications are not only popular sources of social criticism but also of great interest to people. My analysis of representations of gender and sexuality in popular culture were informed by interviews with people working in mass media and popular culture, including at a daily newspaper, at a radio station, for magazines, and in the Ugandan entertainment industry.

Youth Love Letters

As scholars of youth sexuality have noted, tapping into the intimate lives of youth presents a methodological challenge. Sharon Thompson (1984) reflects on her own difficulties researching sexuality among adolescent girls in the United States:

> If there are more reluctant interview subjects, I have never encountered them. Puberty, like pregnancy, is a secret the body cannot keep forever, but to the extent that language constructs physical experiences—makes them real, gives them shape, limits, and significance—pubescents exercise their right to remain vague, amorphous, unshaped and unlimited by words, concealed: if not to repress, then to keep private, personal, their own. Their silence struck me as an act of self-possession. (350)

Fortunately for me, youth in Iganga were not particularly self-possessed, and in fact many were very humble, insecure, and unsure about their romantic relationships and status with their sweethearts. Still, they were inhibited in their discussions with me. On a developmental level, many are still developing the ability to critically reflect on and articulate their feelings about emerging social and biological changes occurring to them. Young people typically expected to sit quietly as I gave them advice or lectured about the dangers of sex—a hierarchical social relationship they had been conditioned to accept. My questions were answered with nervous giggles, coy smiles, and amazement; some youth were interested in and amused by my questions, while for others my interest in their romantic lives seemed odd. Interviews with youth were useful but by themselves produced an incomplete picture of youthful sentiments.

Sam's love letter and particularly the conversations it enabled made it clear that the cherished romantic missives would provide an ideal window into youth romance. In 1998 I collected over one hundred letters, and in 2002 I collected about two hundred more. In Part III of this ethnography, I elaborate on the process of collecting the letters and discuss in detail what the letters tell us about emerging youth romantic subjectivities and culture within the context of economic and social constraints. I examine these letters as "sites of emergent consciousness . . . in which new kinds of self and collectivity," or in this case romantic consciousness, are created (Barber 1997:6).

Folklore: Gossip and Tales of Long Ago

Whereas people may not easily discuss their own sex lives, they quite eagerly speak about the sexual escapades and misfortunes of others. These tales of others often follow the Basoga convention of advice-giving, an indirect communication style in which a person tells an unfortunate story about someone else and ends with a phrase such as "therefore, it is advised for people to . . ." In everyday communication settings these morality tales, as I call them, are an important speech event and source of entertainment. Tales of others' misfortune not only reveal the ways that people understand and attempt to regulate the sexual behaviors of those listening, but also serve as important vehicles for social bonding and exchange (Gluckman 1963, 1968). In cases where I thought my presence would have changed the dynamics and nature of the story told (such as in male-centered drinking groups), an assistant who was more appropriate for or familiar with that setting would collect the gossip, with the permission of participants. Settings we frequented included drinking spots, kitchens, schoolyards, transportation stations, and household compounds. Interestingly, some stories people shared as being "from a neighboring village" turned out to be national news stories most likely heard over the radio and retold in Iganga as if they were local events, signaling the power of the media in shaping narrative formats and opinions. My assistants and I also collected popular Basoga folktales and general stories about the past concerning sexual relations, some of which are discussed in Chapter 7. Some of these stories are well-known Basoga legends and fables that are transmitted between generations; others are based on actual but reinterpreted past local events that an elder told to illustrate his or her point.

Participant Observation

Participant observation remains the cornerstone of ethnography, for it best allows an anthropologist to meet the primary disciplinary aim of obtaining a nuanced understanding of the textures of people's everyday lives as they navigate through and interact in local social worlds (Malinowski 1922). Without longitudinal participation in and observation of in daily life, data I collected from other methods would lack the contextual backdrop that is necessary for appreciating how the heightened anxiety surrounding youth sexuality gets folded into the current regulation of youth romance. Living with a host family in Bulubandi Village during my initial research stint facilitated my entry into the community and greatly aided my understanding of the sexual economy and meanings. About ten months into my initial research stay I shifted to living in my office in Iganga Town, giving myself easier access to other villages and a neutral place to meet with and interview young people and others. After relocating to Iganga Town I realized the extent to which my movements and interactions in the village had been highly supervised—not maliciously, but rather for my "protection," since my concerned host and other neighbors wanted to make sure that as a young unmarried and foreign woman I did not accidently venture to "dangerous" places or have to deal with less than reputable characters.

Community-Based Participatory Research (CBPR)

Based on Brazilian postcolonial theorist Paulo Freire's theory of critical pedagogy and his notion of *conscientization* (or, critical consciousness), community-based participatory research (CBPR) or participatory action research (PAR) is designed to actively engage participants in the research process through structured, small-group activities that are followed by reflection, a large-group discussion, and eventually community collective action.[24] I had initially learned and used PAR as a small business advisor with the US Peace Corps in Kenya and found the techniques useful in gaining insight into aspects of local life that were taken for granted, such as gendered division of labor or assumptions about gender. Anthropologist Brooke Schoepf and others have called for more such research, explaining that "action-research enables anthropologists to combine theoretical concerns of the discipline with humanist concern for the survival and empowerment of the individuals and communities studied" (Schoepf 1995:38).[25] Action research and community-based participatory methods can thus attempt to address characterizations of research as a neo-colonial enterprise in which Africa and other poorer countries and communities serve as laboratories for advancing the careers of Westerners and the elite (Obbo 1995).[26] Although CBPR is far from dismantling the inequalities that underlie continued dispossession of poor communities and shape the research process, it seeks to engage participants in ways that provide space for reflecting on the roots of their marginality and determining their own set of individual and community priorities.

A technique we found useful in research among youth was picture drawing (Figure I.7). To gain adolescents' gendered perspectives on sexual dilemmas, we asked them to visually depict a story about a common issue faced by their respective gender and age group, such as a typical versus ideal progression of a youth relationship or how young people learn about sex at different ages. The storyboards provided an opening for students to discuss among themselves obstacles for achieving their ideals and strategies for overcoming those obstacles. Other action research techniques I used with youth included essay writing, debating, and role-playing.

Particularly useful in understanding the social production of space and sexual geographies was community mapping, in which residents created a map and indicated spaces such as those associated with "bad" morality and "good" moral behaviors, or spaces meaningful for youth romance. Historical trendlines with older residents—in which age-segregated groups charted changes and fluctuations in an aspect of sexuality or social life—offered an entry into group and individual discussions of how local changes were shaped by larger political, economic, and social occurrences (Figure I.8). Life cycle reproductive charts allowed older people to reflect on how their life stages corresponded with their sexual and reproductive experiences and cultural expectations. I used participatory methods primarily as an entry into research and participants' subjectivities and worldviews, and, as is the case with focus-group discussions, results cannot be taken as an end point of ethnographic research or the development process.[27] Whereas the overall aim of CBPR is community empowerment achieved by strengthening a community's ability to mobilize resources and agitate for change, like many academic researchers I regrettably came nowhere near achieving these goals, for doing so takes a dedicated and longer-term focus than academic research provides and values.

Household and Other Surveys

Household surveys were conducted on all the 423 households in Bulubandi Village that were identified during community mapping activities during my initial research stint from 1997 to 1999. As explored in Chapter 2, household surveys and in-depth follow-up interviews with a cross-section of households built for us an understanding of demographic distribution and trends in household composition, wealth distribution, marital patterns, and the religious, ethnic, and age composition of the village. In

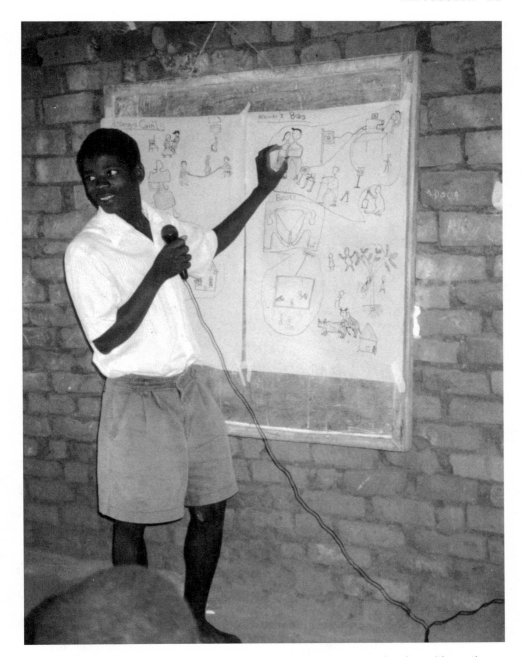

FIGURE 7. Community-based participatory research method, picture-drawing with youth

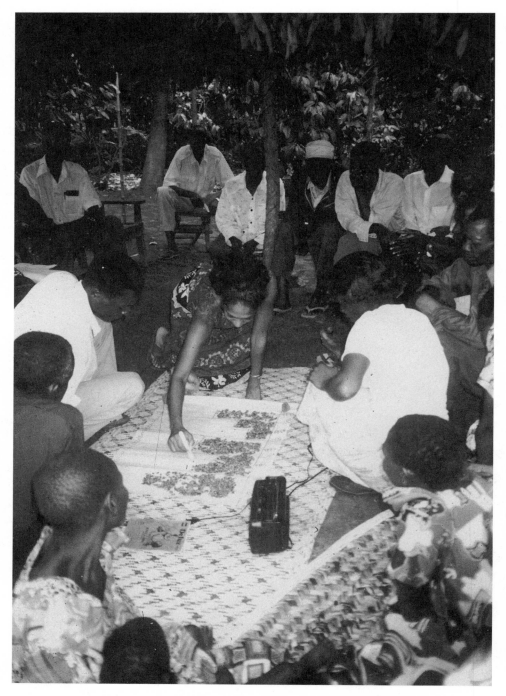

FIGURE 8. Community-based participatory research method, trendline with elders

addition to providing us with a quantitative snapshot of a village during a particular time and residents' perspectives of these changes, the surveys and interviews also helped us identify possible people to interview in depth. I also conducted a survey among youth about sexual practices (such as age of sexual debut and number of sexual partners), knowledge and attitudes about sexual health and sexuality, and methods or sites of knowledge acquisition (such as the media, friends, school, and HIV campaigns).

Research Assistants and My Identity

My assistants have been indispensable, both in gaining access to people and communities and conducting research. Over the years a core group of four assistants have helped with conceptualizing and implementing various research projects, though the number of assistants involved in each project has varied—ranging from two to eight full- and part-time assistants—depending on the specific purpose of my project and their individual availability. They all speak Lusoga fluently, and my main assistants for this project were considered youth or young adults at the time of research. They helped with a range of activities, including identifying people to interview, conducting household surveys and preliminary interviews, acting as cultural interpreters at ceremonies and events, showing me around, teaching me Lusoga, assisting with participatory activities, and generally serving as contacts to various communities and individuals. More than anything, my team and I spent a lot of time informally talking about and analyzing research topics, venturing to different places around Iganga, and visiting their friends and families, as well as members of other social networks such as churches and civic associations. They also read various manuscripts from this project, giving feedback on my interpretation and representation of the data we collected. In between research visits, I have been able to maintain contact with assistants and other friends in Iganga via e-mail and phone, which has allowed me to keep up with their lives and with developments in Iganga.

I end this section by briefly commenting on how my own identity may have influenced interactions with residents. Regardless of my hesitation in turning an ethnography into a navel-gazing project, I include this discussion because lingering behind any critical reading and classroom discussion of ethnographic texts is the issue of how the researcher's identity shaped the data collection and interpretation. I can say that my identity as a woman from the United States of mixed ancestry (an African American mother and a father from Gujarat State in India) who was unmarried and without children for much of this research certainly did influence my research possibilities, the types of people to whom I had access, and what people told me.

For researchers conducting projects in formerly colonized places or among disenfranchised groups, the power differentials between the researcher and the communities—a consequence of European colonization reproduced through contemporary global capitalism and governance—are of particular importance. Like other foreigners, I was given special treatment locally but was also asked regularly for money to help pay for school fees, medical services, taxes, and the like (though I likely received neither special treatment nor requests for assistance to the extent that they are directed at white men). I often did assist with small requests. Apart from those closest to me, my general practice was, instead of giving to individuals at the end of my research, to offer a gift to the community as a whole or to help link them to a resource that could further develop their project. A car is often another source of anxiety for researchers—while it allows one to get around, it also heightens the visibility of economic differences between residents and the researcher. I decided not to get a car. Not having a car forced me to integrate into the Iganga peoplescape as I walked or used bicycle or motorcycle taxis alongside other residents and my research assistants.

My race and ethnicity was often a topic of interest to people in Iganga and in Uganda generally. In Uganda I am considered a *kyotala* or a "mixed-race" person, and of a particular mixture that is common in the eastern region of Uganda, given the legacy of British colonial use of Indian indentured laborers in the early 1900s to build the railroad, as well as a later wave of immigrant Indian business operators. As many of the early Indian male laborers and immigrants did not bring wives to Africa, they had relationships with black women, producing a *kyotala* population that in some areas of Uganda formed their own social networks and residential areas. When I initially arrived in Iganga, many black Ugandans assumed that I was either a *kyotala* or a *Muhindi* (literally "Hindu," or Indian), but as word spread and people began to see me around town, I became identified as black American. Recognizing the power of one's own identification in shaping the perception of others, one of my longtime research assistants commented, "We see you as black because that's how you see yourself. But in reality, you are not." Her comment highlights a continuum of racial categories and an awareness of historical complexities and shifting realities of race and ethnicity that are often flattened out in the United States's politics of race. My race and ethnicity often allowed me to venture to places around Iganga and especially Kampala without attracting too much attention. My presence in evening social spaces was particularly interesting. While my ethnicity allowed me to fit in more easily (than, say, a white woman) or at least not to stand out, I at times became an object of gaze because my age, gender, and assumed higher socioeconomic status raised curiosity about what brought me to places I should have been told to avoid. Venturing to such places did not necessarily ruin my reputation in Iganga, however, and eventually my presence became the norm and no longer drew so much attention, allowing me to enter social settings with less disruption to the flow of interactions.

Finally, on a more political note, being black also invited conversations about shared experiences between blacks in Africa and those in the United States, including histories of domination, poverty, criminalization of blackness, survival, and cultural creativity in the face of adversity. Like other feminist scholars of color, I am also acutely aware of the propensity of the West to attribute the "problems" of darker-skinned women to the men in their lives (whether fathers, husbands, or bosses), patriarchal government officials, masculinist militaries, or sexist religion leaders. This demonization of men in poorer communities and, hence, the practice of locating the source of women's oppression as being generated *within* her own community have allowed international efforts and the media to downplay or ignore the role that global capitalism and politics and histories of outside intervention (from the colonial period to contemporary HIV and gender equality programs) have played in structuring local configurations of gender and power. No doubt being a feminist and critical theorist of color certainly shapes the questions that guide my collection of empirical data and influences my epistemological understanding of how various inequalities operate in Iganga, Uganda, and globally, much as the identity and positionality of white men, or other intersectional identity, play roles in their ways of seeing and interpreting the lifeways of others.

The Organization of the Book

This book is organized into three parts. Part I is about Iganga's long history of the dispersal of kingroups and the anxiety it has caused through the eyes of elders; Part II is about the emergence of the sexual public sphere and interventions around youth sexuality; and Part III is about the counterpublic of youth romance and love letters. In Chapter 1, I lay out the theoretical framework of this book. I draw from Jürgen Habermas's insights into the emergence and functioning of the public sphere, Michel Foucault's theories of surveillance and regulation, and more recent work on the counterpublic as a site for resistance, creation, and contradiction by scholars such as Nancy Fraser, Lauren Berlant, Michael Warner, and Cathy Cohen. Part I ("Things keep changing"), which includes Chapters 2 and 3, introduces the reader to the ethnographic setting while tracing the changes and continuities in gender and sexuality that have shaped the sexual economy in Iganga. Within the context of economic precarity, social uncertainty, and anxiety, the freely floating *nakyewombekeire* has become a discursive signifier for residents' critiques of immorality and cultural dislocation. Each of the three chapters in Part II ("Publics") examines a different intervention or moral authority aimed at regulating youth sexuality, paying particular attention to how these interventions get localized (in often unintended ways) when refracted through Iganga's specific history, cultural conventions, and sexual economy. The interventions explored include Uganda's AIDS industry (Chapter 4), sexuality education (Chapter 5), and the age of consent law (Chapter 6). Part III ("Counterpublic") shifts from the localization of public moralities into the counterpublic world of youth romance, and broadly argues that love letters offer a unique window into how young people engage with the public sphere in forging their gendered romantic subjectivities and aspirations while remaining aware of the reality of social uncertainty, economic precarity, and reputational risks. In the Conclusion, I return to the story of Agnes and Sam. I trace their stories ten years later to demonstrate that while the scale-up of antiretroviral therapy (ART) has brought hope, it has also exposed existing and new forms of inequalities. In debunking the culture of poverty thesis and the concept of fatalism that subtly underlie programs and policies targeting disparities among the poor, the Conclusion illustrates that a critical anthropology of interventions can uncover how efforts to ameliorate suffering are linked to poor outcomes, persistent inequalities, and the unfolding of counterpublic community responses—such as, in this case, refusal to being further pulled into regional and global marketplaces of interventions, commodities, biomedical fetishes, and moral ideologies.

Youth became social category (attention)

Biological citizenship: the demand for, but limited access to, social welfare based on medical, scientific, and legal criteria that recognize injury and compensate for it

CHAPTER 1

Going Public

The Virus, Video, Evangelicalism, and the Anthropology of Intervention

> Like the effects of industrial pollution and the new system of global financial markets, the AIDS crisis is evidence of a world in which nothing important is regional, local, limited; in which everything that can circulate does, and every problem is, or is destined to become worldwide. (Sontag 1988:180)

> Our government has had no qualms about being frank to our people on issues of a national catastrophe such as the AIDS epidemic. When we came to power in 1986, the problem had already spread to most parts of the country. We opened the gates to national and international efforts aimed at controlling the epidemic. Unfortunately, despite my government's efforts and the high level of awareness among the population, the AIDS epidemic is becoming more and more serious in Uganda. However, this awareness has, over the last few years, started paying off. (President Yoweri Museveni's speech at the first AIDS Congress in East and Central Africa, Kampala, 1991, cited in Museveni 1992:253)

Like all interventions—whether social, legal, economic, military, technology, or public health—designed to engineer the direction or outcome of a society, Uganda's aggressive AIDS control efforts have had profound effects beyond the primary aims of abating the spread of HIV and alleviating the suffering of those infected and affected.[1] With the coming of the HIV epidemic, sexuality in Uganda as elsewhere took on new meaning and urgency. A critical anthropology of interventions reveals how HIV efforts have also contributed to the formation of new public spaces of dialogue and how these competing moralities about sexuality, gender, and the body get absorbed into local communities and their existing tensions. Uganda's internationally recognized and funded AIDS industry thrust talk about sex and sexuality into the public domain in ways that had not been previously encountered in the country, and in many places disrupted what had been considered appropriate and age-specific social spaces for such discussions. It is these social effects of HIV-related interventions—or, the "going public of sexuality"—that form a crucial backdrop for my examination of youth sexual culture in contemporary Uganda and the anxieties surrounding it.

Woven throughout this ethnography are two larger arguments about the consequences of interventions that intensified the going public of sexuality in Uganda.

30

First, Uganda's HIV control efforts, which were initiated in the mid-1980s, leaned on biomedical moral authority to begin what at the time was a globally unprecedented, aggressive campaign to educate the population about acts associated with the new sexually transmitted disease, giving rise to and legitimizing the public discussion of sex. The state-sanctioned public sphere of sex talk was soon populated by the mass media and other commercialized sectors, and helped mobilize the socially conservative counter-movement within the Pentecostal church. Museveni later reflected on the HIV epidemic in his autobiography, writing that the epidemic "opened the gate" for public discourses about sexuality and sexual relationships (1992:275). Second, in the process of "analysis, stocktaking, classification, and specification" of sexual practices and risk, the AIDS industry has worked to delineate and codify the population into tangible risk groups and to define the assumed characteristics of each group (Foucault 1990:24). Public health, along with other discursive regimes such as the law and the mass media, has contributed to making "youth" a more legible social category as each sector pursues its respective project and form of intervention. Understanding the conditions and implications of the going public of sexuality in Uganda is crucial for exploring, as I do in this ethnography, community-level consequences of and responses to bringing intimate relations and the sexuality of individuals into a newly configured public space. This codification and increased surveillance served to heighten not only public awareness of youth as a distinct social category, but also the moral anxiety surrounding youth sexuality. Through these transformations in the public sphere that make youth sexuality hyper-visible and incite anxiety, young people are not silently acted upon. Though structurally and economically marginalized, young people creatively appropriate and recast these same discourses as they participate in meaning-making and in imagining future possibilities in Uganda. As Mamadou Diouf observes, "the condition of young people in Africa, as well as their future, is heavily influenced by the interaction between local and global pressures: the fragmentation or dissolution of local culture and memory, on the one hand, and the influence of global culture, on the other" (2003:2)

The Marketplace for Sexual Moralities

In *The Structural Transformation of the Public Sphere: An Inquiry into a Category of Bourgeois Society* (1991), Habermas argues that the public sphere emerged as a transformative space for dialogue and debate in civil society and outside the operations of the state. Written partly in response to what he saw as pessimism in prevailing Marxist theory, for which the state existed as an authoritarian regime serving the interests of capitalists, Habermas chronicles the emergence and evolving constitution of the non-state public sphere from the seventeenth to the early twentieth centuries in northern Europe as a space for rational, public debate and discourse among educated citizens. This public sphere was both a physical space (such as coffee shops and salons) and a public discourse (such as letters, newspapers, and the media), becoming an important potential "mode of social integration" for various segments of social life (Calhoun 1992:6). Yoweri Museveni's coming to power in Uganda in the mid-1980s after twenty-five years of postcolonial state limitations on trade, speech, and human movement ushered in a new era of free mobility for goods, people, and information, facilitating an increase in the "traffic in commodities and news" (Habermas 1991:15). The emergence of the HIV epidemic along with international (humanitarian and research) interest in tackling the new disease set the stage for the creation of a public sphere around sexuality.

However, it is an oversimplification for the Western media and researchers to say that the HIV awareness campaigns "broke the silence" surrounding sexuality, implying that prior to HIV awareness campaigns there was no discussion (or at least candid discussion) of sex in Africa. As in most societies around the world, communication about sex indeed existed in Uganda in culturally appropriate and coded ways that may not be immediately obvious to outsiders. The idea that HIV campaigns "broke the silence" is not only a misrepresentation but also forecloses an investigation into how communities *did* and *do* communicate about sex, what *is* communicated, and what the deliberate acts of concealing and revealing can tell us about fractures in the ideal sexual culture. Instead of viewing the HIV campaigns as breaking the silence on sex, I argue that the country's well-funded public health efforts set in motion and legitimized a rapid "going public" of sex talk that already existed in culturally appropriate and kinship-based spaces. Before the creation of the AIDS industry, sex could be considered what anthropologist Michael Taussig calls a "public secret" or "that which is generally known, but cannot be articulated"—a secret around which communities remain willfully and publicly silent, at least at the wider social level, but around which they have their own lexicon and set of codes that are communicated in particular designated spaces (1999:5). Arguing for the notion of secrecy rather than silence, Philip Setel writes, "Given this pervasive secrecy it is not difficult to see how the emerging AIDS epidemic was like turning on the lights in a room long kept intentionally dark" (1999:103). I would push this a bit further.

"Going public" has temporal and spatial dimensions. Sex talk existed but had been heavily coded and relatively confined to socially-sanctioned age/sex groups and with the "room long kept intentionally dark." Spatially, the AIDS industry helped elevate discussions of sex from the level of space-specific and coded talk to a public level where sex became subject to wider debate and witnessing, and where the conversation was extended to previously excluded members. In other words, what changed was not that people were now talking about sex, for it was indeed an important topic of discussion in Iganga long before HIV campaigns. For instance, sexually explicit songs performed during Basoga twin-naming ceremonies or, as explored in Chapter 4, intergenerational sexual learning between a betrothed girl and her paternal aunt played major roles in the transmission of ideas about sexuality. Rather than a rupture in which sexuality became a topic for discussion, what the AIDS industry offers legitimacy to, increases the visibility of, and invites wider participation in is the *public* circulation of discourses of sexuality. The permeability of spaces and locations further characterized the public sphere as an arena of participation not only for the educated or middle-class but, to some extent, for the masses who consumed these public ideas and commodities. Important here is that "public discourse must be circulated, not just emitted in one direction" (Warner 2002:71). In the circulated discourse, recognizable "catchphrases," Warner observes, "suture it to [everyday] informal speech, even though those catchphrases are

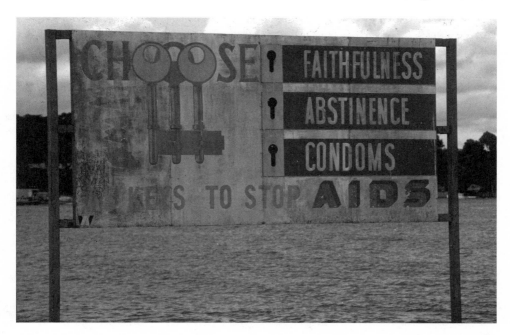

FIGURE 1.1. ABC (abstinence, be faithful, and use condoms) billboard, built in the late 1980s

often common in informal speech only because they were picked up from mass texts in the first place" (ibid.).

Mass-mediated technologies led to a reconfiguration or rearrangement of social categories, or as Lawrence Birken (1988) observes, a "democratization of sexual information," in which a genderless and ageless public consumes an abundance of images (see also Frederiksen 2000). In Uganda, this has meant that the sexual learning of young people shifted from kin networks to the public sphere, further threatening the already fading system of sex education for youth. The proliferation of sex talk in the public sphere broke down preexisting generational and gender lines that determined appropriate access to information and discussions about intimacy and sexuality. Billboards about condoms or sexual networking, for instance, are visibly accessible to all ages and genders at all times, regardless of culturally specific ideas about the rolling out of sexual learning. This seemingly indiscriminate presence of sex in public—the democratization of sexual information—makes many older residents uncomfortable and lies at the heart of critiques of contemporary public sex culture. Importantly, as Warner points out, engaging with the public sphere in which circulation and reflexivity are key requires little individual investment, for "merely paying attention can be enough to make you a member" (Warner 2002:53). Because membership into public sex talk is not exclusive and because public health campaigns are considered an extension of state services (regardless of the funding sources), HIV campaigns became prime targets of scrutiny by an increasingly vocal group of social conservatives. Campaigns were routinely accused of encouraging promiscuity by offering ways to make sex safe (as opposed to discouraging sex altogether). One early campaign was the first condom

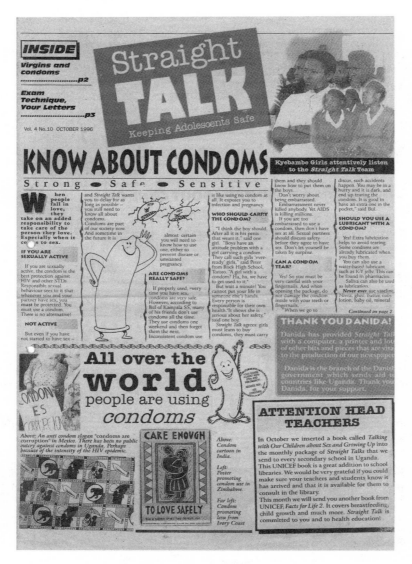

FIGURE 1.2. *Straight Talk* condom campaign, 1996

promotion for youth, which appeared on the front page of the widely circulated and praised *Straight Talk* newspaper insert (Figure 1.2).

In addition to the medico-moral authority that legitimized sex going public, Museveni's economic liberalization policies provided the foundation and incentives for private industry and media outlets to flourish. In the authoritarian periods before Museveni, the state had exercised its power through the control of media and transportation networks, constraining the movement of information and people around the country. The infamous troops at road checks who harassed and stole from citizens created a situation in which the flow of goods and information "remained strictly regulated, serving more as instruments for the domination of the surrounding areas than for the free commodity exchange" (Habermas 1991:15). Museveni's project of "disciplining" the military and police led to a decrease in threats and acts of violence against citizens and facilitated an opening up of movement. The same long-distance road networks that carried HIV throughout Uganda and east Africa a decade earlier now freely carried the exchange of goods, information, and people, resulting in the familiar intertwining of sexual and capitalist geographies. For example, retail shops marketing modern love, romance, and sexuality in products such as clothing and self-help books were able to flourish under Museveni's regime.

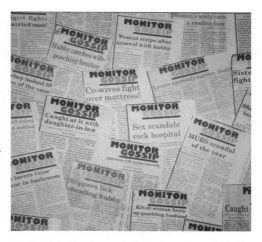

FIGURE 1.3. *Monitor* gossip columns, mid-1990s

A group of young people whose parents had fled Uganda during the political turmoil between the 1960s and early 1980s were instrumental in the formation of popular media and the commercial sector. Returning to Uganda, members of this elite "bentu" class (as in "been to" London or the United States and back) brought into Uganda's burgeoning public sphere new media genres, commercial establishments, and messages that linked sexual pleasure and desire with being modern and global. This is not to say that the media, public health, or other sectors had not provided such messages previously, but rather that the calming of the previous civil unrest and the urgency of HIV led to an opening up of Uganda and intensified the publicness, purpose, and legitimacy of sex talk.

Uganda's globally traveled bentu had seen how the commercialization of pleasure elsewhere in the world was profitable. The bentu played a major role in how global aesthetics and ideas about modern sexuality have been incorporated and adopted into diverse Ugandan social landscapes. If we accept Arjun Appadurai's 1996 theory of a new global cultural economy, which, he argues, "cannot any longer be understood in terms of existing center-periphery models," then the importance of the bentu as cultural brokers who brought ordinary Ugandans to the center of internationally influenced meaning-making becomes clear (32). Their pursuit of entrepreneurial possibilities led to the entry of magazines, radio programs, newspapers, and advertisements into the newly legitimate public conversation of sex, capitalizing on citizens' desires to engage with ideas, goods, and discourses circulating in the global marketplace (Figure 1.3). The growth of this sector is particularly visible in the controversial but popular tabloids, which offer people sensationalized news about scandals and sex. As journalist Xan Rice writes in the *Atlantic*, "although Uganda's leaders like to portray themselves as the guardians of a deeply conservative, Christianity-based culture, Uganda has developed what is perhaps Africa's most sensationalist, predatory, and lurid tabloid press" (2011).

For most youth in Iganga, however, the images that inform their romantic imagination remain economically and socially unobtainable realities, and gender relations still remain largely based on historically produced inequalities. Similarly, reflecting on the mass media in Egypt, Lila Abu-Lughod calls into question the ability of the media to create democratic information flow among women in her study, creating instead a state of social delusion: "The media produces a false sense of egalitarianism that distracts from the significant and ongoing problems of class inequality in Egypt" (1995:53). In Uganda, this dissonance between the constrained realities of everyday life and the lofty promises of modern love adds to the increasing anxiety surrounding youth romance, with older people in Iganga fearing the consequences of young people's pursuit of the unobtainable.

In sum, Museveni's liberalization policies and disciplining of state police and the emergence of the bentu class ushered in a vibrant media and commercial economy that allowed the general public to consume various images and messages about sex in daily newspapers, radio shows, billboards, magazines, advertisements, and gossip columns. Public health conceptions of individualized sexual responsibility and risk initially shaped the public space of sex talk in Uganda, but that quickly changed as alternative dominant discourses emerged. While the AIDS industry and the public health sector circulated discourses of risk and death, the commercial sector, and particularly Uganda's burgeoning mass media, brought onto the public stage the topics of pleasure, love, and desire. What was created was a lucrative "marketplace for sexual information" (Parker and Gagnon 1995:7) that produced multiple messages about sex for an eagerly consuming, though differentiated, public.

Surveillance, Regulation, and the Incitement to Discourse

Whereas for Habermas intellectuals and entrepreneurs who create and participate in the public sphere provide opportunities for social transformation, Michel Foucault would suggest that these people of power are far from benign agents of social change; rather, through their collective participation, these people with influence deploy new forms of specialized authority that reinforce control over ordinary citizens and society. Foucault's general understanding about the relationship between power and those who produce knowledge leads him to conclude that the professionalization of intellectuals stimulates the emergence and refining of tools of social domination and control over populations and bodies, not the freedom of the masses. In *The History of Sexuality: An Introduction*, Foucault argues that in northern Europe, the eighteenth century was the age of the development of *scientia sexualis*, the sciences of knowledge about sexuality (namely, medicine, religion, criminology, and population sciences). The emergence of sciences of sexuality led less to "*a* discourse on sex than . . . a multiplicity of discourses on sex produced by a whole series of mechanisms operating in different institutions" (1990:33; Foucault's emphasis). There was "a dispersion of centers from which discourse emanated, a diversification of their forms" (34). The "explosion of distinct discursivities" of sex occurred such that official discourse about sex was no longer the exclusive domain of Catholic confessionals, as it had been previously. Catholicism's moral authority on sexuality began to weaken in the nineteenth century with the rise and professionalization of medical and population sciences, with each profession producing and training people in its specific tools and language that were aimed at documenting and analyzing data on the sex lives of its clients. The confessional as a hierarchical communication activity between clergy and laymen spread from the Catholic Church to the emerging centers of knowledge, becoming the method through which clients revealed their sexual idiosyncrasies and "deviances" to a new cast of professionals. Through the practice of the confessional, systems of data collection emerged for the nascent fields of science such as psychiatry, population sciences, and medicine (see also Nguyen 2010).

This proliferation of scientific centers of knowing created various discourses (or sets of knowledge) on "proper" sexuality through the "processes of normalization" and its counterpart, the social construction of the deviant. The creation and circulation of truths about normal and deviant sexuality provoked "the urgent need to keep it under close watch and to devise a rational technology of correction" and surveillance (Foucault 1990:120). Hence, the anxiety around sex: the more sex is regulated and deemed illicit, the greater the interest in it. As Foucault argues in his oft-cited chapter "The Incitement to Discourse," this process of normalization did not diminish talk about the sexually illicit and deviant. Rather, newly forming *scientia sexualis* and narrowing of categories of normalcy "radiated discourses aimed at sex, intensifying people's awareness of it as a constant danger, and this in turn created a further incentive to talk about it" (31). These new forms of knowledge led to "a policing of sex: that is, not the rigor of a taboo, but the necessity of regulating sex through useful and public discourses" (25; see also Weeks 1982). In other words, the professionalization and the rise of technologies of sexual surveillance and regulation aimed at cataloging sex into categories including normal and deviant worked to incite—rather than limit—talk about sex.

Capitalism, Foucault argues, further inspires a "series of interventions and *regulatory controls: a bio-politics of the population*" in which technologies were developed to ensure "the controlled insertion of bodies into the machinery of production" and the disciplining of those bodies (1990:139, 141; italics in original text). It is here that historians of gender in Africa have found Foucault's insights particularly useful, for example, in understanding how the regulation of reproduction, sexuality, and gender played a crucial part in establishing and maintaining colonial rule in Africa (Vaughan 1991; Jeater 1993; Hunt 1999; Jackson 2005). Didier Fassin argues that projects of power (such as humanitarian efforts or HIV control programs) are not simply about the regulation and governing of a population, as suggested by Foucault, but also constitute a "politics of life," or "the evaluation of human beings and the meanings of their existence" in which there is a "dialectic between lives to be saved and lives to be risked" (2007b:500–501). HIV interventions act as the politics of life in the *selection* and *criteria* of determining those deemed to be the target of saving (deciding which patients should receive antiretrovirals or what disaster to focus on) and in how those in need of saving are represented (the ultimate vulnerable sufferer falling into despair without external assistance). In the process, however, other causes or people are left aside when they are not selected for saving or for public representation. The emerging publics in Uganda can be understood as systems of control and forms of disciplining or instilling new moralities onto gendered bodies and sexualities. The abundant popular and public health messages about sexuality in Uganda are powerful in shaping the meanings and personal significance of people's sexual realities and experiences. An example is the shift in the early 2000s to identifying segments in Uganda with immoral behavior (such as unfaithful adults) who needed to be disciplined through new ways of thinking. Although the discourses are not totally transformative, nor do they replace existing ideas, they nevertheless do provide Iganga residents possible ways of understanding their own and others' experiences and are particularly important in shaping what is considered to be the "norm." Moreover, the motivations and techniques aimed at controlling the sexuality of young people are underlined by economic incentives and class-based motives. Such is the case with local use of Uganda's defilement law and, in particular, the ease with which certain cases move through the judicial system, such as those involving a poor and younger alleged male perpetrator or an alleged female victim from a wealthier family.

In general, I find Foucault's overall argument compelling, as organized discourses about sex in many ways did lead to a simultaneous incitement to discourse and a greater regulation of sexuality in Uganda. Yet, in addition to demonstrating how discourses in Uganda regulate or replace local beliefs, a critical examination of daily life also shows that the increased circulation of sex talk provides people in Iganga with condensed codes and competing ideas for debating and claiming moral authority. My central question regarding the public discourses of public health campaigns and the mass media is twofold: (1) how is the democratization of sex talk used to create and enforce ideas about morality and youth sexuality, and (2) what are the homemade responses and deployments of local, national, and global flows of sexual imagery, discourses, and ideas—both those of romance and those of regulation—that circulate with increasing ease around Uganda?[2]

Sexperts, Therapeutic Genres, and Controversies of Pleasure

Uganda's aggressive HIV control efforts and the subsequent proliferation of sexual images and messages have played an important role in the creation of a national sexual identity. The national identity is a merger of conservative interpretations of Christianity (greatly influenced by the recent and visibly growing charismatic evangelical Pentecostal movement), reinventions of "traditional" African sexuality (based on well-defined gender roles and kinship obligations to reproduce), and public health ideas about rational decision making and individual responsibility. This national sexual identity revolves around a middle-class, heterosexual, and monogamous couple with not too many years or educational levels separating them (or, in other words, nearing an egalitarian or companionate union). The mythical national sexual citizen is circulated in public speeches and sermons, public health campaigns, the media, and advertisements, and is reproduced in local settings. However, as Lauren Berlant and Michael Warner observe in their article "Sex in Public," an inherent contradiction of a hegemonic national sexuality is that it is virtually impossible to achieve, given people's everyday realities and the wider sociopolitical context, which encourages a different set of sexual liaisons and sexualities. These "daily failures" of a hegemonic sexuality and partnering, Berlant and Warner suggest, expose the "cruelty of normal culture even to the people who identify with it" (1998:556).

Although in Uganda the disconnect between the national ideal and reality (in which structural conditions make it virtually impossible to achieve the ideal) in most cases does not amount to the public shock or feelings of inadequacy that Berlant and Warner suggest in their work on the United States (except, perhaps, the recent visibility of the gay debate), the disconnect at least in heterosexuality does provide an opportunity for creative interventions to emerge. These "daily failures" of Christian doctrines of monogamy, premarital female chastity, historically based male sexual privilege, and—more recently—rigid heteronormativity provoke "a whole public environment of therapeutic genres dedicated to witnessing the constant failure" (556).

The bentu and other popular cultural producers have filled this gap by offering therapeutic genres in Uganda (such as gossip columns or call-in radio shows) that not only allow people to work through individual anxiety about their failed moral competence, but also provide a platform upon which people are required to display an appropriate amount of shock and scorn when the national sexual myth fails so dramatically—a reaction invoked in order to keep that myth alive and well (ibid.). The emergence of a cast of "sexperts" in Uganda has helped citizens achieve a modern premarital sexuality—one that began to privilege, though not completely, individual desires and pleasures over the historically important kin-based web of social relationships. Sexperts have become a new professionalized class whose members, alongside public health workers, diagnose sexual problems and offer advice on how to achieve the desired norm. The contradiction presented to citizens is pursuing of modern sexuality while simultaneously remaining rational-health droids.

The proliferation of sexualized media has drawn extensive criticism from groups who claim that its images are fueling promiscuity and immorality. As the criticism and controversies over images in the media have grown, so too have the interest in and availability of sexual media and the popularity of the commercialized sexpert. The moral wars have escalated. The host of a call-in show on what was considered Uganda's hip radio station received harsh criticism for using sexually explicit terms such as "penis," "vagina," "sexual intercourse," "orgasm," and "cum." In defense, the host, who was also the station manager, explained that the aim of the show was to "keep people alive" by discussing HIV and sex honestly and encouraging people to discuss sex with their partners, hopefully resulting in more responsible sexual choices. The show, he argued, was not vulgar but educational and transformative. Using the language of youth was his way of reaching youth and educating them about their bodies and safer sexual practices. But the Buganda Kingdom, part owner of the station, was not convinced. Fearing that inaction would translate publicly to condoning such obscenity, the Buganda Parliament cancelled the show to avoid tarnishing its relationship with religious leaders and its own moral reputation. The Buganda Parliament publicly stated that it did not want its name associated with promoting sexual vulgarity to an audience of innocent, young people.

By the mid-1990s, soft-sex magazines had introduced color images of young, sexy cover girls into the public sphere; inside, the magazines had black-and-white pullout centerfolds and "real life" short stories about lurid sexual affairs and erotic fantasies. Public controversy erupted when one magazine featured a cover on which the camera

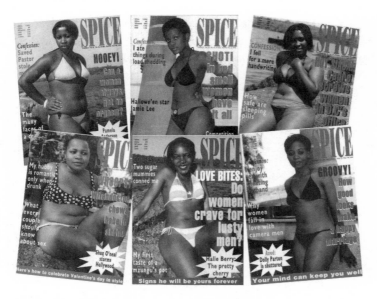

FIGURE 1.4. *Spice* magazine cover girls, late-1990s

angle captured a bit of the cross-legged cover girl's panties. This indecency sparked a flood of letters to the daily newspapers and widespread scrutiny of the sexually ex- plicit covers and content of the magazines. Religious leaders and, later, members of parliament tried to get the magazines banned, but President Museveni was opposed to censoring the media and claimed that freedom of speech was essential for democracy, a position he would later change when it came to issues of same-sex relationships (BBC 2004a). "Before that cover," explained the university-educated editor during an inter- view, "no one said much about our magazine although there were definitely uneasy feelings about what we were doing. Now it is thought to be a dirty magazine." As we spoke, a Koran and Bible lay among the eclectic collection of reference books on his desk. Since being labeled "dirty" and "vulgar," that magazine's and other publications' cover girls have become more scantily dressed, frequently in bikinis or in a suggestive pose (Figure 1.4). Many residents assert that these publications have gone too far, with titles such as "Piss Makes Me Horny," "Housewife Had Bedded 5000 Men, Wants More," "Teen Girl Screws Man in Her Father's Bed," "I Fantasise about Being Raped," and "Miracle Doctor Cures with His Dick." The target of much controversy and atten- tion, their popularity has soared. From the controversial *Red Pepper* tabloid reporting on infidelities of public figures and clandestine lovers on the back streets of Kampala to the December 2014 release of Uganda's first LGBTI publication, *Bombastic*, amid the fervor of the Anti-Homosexuality bill, the tabloid culture occupies a prominent space of transformative and transgressive sexual expression in the country's public sphere. Today, such publications are highly visible in urban pedestrian landscapes throughout Uganda as street vendors eagerly display and frequently wave around the provocative cover photos, scandalous headlines, and fantastical stories.

The Counterpublic: An Alternative Space
for Youthful Expression and Affective Imaginings

Berlant and Warner note that people who fail to achieve or are unable to access the national sexual identity, even after receiving "therapy" or messages about how to achieve the mythical norm, might participate in the formation and sustaining of an alternate community or "counterpublic" based on their transgressive but shared sexual reality. The notion of a subaltern counterpublic was proposed by scholars who appreciated Habermas's attention to the functioning of civil society but who were unsatisfied with his handling of nonelites' or marginalized communities' participation in the creation of alternate lifeways and meaning-making. In Nancy Fraser's influential 1992 article, "Rethinking the Public Sphere: A Contribution to the Critique of Actually Existing Democracy," she posits that feminists have formed a counterpublic: "On the one hand, they function as spaces of withdrawal and regroupment; on the other hand, they also function as bases and training groups for agitational activities directed toward wider publics" (124). More recent reformulations of Habermas turn attention to the nondominant "counterpublics" as an alternate "world conscious of its subordinate relation" (Berlant and Warner 1998:558). They extend Habermas's initial use of public—which signaled a discourse of the bourgeois, educated class that existed outside of the state—to include a "plurality of competing publics" that emerge from a variety of often divergent social groups and movements whose members find they "have no arenas for deliberation among themselves about their needs, objectives, and strategies" (Fraser 1992:122). However, as Cathy Cohen highlights in her analysis of "indigenous moral panics" within the African American community, segments of subgroups call upon a moral authority in attempt to protect their prestige, status, and mobility. Within the counterpublic world of youth romance this results in an internal policing and an engagement with a politics of respectability that serves to further stratify youth (C. Cohen 2009).

In Part III of this ethnography, I take the exchange of love letters among young people in Iganga as creating a "parallel discursive arena" of "agitational activity" through which youth "invent and circulate counterdiscourses to formulate oppositional interpretations of their identities, interests, and needs" (Fraser 1992:123). Warner writes that whereas "dominant publics are by definition those that can take their discourse pragmatics and their lifeworlds for granted . . . counterpublics are spaces of circulation in which it is hoped that the poesis of scene making will be transformative, not replicative merely" (2002:88). As we see with love letters, however, youth combine their invented discursive repertoires with ones borrowed and reworked from the dominant spheres to create a new romantic lexicon. But unlike Fraser's subaltern feminism and Warner's queer world, many heterosexual participants in the youth counterpublic eventually will transition into the dominant public, setting both spheres in constant re-creative motion. It is precisely adults' intimate knowledge of and past experiences with the counterpublic world of youth love letters—for they were once subaltern participants in it—that makes adult regulation of youth romance so intense. In examining love letters and youth romance as a counterpublic to adult regulatory publics, this ethnography considers how young people create and express gendered sentiments of affection through their love letters and, in doing so, regulate or monitor their own sexual behaviors as well as those of their peers. Youth romance is both a site of imagining desire and a site for reproducing gender and other inequalities. As an imaginative space, it is a site of infinite possibilities where young people grapple with and work out contemporary issues in ways that give us, the reader and researcher, insight into what Uganda's future culture of intimacy and gender might look like.

Theoretical Lineages and Contributions

In addition to investigating the effects of interventions that enabled the going public of sexuality and competing moralities, this book engages with three bodies of literature—anthropological and humanistic research on HIV and sexuality in Africa, feminist theories on love and romance, and studies on youth as agents of change. I provide readers with brief overviews of the historical developments in each body of literature in order to situate the analytic approaches taken in this study.

Sexuality and HIV in Anthropology and in Africa

The 1981 emergence of the HIV epidemic brought new urgency, motivations, methods, and attention to the study of sexuality and gender. This urgency has inspired greater creativity in the study of sexuality, but has also brought to the surface tensions among various disciplines' aims, assumptions, and methods. An early divide existed between traditional public health and behavioral research approaches and more humanistic disciplines. The former tended to rely on population-data and cohort studies to understand the social determinants of health, determine causal relationships, and eventually design programs and policies to control the epidemic. When the epidemic emerged, anthropologists and other scholars interested in sexuality and gender in everyday life focused on refining methods and theories used to understand sexuality and gender within the epidemic as being socially constructed and embedded within shifting social, historical, and ideological landscapes (Herdt and Lindenbaum 1992; Brummelhuis and Herdt 1995; Farmer, Connors, and Simmons 1996; Parker 2001; Parker and Gagnon 1995; Schoepf 1988; Bond, Kreniske, and Susser 1997). There have been numerous calls to break down the differences between the behavioral and humanistic approaches and move toward interdisciplinary (or, more recently, transdisciplinary) approaches, but general disciplinary differences and priorities persist. This book builds on humanistic and anthropological approaches to sexuality, gender, and HIV, and therefore my discussion focuses on developments in those disciplines.

Early in the epidemic, cultural theorists highlighted the ways in which both media and scholarly representations of the disease tended to reify existing fears and prejudices about affected communities, shaping how the epidemic overall was understood in the minds of the general public and often leading to denial and blame. Cultural theorists demonstrated that AIDS was not only a biological or medical condition but also a discursively constructed social phenomenon, or what Paula Treichler (1987) has called an "epidemic of signification." The epidemic, according to Treichler, was represented in racialized, gendered, and sexualized ways in news stories, speeches, conference proceedings, and donor reports, generating a new reality of the disease (1987, 1999). Scholars working in Africa argued that AIDS was commonly portrayed in the Western media as a distant disease of the sexually or racially exotic "other" through the language, metaphors, and visual images used to discuss the epidemic (Lyons 1997). Such characterizations create an image of a dirty and deservingly infected and at-risk population, serving to further stigmatize and invoke fear of already marginalized communities, including in the early days of the epidemic gay men, injecting drug users, Haitian immigrants to the United States, and people in Africa (Parker and Aggleton 2003; Sontag 1988; Watney 1989; Patton 1990, 1997, 2002).

By comparing European responses to STDs in colonial Africa to contemporary Western responses to HIV in Africa, historical work has shown how discourses on HIV contained the same racist stereotypes as those that shaped responses to syphilis, a disease that colonial health officials believed to be the result of inherent African promiscuity and immorality (Lyons 1999; Setel, Lewis and Lyons 1999). Scholars have highlighted how media depictions of the primarily sexually transmitted disease in Africa drew from and reinforced colonial-based and racist notions of a dark, diseased, and savage continent (Oppong and Kalipeni 2004; Craddock 2004). Media images of emaciated black bodies fit easily with neoliberalism's paternalist attitude toward the global South, giving rise to a troubling yet familiar message: that of Africa as a place of rampant sexual promiscuity and immorality, *still* in need of Western assistance to save Africans from their own self-destruction. And this saving was to be accomplished by introducing Western morals, sensibilities, and biomedical understandings of the body, including proper sexual relations. The publicity surrounding and aid given to the cause of HIV in Africa proved to be a double-edged sword—Africa received economic and technical assistance while simultaneously (and necessarily) being constructed as backward or in a state of complete helplessness.

The media was not the only target of accusations of racist portrayals of HIV in Africa. Scholars already involved in research on sexuality or reproduction in Africa turned their findings from other studies into models for understanding the epidemic. Joseph Oppong and Ezekiel Kalipeni wrote that some scholars "constructed theories based on the eccentricities of African sexuality" and in some cases "outright racial determinism" (2004:49). Particularly concerning were works that linked Africa's epidemic to cultural practices that were portrayed as definitive and never changing, such as William Rushing's claim that in Africa "having multiple sexual partners is a common cultural practice" (1995:60). Rushing and others based their conclusions on an article by widely known demographer John Caldwell and his collaborators (1989). In the article, Caldwell, Caldwell, and Higgins argued that "a distinct and internally coherent African system embracing sexuality, marriage, and much else" was fueling Africa's high HIV and fertility rates (187). The authors contrasted what they called a "Eurasian sexuality" model (which revolved around female chastity and intense supervision) with a model of "African sexuality" (in which sex was conceived as an activity "much like eating and drinking" and permissiveness led to widespread sexual networking) in order to explain why sexual health outcomes on the two continents differed. Like other authors proposing an overarching theory of a monolithic African sexuality, Caldwell and his team were criticized for cherry-picking their evidence from previous studies that were not focused on sexuality (Le Blanc, Meintel, and Piché 1991), decontextualizing data from their historical and structural conditions, and particularly ignoring the effects of colonialism (Ahlberg 1994); the reasoning of Caldwell, Caldwell, and Higgins also narrowly equates morality with Christianity while ignoring indigenous systems of morality and rules of sexuality (Heald 1995). This piece for many served as a reminder of the necessity of historically grounded and contextually specific research for understanding contours of the epidemic in Africa as well as globally.

Another group of anthropologists cautioned about the limits of the narrow epidemiological categories of risk that guided HIV policies and programs (Packard and Epstein 1991; Kane 1993). These critics maintained that the concept of risk groups was inadequate in understanding Africa's epidemic given the region's generalized epidemic (meaning that more than 1 percent of the adult population was infected and that the illness was not confined to any particular behavioral group). Their work suggested that the notion of risk categories not only decontextualized risk by locating vulnerability at the individual level and masking structural inequalities and factors but also ignored the permeable boundaries of these categories. For example, as Karen Booth observed, women were defined as either innocently infected mothers or virus-carrying sex workers, precluding the reality that, out of economic necessity, some women might belong to both categories or slide between them at any particular moment (2004:56–57). Other criticism arose about the development practice of dividing the world into types of epidemics. The disease cartography suggested that the developed world had a concentrated epidemic that was contained within specific risk groups, whereas sub-Saharan Africa had a generalized epidemic that was uncontainable and spread throughout society. This division led not only to a stigmatization and undifferentiation of risk groups in the West, but to a further exoticization of the epidemic in Africa. A more recent work examining the relationship among medicine, science, and research is Johanna Crane's *Scrambling for Africa: AIDS, Expertise, and the Rise of American Global Health Science*, in which she examines the politics of research collaboration between Africa and the West and the global production of knowledge (2013).

Chronicling shifts in the focus and politics of anthropologists' work on HIV in Africa, George Bond and Joan Vincent (1997) observed that the first generation of anthropologists working on HIV in Africa were often PhD graduate students who became "handmaidens" to biomedical and epidemiological researchers. These young anthropologists were funded to be cultural experts, taking stock of the variety and frequency of sexual practices and beliefs, just like anthropologists who had been deployed to the unexplored interior of Africa to collect information for the colonial administration. The second generation of anthropologists, Bond and Vincent observed, moved away from collecting data for behavioral studies and began bringing to the study of HIV the same critical social theory and nuanced ethnographic methods that the discipline used to explore other social problems (86–90). This now well-established body of ethnographic work focused on HIV and AIDS as situated in complex social and economic contexts and webs of inequalities, an approach often called "political economy" or "critical medical anthropology" (e.g., Ankrah 1991; Bond, Kreniske, and Susser 1997; Brummelhuis and Herdt 1995; Farmer 1992, 2001; Herdt and Lindenbaum 1992; Schoepf 1992, 1995; Singer 1997; Campbell 1997; Parker, Herdt, and Carballo 1991; Scheper-Hughes 1994; Setel 1999; McGrath et al. 1993; Smith 2014).

Finding analytic inspiration from this Marxist-informed political economy approach in anthropology (see Roseberry 1988; Ortner 1984; Wilk and Cliggett 2007), critical medical anthropologists have paid close attention to the material and historical conditions and inequalities that structured the lives of people in Africa and that shaped the spread of HIV around the continent. They sought to shift the paradigm away from a narrow view of the epidemic as merely the result of sexual habits and toward a wider understanding of how conditions and histories of global and local economic inequalities, labor migration with spousal separation, high geographic mobility, armed conflicts and insecurity, and disruptions of local marital and kinship systems provided ideal conditions for the epidemic to flourish. Jennifer Cole and Lynn M. Thomas summarize the shift toward the political economy approach: "Most anthropological research on AIDS and sexuality has deliberately eschewed broad cultural generalizations, fearing that such analyses simultaneously blame the victims and dehistoricize the causes of the epidemic. Instead, scholars have demonstrated how pervasive poverty and other forms of structural violence shape sexual practices" (2009:9).[3] This ethnography builds on a political economy approach in its understanding of sexuality and HIV in Iganga for, in addition to providing a more holistic understanding of the epidemic, it also reflects the way residents themselves understand HIV and changes in youth sexuality as embedded within a complex web of change and globally inflected historical disruptions. Examinations of economic underpinnings and inequalities shaping structures of vulnerability and risk are important not only for dispelling popular myths about sexuality in areas highly affected by HIV, but also for designing appropriate and sustainable policies and programs to combat HIV. However, as Cole and Thomas argue, vulnerability and sex-for-money relationships represent only one aspect of people's experiences with sexuality and "such accounts once again background the role of emotions in intimacy" (10).[4]

The Anthropology of Romance, Love, and Intimacy

Over the past several decades, romance, love, and intimacy have become productive areas of research. Since the earlier works of Bronislaw Malinowski (1927; 1929) and Margaret Mead (1928) that challenged European assumptions of lust-based sexuality among colonialized people as well as the universalist ideas of the Oedipus complex and *sturm and storm* (respectively), anthropologists today stress that love and romance as part of sexuality are not particular to the West but are found in various iterations throughout the world. The topics of romance and love have gained currency as a way for scholars to examine how people, in their intimate relations with others, interact with modernity, globalization, economic monetization, demographic shifts, and moralizing discourses. Literature on love and romance can be broken into two analytic tendencies—a social evolutionary approach and a critical gender theory or feminist perspective. Much of the social evolutionary literature on love is undergirded by a main (and often unstated) assumption of a unilinear progression between levels of intimacy and social development such as literacy or technology. A text that can be interpreted as leaning on an evolutionary framework is Anthony Giddens's *The Transformation of Intimacy: Sexuality, Love and Eroticism in Modern Societies* (1992). Giddens documents historical developments in love and intimacy, positing that in premodern societies intimate liaisons are grounded in systems of kin-based sexual pairing. It is the rise of capitalism and literacy that occasions the rise to "romantic love," which eventually gives way to "pure love," in which the individual and self-identity are central (38–40).[5] The implication, whether intended or not, is that monogamous companionate love originates in the West among people with greater economic means and literate abilities, fairly recently spreading to the elite in the global South, and becoming an aspiration of the lower classes around the world with the increased circulation of consumption-based romance. Jack Goody, while critical of Giddens's causal link between the rise of literacy (as demonstrated particularly in the popularity of novels) and romantic love, falls back on the idea that romantic imagination is absent in Africa: "In Black Africa generally one does not find much development of a discourse of love" (1998:119). As I demonstrate in this book, however, elders' life narratives are replete with notions of love and romance, and an analysis of love letters shows the complexities involved in youthful romance today.

Another analytic approach to love and the one taken in this book—the political economy of love—rejects the idea that romantic love and companionate relationships have emerged from a homogenous process and represent an advanced stage of social development. Rather than setting out to categorize types of relationships and locate them on a unilinear scale of progress, this alternative approach seeks to tease out how the meanings, significance, and forms of relationships depend on historically specific political, economic, and social processes. This history- and context-specific approach has emphasized the notion that people's romantic experiences are profoundly shaped and given meaning by the material and social conditions around them (Ahearn 2001; Rebhun 1999; J. S. Hirsch and Wardlow 2006; Cole and Thomas 2009; Collier 1997; Kendall 1996; Padilla et al. 2007; Adrian 2003; D. C. Holland and Eisenhart 1992; Constable 2003; Brennan 2004; Lutz 1988; Lutz and Abu-Lughod 1990). This work situates local and historical transformations in intimacy within the monetization of the economy, Christian missionizing, and the weakening of kinship bonds in favor of civil affiliation and as intersecting with the globalization of discourses and the ideologies of love. Scholars argue that while there may seem to be a trend toward an individualization of intimacy, there is no obvious or predetermined way in which these liaisons and their significance take shape locally. In other words, while recognizing that globalization and capitalism have occasioned material and ideological similarities in modern love and romance, anthropologists interested in the relationship of the dialectic between structure and agency demonstrate how local realities shape the configurations and meanings of intimacy and emotion.

Far from the earlier anthropological approach of "cultural relativism," which attempted to move away from an evaluative judgment about cultural differences and to emphasize instead that variations among societies and values are different but equal, this more recent context-specific approach pays attention to the *conditions* that shape, sustain, promote, or transform practices of intimacy. While acknowledging that specific practices and discourses of love vary around the world and through time, scholars have generally agreed that companionate liaisons are characterized by some degree of individual choice (as opposed to unions arranged by kin groups), affective bonds, trust and communication, intimacy, and a mutual investment in a larger marital or relationship project (see Simmons 1979; Skolnik 1991). Interest in the global trend toward an idealization of companionate relationships has led to a body of social histories of intimacy that bring attention to how wider economic changes, social policies, and greater distinctions in class boundaries have shaped (often in unpredictable ways) normative forms of sexuality and gender and as a result have further stigmatized communities or groups that do not conform to the phony morality of monogamous heteronormativity (Warner 1999; D'Emilio and Freedman 1988; Bailey 1988; Povinelli 2006). Other scholarship on romance has provided useful ways of considering how popular cultural images of romance and love have challenged and created social conflicts over what it means to be a modern lover (Larkin 1997; Boden 2003; Fuglesang 1994).

Particularly influential in these critical gender theory or feminist approaches is Friedrich Engels's 1884 treatise *The Origin of the Family, Private Property and the State* and his proposition that the privatization of property under capitalism may engender women's subordination as wealth becomes consolidated in the hands of male household heads while wives and children are relegated to the roles of dependents and household laborers. This Marxist-inspired perspective highlights how the persistence of gender and class inequalities shapes the experiences of men and women in companionate relations in such a way that romance and love might reproduce rather than disrupt women's subordination, as one might expect (Illouz 1997; Radway 1984; Holland and Eisenhart 1992; Sobo 1995; Wardlow and Hirsch 2006; Bastian 2001). For instance, women might choose to accept or willfully ignore their husbands' infidelities as a way of protecting their reputations and presenting themselves and their marriages as "modern" and "monogamous" (Parikh 2007, 2009; J. S. Hirsch, Wardlow, Smith, et al. 2010). Yet, as Wardlow and Hirsch warn, "to think about couples only in terms of power . . . is to miss the fact that men and women may also care for the conjugal partners with whom they are simultaneously involved in daily battles over bodies, power, and resources" (2006:3).

In this book, I build on this feminist approach to love and intimacy by locating the gendered and class dynamics of contemporary youth sexual culture in Uganda within broader historical, social, and economic transformations and inequalities that shape the lives of young people and their families. I am interested in how relationships such as Sam and Birungi's are situated within Iganga's sexual economy—or, as I discussed earlier, the complex exchange system that is not entirely economic (such as the relationship between sex and money) but that also weaves together structures of affect (such as sentiment and emotion) and symbolic meanings (such as the significance of elaborate wedding rituals).

As I argue in the case of Iganga, it is not that romance or companionate love is new in Uganda, for narratives of companionate love and romance are a common feature in the older men's and women's life histories that I collected as well as in Basoga folktales and songs. What has changed is "the way people evaluate their experiences of love and marriage in relation to this emerging global ideal" (Wardlow and Hirsch 2006:4). As Jane Collier (1997) suggests, we should not misread a discursive shift as a shift in desires or lived experiences. In addition to discursive shifts, a shift in actualization has occurred. As we saw in the Introduction, Sam's romantic desires were thwarted by social and economic uncertainties that interact with gendered access to resources. Hence, as in the past, turning a romantic premarital relationship into a marriage or more permanent relationship is often complicated by other social forces, such as kin obligations, status, and class. The difference is that unlike their grandparents, young people in Iganga do expect (sometimes to their great disappointment) that their future marriage will come from one of their romantic relationships, or at least from their own selection of a mate. The youth with whom I interacted also would prefer that their romantic relationships not be shrouded in such secrecy and that their youthful courtship encounters could more comfortably enter into the public arena, though their current circumstances of being dependent on and under the constant supervision of disapproving adults at home and school do not permit this (see also Haram 2005; Harrison 2008; Mutongi 2000). On the other hand, elders' concerns about the increased publicness of desire-seeking youth are exacerbated and justified by the equally visible category of *nakyewombekeire*, who represent the ultimate consequence of modern romance.

Youth and Moral Anxiety

In Uganda, as around the world, the past century has witnessed a gradual prolongation and codification of the life stage of "youth," which has led to an extension and social recognition of the period between childhood and adulthood. The prolongation of this stage has brought further policy and scholarly attention to the social experiences and problems faced by this growing group of unmarried and often unemployed young people. For a long time anthropologists argued against the tendency of treating adolescence as merely a transitional life stage or a liminal state through which children pass on their way to adulthood (Mead 1928; Whiting and Whiting 1975; Herdt 1981). The conceptualization of youth as a passing ground on the way to adulthood has been replaced by an appreciation of the role of youth play as cultural producers who, through their practices, have appropriated and created new cultural forms and offered social critiques of their own economic and political marginalization as well as of oppressive practices in their societies in general (S. Hall and Jefferson 1976; Hebdige 1979; Rose 1994; Amit-Talai and Wulff 1995; Gable 2000; K. T. Hansen 2000; Casco 2006). Similar to theories of counterpublics, this literature often points out how these young agitators for change assert their challenges to hegemonic authority by appropriating and reworking global and regional cultural forms and ideas, making them their own creations. To borrow from Deborah Durham, in this book I take youth as "social shifters," drawing attention to them both as "indexical," located within wider social relations of power, authority, and responsibilities, and as "referential," highlighting their "reactions to and agency within a larger society" as they actively shape the public sphere despite their often marginalized positions (Durham 2004:592–93; see also Honwana and De Boeck 2005; Dolby 2006).

Analysis of youth in sub-Saharan Africa has been complicated by the distinction between age-grade systems, which are found among many ethnic groups, and Western-influenced ideas about life stages, which are often promoted through formal education, laws, and other colonial institutions (see, for instance, Evans-Pritchard 1940). While the former is based on and solidified through social networks and lines of authority, the latter is more closely linked to chronological age and wider social, economic, and legal projects pursued by the colonial and postcolonial states. Ethnographers working in precolonial and colonial Africa observed the importance of age-grade sets, commonly formed through initiation ceremonies, in establishing and maintaining inter- and intra-generational networks, relationships and hierarchies, and gendered adult status and bodies (Fortes and Evans-Pritchard 1940; Evans-Pritchard 1940; Richards 1956; LeVine and Sangree 1962; Mbiti 1973). During the colonial era the age-grade system did not necessarily disappear, but alongside it emerged the colonial-based idea of belonging to the life stage of adolescence (Baxter and Almagor 1978).

Historians and anthropologists have emphasized the fact that the extension and codification of youth as a life stage is an ongoing processing, taking on different configurations and occurring at different rates around the world depending on wider political, economic, and social contexts. However, in general they have noted that the creation of "youth" has been occasioned by formal education, delays in marriage and reproduction, transformations in the labor market and regulations, high rates of unemployment, international development and policy agendas surrounding the notion of children's rights, and commercial marketing and consumption practices (see Durham 2000; Thomas and Cole 2009; Cole and Durham 2006; Stambach 2000; Hutchinson 1996; Cole 2004). Scholars of youth have also highlighted the gendered and class nature of adolescence. A young girl was expected to marry soon after reaching menarche, partly to avoid the shame of getting pregnant while in her father's home, as premarital pregnancy would bring both social stigma and economic burden to the girl's natal family. Also, formal education and colonial youth-based groups were created initially for the sons of elite Africans in order to create a future generation of government and civil servants (Parsons 1999). Only later was colonial attention given to educating or domesticating girls, mainly to become potential wives of elite African males, facilitating the creation of the social category of adolescence for girls.

International humanitarian efforts have worked to further codify and problematize the category of youth. Emerging from international efforts to help rebuild European economies and prevent the spread of communism after World War II—like the US's Marshall Plan—such programs eventually evolved into what we now call international development. Humanitarian aid programs and development agencies in general define population categories that researchers, planners, and policy makers use to collect data and understand risk, and for which they design targeted programs (Escobar 1995; Ferguson 1990; Patton 1996). In contrast to the initial years of the AIDS epidemic in the United States, where the behavioral categories of "men who have sex with men" (MSM), injecting drug users (IDUs), and hemophiliacs emerged as categories of risk as defined by surveillance bodies, in Africa the initial categories were more occupationally driven, with long-distance truck drivers, commercial sex workers, and highly mobile populations (such as migrant workers or military combatants) identified as risk groups. By the second decade of the epidemic (when the epidemic was clearly generalized), global attention on Africa's epidemic turned to the broader concern of African women's and girls' sexual vulnerability as fueled by African (and, as more recent scholarship highlights, global) patriarchal structures (Obbo 1995; Schoepf 1997).

A major concern of this literature is how a society or community deals with a growing population of socially active and independent but frequently economically marginalized and hence dependent group of young people who are eager to, but cannot fully, participate in the marketplace of work and consumption. Economic uncertainty and crisis around Africa in more recent times, coupled with the shift away from agrarian-based economies to market-based ones, has left a large portion of young people, like Sam in the opening vignette, unemployed or caught in temporary work assignments, making it increasingly difficult for young people to transition into independent adults (see Durham 2000). These "idle" young men and sexually "precocious" yet "vulnerable" young women garner much attention from policy makers who seek to abate negative outcomes caused by this population. Within Iganga, while "idle" young men represent general social decline or stalled social advancement, the female counterpart is the "free young woman" who is left in a liminal state of belonging by economic realities, suspended between her natal family, who can no longer financially support her, and a pool of young men delaying marriage because of the lack of resources necessary and expected for modern matrimony. The problem of youth sexuality is expressed in the changing notion of the social category *nakyewombekeire*, the women Sam frequented after his heartbreak from Birungi (see also P. J. Davis 2000; La Fontaine 1974; Hodgson and McCurdy 2001). Once used to refer to older, unmarried, or independent women, today *nakyewombekeire* is more commonly a derogatory term for younger women who appropriate control of and profit from their own sexuality and romantic desires. Together, these idle young men and free young women create a socially suboptimal condition of prolonged economic dependence and thus prolonged adolescence.

PART I

"Things keep changing"

Histories of Dispersal and Anxiety in Iganga

[handwritten at top: Disease, urbanization and migration have uprooted people from their *maka and thus taken them away from the "protection and moral economy" it provides]

[handwritten: Anxiety towards sexuality ↑ in unmarried adolescent males]

[handwritten: maka = where a person's soul and intimate attachments belong]

CHAPTER 2

Demographic Shifts, Free Young Women, and Idle Adolescent Men

Eric Wolf (1982) suggests that local histories play a critical role in how contemporary problems take shape and are understood by communities. Capturing this perspective requires that we shift our gaze away from the traditional history "from above" as codified by elites through official colonial or government records, and instead refocus our attention on historical narratives "from below" as generated by communities affected. Histories from below that take seriously residents' understandings of the past can reveal how community responses, which may be interpreted from above as evidence of backwardness or timeless cultural habits, may in fact be logical and creative adaptations for coping with uncertainty and change (see Whyte 1997). A community's process of constructing historical narratives about how things came to be as they are can be understood as an act of reclamation, the development of a collective consciousness, or small acts of resistance against fully accepting dominant narratives, expressing awareness of oppressive conditions that are beyond a community's control (see Scott 1985). In addition to providing alternative narratives to official and meta-narratives, the *process* of local history making is itself a contested site through which individual community members draw upon various forms of authority to make claims not only about the past but also about how the present ought to be.

This chapter and the next introduce the ethnographic setting of this book. This chapter draws from elders' historical narratives, which reveal how they understand their recent past as one of constant change that has been occasioned by environmental transformations, the penetration of capitalism, state intervention, political conflict, and technological advances. Elders capture this constant change with the Lusoga saying "Ebintu bikyuka kyuka" (things keep changing), which equally reflects their feelings of powerlessness amid wider changes. Of particular importance in this sea of change is the concept of belonging to a *máka*, loosely defined as the cosmological place where a person's soul and intimate attachments belong. For a long time, forces such as disease, migration, and urbanization have occasioned the gradual and sporadic uprooting of people from their *máka*, scattering families and individuals around the region and causing a general moral unease. More recent social and economic trends experienced locally have led to the dislocation of adolescent males and *nakyewobekeire*. Hence, before the coming of HIV, this uprooting of youthful bodies from the protection and moral economy of the *máka* had contributed to the increased anxiety surrounding youth sexuality.

The *Longue Durée*: Modernity, Change, and Disease

Historian David Cohen wrote, "The colonial era in Busoga was marked by tremendous demographic upheavals. . . . In many cases, people have left their traditional lands. Peoples have migrated into Busoga in large numbers in this century, carrying with them the traditions and cultures of other lands" (1972:24). The collective memories of elders I interviewed who were born between 1905 and 1957 mirror Cohen's description of demographic upheavals in the region. Elders' narratives of the *longue durée* (long-term historical structures) reveal that the emergence of HIV was just another moment in what they view as a longer history of disease and devastation brought on by wider economic, climate, and demographic changes. These changes have greatly affected how kinship groups organize and have authority over their junior members, particularly as the security provided by kinship affiliation has gradually diminished over time. A brief look at this *longue durée* through the memories of older people provides a useful perspective into contemporary anxieties about HIV, interventions around it, and the bodies of those at risk.

With great vividness and dramatic flair, a group of elders in the small brick-making village of Busowobi, about a forty-five minute *boda-boda* (bicycle or motorcycle taxi) ride from Iganga Town, used the lens of disease and demographic shifts as a way of chronicling the history of the region. They explained how various diseases entered into the community; some shared memories of public health interventions to control the epidemics; others detailed the responses of the government, relatives, and neighbors. Busowobi elders began their history by recalling two deadly waves of sleeping sickness—the first in the early 1900s, the second in the middle of the century—that decimated their region. They detailed the colonial government's eradication plan, which involved forced evacuation in southern Busoga along the shores of Lake Victoria where the tsetse fly (the vector) bred. The evacuation policy was controversial and drove hundreds of thousands of residents from their homeland and dispersed them throughout Busoga and neighboring regions while another third of the population, an estimated 250,000 people, died (D. W. Cohen 1972; Musere 1990; Fèvre et al. 2004). For some of the residents, this evacuation set off a dispersal of clans and kin groups into smaller units. Families lost touch with their initial *máka* as smaller kingroups tried to reestablish elsewhere in the region. The dispersal of the population and breakdown of the *máka* led to the spread of sleeping sickness and other diseases to uninfected populations.

Elders attributed the arrival of other diseases to the "opening up" of their area and the increased connection of their area to previously foreign worlds. Their collective stories of the plague (*kawumpuli*) in the 1920s provide an example that closely resembles their thoughts about the arrival of HIV. An elder named Joseph remembers the plague coming with the expansion of the East African railways into Busoga and the arrival of British capitalists, Indian railway laborers, and eventually commerce. He had been assisting his uncle in building his coffee business into one of the largest providers for a well-known Indian merchant in town when people started to die of a mysterious new disease. A noticeable population of black rats (*nsolima* or *Rattus rattus*) appeared and began eating the cotton seeds that were stored inside people's homes and in household ginneries. Joseph's uncle was particularly hard-hit by an invasion of black rats. "White men dressed in shorts" used African interpreters to tell farmers that the increase in illness and death was because of a disease carried by the rats. However, instead of halting the farming of cotton, the British introduced new incentives to increase cotton production as global demand for cotton surged. Other colonies also increased cotton production to take advantage of the global demand, leading to a great surplus of stored cotton, even more rats, and more frequent occurrences of *kawumpuli*.[1]

The public health policy to eradicate the plague involved a rat destruction program in which residents were given money for every rat tail they brought into the District Health Office (see Vaughan 1991:41–43). People began to invade others' property and traps in search of *nsolima*, as the new public health program made rat tails a more reliable source of income than cotton. Pilfering traps and stealing rat tails became a way of surviving. Joseph's uncle's business declined as his workers started becoming ill and neighbors began stealing cotton and other household property while searching for the profitable rat tails. Years of intensive cash cotton farming also had a devastating effect on the land. The soil was depleted of minerals, leaving acres of land barren and unable to produce even simple household food crops. Eventually Joseph's once wealthy family had to relocate to the area where Joseph now lives. "*Kawumpuli*," he recalls, "was far worse than AIDS. It killed so quickly and terribly. *Nsolima* infested a home when everyone left for farming, and neighbors began stealing from each other, so the only solution was to keep someone there and sacrifice farm labor." Similar stories of structural change and disease were told about a smallpox (*kawari*) epidemic, a second and more virulent wave of sleeping sickness, and eventually the arrival of AIDS into their respective villages, a topic I examine in greater detail in Chapter 4.[2]

When reflecting on Uganda's post-independence era, elders shift their memories from agrarian-based diseases to the series of national political power struggles that had profound economic consequences. The social euphoria of the country's peaceful liberation from the British in 1962 was followed by more than twenty years of political unrest. In 1966, the first post-independence president, Milton Obote, won a battle for power against the king of Buganda, at that time the most powerful kingdom in Uganda. The king went into exile, and Obote was in turn overthrown in 1971 by one of his army commanders, Idi Amin. Amin's subsequent reign of terror, which lasted until 1979, left a collapsed public sector, a looted private sector, a thriving *magendo* (smuggling) economy, and a pilfering of Indian-owned businesses after their expulsion in 1972. Then, in 1980, after a series of short-term rulers, Obote returned to power. According to residents in Iganga as well as many scholars of Uganda, the Obote II regime exacerbated political tensions, distrust, and violence even more than Amin's had, causing deeper divisions within communities. Years of residents struggling to consolidate local political power had taken a toll on the area, leaving villages around Iganga even further divided, as neighbors were highly suspicious of each other and families had fractured political loyalties.[3] In 1985, Obote was deposed by Tito Okello, and six months later Okello was overthrown by Yoweri Museveni and his National Resistance Movement (NRM) in 1986. The NRM's five-year bloody guerilla battle in the Luwero

Triangle appeared to have ended the twenty-year period of political and civil insecurity, and to have ushered in what some residents call "Uganda's second independence."[4]

But that euphoria too was short-lived. The guerilla war left a host of orphans in the central region, and a new illness was spreading both there (where Museveni's troops had fought) and along the border with Tanzania (where fighting and trade had occurred a bit earlier), as well as traveling throughout the country. The disease, the president warned, was disproportionately affecting young adults and wealthier people. What had initially looked like Uganda's reentry into the global economy and political stability turned out to resemble much of the past, with the presence of death, forced movement of people because of civil unrest, disease, or limited economic opportunities, and intensified class and gender inequalities. Hope in Uganda once again was tempered, this time by the sobering reality of a quickly spreading deadly epidemic.

The keen awareness that residents have of how their rural community is intricately connected to historical patterns of disease, ecological changes, and political transformations is, simply put, quite remarkable. *Ebintu bikyuka kyuka* (things keep changing) signals not only their recognition of constant structural changes but also the necessity of adapting to those changes. I now shift from the broad brushstrokes of the *longue durée* to a contemporary focus on demographic changes and tensions structuring the lives of residents. I begin my exploration of key demographic categories with a brief discussion of the research method we used, social mapping, which allows for the organic emergence of key points of contention (as well as agreement) in the demographic, social, and physical landscapes.

Mapping Bulubandi Village: Method and Social Legibility

Several people took me on tours of Bulubandi Village during my first weeks there, introducing me to people and pointing out key features. Disoriented from the tours and unable to navigate the maze of winding footpaths through banana plantations on my own, I decided to adopt the participatory development method of community mapping, not only to make the village more legible to me but also to introduce myself and my research to residents. With the assistance of a few residents, I broke the village into five regions, mainly along physical markers, including such as a swamp, change in vegetation, or a main pathway. A group of young people who would eventually become my assistants helped me facilitate a series of mapping activities in each of the five regions, during which participants engaged in a map-drawing activity. We divided participants into groups by sex and age to see if differences emerged between men and women, and between young and old. These gendered and age reflections are scattered throughout this book. After drawing a map of their subregion, residents indicated different houses and the names of the household head, drew circles around households connected by kinship or other important social relationships, and indicated what they considered to be important geographic features and resources, such as paths, buildings, public meeting and event places, and water collection sites.

Almost more important than the production of a physical map of Bulubandi, the *process* of community map-making gave me an emic (or, insider) insight into cultural

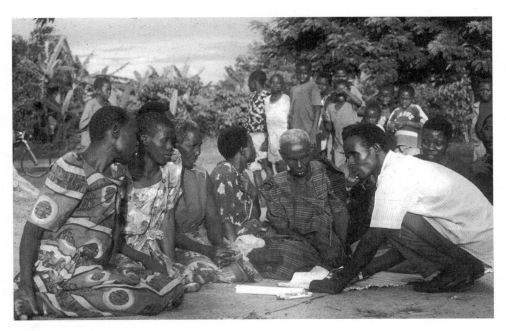

FIGURE 2.1. Household survey with an extended family

norms, epistemological categories, and the ways in which people's lived experiences conformed with or deviated from their ideals. Through the mapping activities, I also started to become familiar with residents' perceptions of geographies of risk and sexuality and of Iganga's sexual economy.[5] While the community maps provided useful data about the sexual geography of Bulubandi and the diversity among households, more specific information about each household was gathered through a household survey conducted with at least one member. Unexpectedly, household surveys often spontaneously morphed into extended family surveys, during which members from various households would gather to provide or share information. This multiple household participation reflects the kinship connections and social fluidity among households.

In 1998, Bulubandi had 423 households with a total population of 1,918 people, which I later found out is large for a village unit.[6] The age distribution of the village closely reflects that of other rural areas in Uganda where young people make up more than 50 percent of the population and women outnumber men because of out-migration and because some men have multiple households and wives (see Table 2.1). The disproportionate percentage of women and young people also has implications for household production and wealth, both of which tend to decline in a monetized economy, and for women's and children's workloads inside and outside the home. Residents frequently talked about the population explosion of Bulubandi as well as of other peri-urban villages, and the creation of what A. F. Robertson has called in the post-independence era "a community of strangers" (1978).[7] As in other parts of Uganda and in Africa in general, there has been a gradual urbanization of the population as people shift from "deep" rural areas to peri-urban and urban centers. This urbanization,

TABLE 2.1. Population of Bulubandi by age and sex, 1998*

	#	%
Adult men	264	14%
Adult women	399	21%
Infants, children, adolescents	1255	65%
Total	**1918**	**100%**

* Includes full-time residents only. Data in the tables in this chapter collected by the author and her research assistants, unless otherwise noted. All percentages have been rounded to the nearest whole number.

however, has been far from complete, as people retain strong social ties to their home *máka* (as discussed in the next section), forming a pattern of cyclical migration present throughout sub-Saharan Africa.

Belonging: Creating and Undoing the *Máka*

The concept of belonging is central in Basoga ideologies of personhood and identity. Older ethnographies on the Basoga (D. W. Cohen 1972; Fallers 1965) emphasized the roles that the clan (*ekika*) and localized, segmented lineages (*nda*) played in social organization and social identity. While there is no doubt that a person's *ekika* and *nda* are significant social identifiers—for instance, determining whom a person can marry or how property is passed down or inherited—the concept of *máka* signifies a place where a person's soul belongs. *Máka,* as a term of belonging, does not necessarily refer to a physical place, though it can be used that way, as discussed below. In the process of trying to locate a person within the social system, it implies a cosmological space within which a person and the soul are embedded in relation to living and deceased members. Even after a person has physically moved away from a place, the *máka* remains a symbolically critical space. More than the imagined or idealized notion of a "homeland" that is frequently used when referring to displaced groups such as refugees (Malkki 1995) or to people who move to urban centers but claim a rural ancestral place (Ferguson 1999; C. Piot 1999), *máka* requires a person to demonstrate a commitment to and investment in a place through affective practices, either by participating in productive labor or by sending remittances and other resources. Without a *máka* a person and his or her spirit are considered homeless. As one elder stated, "It is where your spirit will go to be buried."

During the mapping activities, when residents were determining independent households and the sex of household heads, two situations repeatedly generated much discussion: the existence of households of *nakyewombekeire* and of unmarried young men. It was the ambiguity of these households that introduced me to the importance of *máka* in a person's identity. For residents these two categories are symbolic of the undoing of the *máka*, and they generate moral anxiety but for quite different reasons. Adolescent males represent social stagnation as a result of economic uncertainty, while *nakyewombekeire* are evidence of potential opportunities and especially of the

TABLE 2.2. Household heads in Bulubandi by sex and age, 1998

	Female		Male		Total	
	#	%	#	%	#	%
Elder	47	11%	41	10%	88	21%
Adult	35	8%	130	31%	165	39%
Young adult[1]	8	2%	116	27%	124	29%
Unmarried youth[1]			46	11%	46	11%
Total	**90**	**21%**	**333**	**79%**	**423**	**100%**
1952[2]	**13**	**5%**	**226**	**95%**	**239**	**100%**

[1]In general, the main difference between a young adult and an unmarried youth is marital status. A married young male may be considered a young adult, while an unmarried young male is a youth.

[2]Fallers (1965:72).

weakened authority of natal families and husbands over women's reproductive and productive labor.

Nakyewombekeire and "Tapping from many sources"

Households with female heads can be a source of great social anxiety and ambiguity for a community. The rate of female-headed households more than tripled in the late twentieth century, increasing from 6 percent in the 1950s (Fallers 1965:72) to 21 percent in 1998 (see Table 2.2). This is no doubt higher in Iganga Town and other urban areas, where women face fewer constraints from families and social stigma and have more options for renting accommodations and entering into women's social and economic networks. Female-headed households are more likely than in the past to contain dependents, which are likely to be children but can also be a woman's younger siblings or relatives; the figures in this category increased from 30 percent in the 1950s to 80 percent in 1998. This can be attributed to women's greater access to economic resources and social independence from either fathers or husbands. Furthermore, some divorced and widowed women choose not to return to their parents' houses for fear of stigma, whether because of being single or because the husband died of AIDS and they too are suspected of having the virus; many choose to start their own household and to buy property in rural areas near towns such as Bulubandi. I suspect the number of single-female-headed households in Bulubandi is also slightly higher than what residents reported. Some households reported a man as the head in an effort to make the children legitimate, but the man did not contribute in any meaningful way to the economic or social well-being of the household. He likely also resided in another place with another, perhaps official, wife (see the story of Nakagolo in the next chapter).

In general, the term *nakyewombekeire* implies that a woman has transgressed gender conventions, and over time it has become increasingly notorious: it has come to be directly associated with not only freedom but also sexual permissiveness (*obwenzi*) as a strategy for advancing. Historically, the term referred to a divorced or separated woman who did not remarry and lived alone either on her father's land or in town, where she could engage in trade. During the boom in the informal economy in the 1970s, the term became associated with single and economically independent women (some of whom never married) who left rural areas for urban settings where they could rent housing, construct fictitious kin groups and social networks, and have increased cash-based economic opportunities. The kin-based patriarchy of rural areas provided little social and economic freedom for women who sought greater independence. Some women saved enough money from trading to become "Dubai traders," or women who flew to the Middle Eastern capital to purchase items to sell in Uganda.

The idea that not living with a husband grants a woman greater freedom is not new, nor is the fact that some women desire to live without a man. For example, Gwala, a seventy-four-year-old woman, decided to remain single after divorcing her fourth husband. Here is an excerpt from our conversation:

SHANTI: Why did you leave your fourth husband in 1974? How old was he?
GWALA: The marriage had become meaningless to me. The long period that I kept attending to my mother made me feel as if I had already divorced from that man. So, even when I tried to go back, I did not have the peace of mind that I was married. I had got used to sort of living an independent life.
SHANTI: When you divorced for the last time in 1974, how did your life change and how were unmarried women viewed by society?
GWALA: I felt very free. I would do whatever I wanted without anyone there to stop me. And as I had started to work again, I got my own money and I felt life was good. Although *nakyewombekeire* are looked down upon by some, they live a freer and lead a more independent life than most married women.

Being a *nakyewombekeire* has fewer negative social consequences after a woman is out of or toward the end of her reproductive years. For younger women, what is at stake is not only their own reputation but the reputation of their natal families. When Gwala opted to live alone she had already satisfied her family's desire for her to remain married during the height of her reproductive years, and therefore she could live as a *nakyewombekeire* with minimal threat to her public respectability and little fear of being rebuked by her neighbors or natal family.

Today, the term *nakyewombekeire* commonly signifies a single young woman who is not attached to her father or husband, and instead lives independently and supports herself in a variety of ways, or what residents call "tapping from many sources" (*okulembeka*; literally "to tap water," as in to get water from different sources, such as collecting rain water as it runs down the roof of a house). In the view of Iganga residents, the *nakyewombekeire* challenges the ideal social organization of gender in which a woman has a "ruler," and instead threatens the structure of her natal family and that of other families because she is a potential lover for married men. Within the local landscape of sexual propriety, a *nakyewombekeire* is a nuisance to her natal family and also to married women in the community. Much of the sexual labeling of women reflects their ability to negotiate rules of gender and sexual propriety. Some women in Iganga who fall outside the local ideals are able to negotiate their respectability through various strategies and maneuvers. As one informant told me, "They are 'no-man's land.' They belong to no one." They are the epitome of a soul without a *máka*, and their increasing numbers pose a grave threat to the earthly and cosmological social orders. This increase in the number of *nakyewombekeire*, perceived or real, is only one aspect of the many social changes that bring concern to residents in Iganga.

Adolescent Males and Social Stagnation

After much discussion, it was decided that forty-six households (11 percent) were independent households of unmarried adolescent and young men (see Table 2.2). The discussions about households of young men focused on when a boy's sleeping quarters should be regarded as an independent household. The general expectation has been that after puberty, land permitting, an adolescent male will sleep in his own quarters, in a dwelling detached from the main house but still within his parents' compound. Sons from poorer families may turn an animal shelter or storage area into sleeping quarters. In wealthier families or in town, the son may maintain a bedroom in a separate part of the main house or have "boy's quarters" in the back of the house, where he will stay when he visits from boarding school. There is no definite point at which a boy's sleeping quarters become a household, but often it has to do with the young man's income-generating activities, the perception of his maturity (often meaning economic and social independence), and his own contribution to building his home. Economically, the young man is expected to support himself when he establishes his own household, although his parents may assist with bridewealth and home construction costs. As a boy matures and acquires some of his own wealth from odd jobs in town or from farming his own crops, he may slowly renovate and expand his sleeping quarters or build a new house on his father's land. He eventually marries or brings in a woman to tend to the domestic chores of cooking, cleaning, and doing laundry, at which point he no longer eats meals with his natal family or calls upon his sisters or mother to clean or do his laundry. But since the process of marriage is now delayed because of schooling and lack of money, this criterion only sometimes applies. Usually a daughter is expected to continue living inside her parents' home until she weds or takes up residence with a man, but this pattern is also changing.

A Demographic Snapshot: Key Aspects of Identity

In this section I discuss the demographic contours of Bulubandi in order to highlight diversity, homogeneity, and the significance of key aspects of identity that residents mobilize at particular times. Although many young people do not immediately identify themselves as members of these categories, the intersection of these identities begins to shape the lives of and opportunities for young people.

Ethnicity

The Basoga are the predominant ethnic group in Iganga, accounting for 84 percent (357) of the heads of household in Bulubandi (see Table 2.3). Ethnic affiliation serves

TABLE 2.3. Ethnicity of household heads in Bulubandi, 1998

Ethnicity	#	%
Basoga	357	84.4%
Iteso	22	5.2%
Baganda	16	3.8%
Samiya	13	3.1%
Other*	12	2.8%
N/A	3	0.7%
Total	423	100.0%

*"Other" includes Gisu (8 households) and Acholi, Ankole, Muromogi, and Musiki (1 household each).

as an important social organizing principle and identity, and people often prefer to marry within their own ethnic group. There are stereotypes and hierarchies among ethnicities, but in Uganda, unlike other countries in Africa, ethnicity has not been used as regularly as other forms of identity (such as religion) to mobilize and sustain political conflicts. Older people remember the historical roots of the elevated wealth and prestige of the Baganda, the dominant ethnic group in Uganda and neighbors to the south of Busogaland. The British colonial government sent Baganda administrators to Busogaland and other parts of Uganda to help establish the colonial system, and granted the Baganda administrators large plots of prime farming land, both as an incentive and to establish their authority over local populations. As a way of entering into the cash economy, Basoga commoners became farm and household laborers for the newly arrived Baganda elite, and a socioeconomic hierarchy based on ethnicity was established. This hierarchy still exists today to some extent at the village level, and can be seen nationally in the status of Luganda as the dominant language. When I first arrived in Bulubandi, the Local Council 1 (LC1) village chair and many of the other elected officials were Baganda, and this group owned some of the larger *ddukhas* (small shops) along the main roadway in the village. Older people hold with pride their Basoga identity, but worry that the younger generation is losing touch with the language and customs and is replacing them with the regionally more dominant Baganda ones.

Religion

More so than ethnicity, religious affiliation has been a source of political and social division within Uganda since the colonial period. Today, religious affiliation continues to play an important part in people's lives, particularly in terms of their public and civic identities, marital preferences, and socioeconomic status. Unlike the 1950s, when Fallers (1969) found 21 percent of the residents classified as belonging to the "traditional" religion (which revolves around the worship of *lubaale*—the local god—and associated spirits), today virtually everyone in Bulubandi is affiliated with one of the world religions, even if he or she is not an ardent follower of an organized religion (such as some elders), and even when a person simultaneously believes in or practices customs

TABLE 2.4. Religion of household heads in Bulubandi, 1998

Religion	#	%	1950s*
Muslim	211	50%	21%
Protestant	167	39%	38%
Catholic	45	11%	20%
Traditional*	—	—	21%
Total	**423**	**100%**	**100%**

*Fallers (1969:45–46). "Traditional" refers to people who have not declared themselves as belonging to a Western religion.

around *lubaale*.[8] In Bulubandi, 50 percent of the households are Muslim, which is a much higher percentage than the 28 percent within Iganga District in general and 12 percent within Uganda as a whole in the 2002 national census. Thirty-nine percent (or, 167 heads) of Bulubandi households are Protestant, and Catholics represent a mere 11 percent (or, 45 heads) of Bulubandi households, as opposed to 37 percent and 42 percent, respectively, in the nationwide survey (UBOS 2006: 30–31). Bulubandi's reversal of the national trend on the population composition of religion is discussed below.

There are several possible explanations for the high representation of Islam in Bulubandi. First, Baganda "notables like Bwagu and Lwanga [had imposed] Islam from above" and, according to elders, Muslim Baganda chiefs assigned to Busogaland recruited converts by promising them land and other favors (Twaddle 1993:235). Another reason for the high percentage of Muslims in Bulubandi is that they tend to dominate two major economic sectors in Iganga Town—transportation and restaurants—which has facilitated a postcolonial history of Muslims buying land and relocating to villages directly outside of town. Muslims are highly active and favored in the transportation sector, as I was repeatedly told by people inside the industry, because of the staunch anti-alcohol stance of Islam and the discipline learned through daily prayers; social networks have played a role in keeping Muslims active in this industry. Their visibility in the food industry, including eating-houses and butcheries, can be partly explained by halal butchering practices, which allow them to cater to a wide customer base (Kayunga 1994). The history of the settlement of Bulubandi—of large plots of land given to Muslim and Protestant families, followed by the migration of other family members—helps explain the religious breakdown of Bulubandi and villages outside of Iganga Town.

The increasing popularity of fundamentalism within both Islam and Christianity has greatly influenced notions of morality and sexuality, particularly among young adults and the professional class. Religion has no doubt influenced notions of morality since colonial days, but the more recent congregational mobilizing within fundamental sects has amplified the role that religion plays in shaping gendered propriety. For instance, Sallie Simba Kayunga (1994:324) notes that in Uganda "a major concern of the Muslim fundamentalists is the reinstatement of women in their 'rightful' place under the control of men." This sentiment about gender relations can be found in Protestant fundamentalist movements as well. At the time I collected household data, I did not think to distinguish between the sects within Islam or between Protestantism and Pentecostalism. In hindsight such an investigation would have been useful for better understanding the various competing claims of moral authority and accusations of immorality.

Within denominations, age and wealth differences between sects are salient, with fundamental congregations tending to be younger and wealthier. Sunni was the largest (and oldest) Muslim sect in Bulubandi and Iganga when we began mapping in 1998. Its membership was older. Residents frequently referred to Sunnis as "African Muslims," signifying their descent from earlier Muslim converts and their following of Basoga cultural customs. It was common to see an older Sunni couple in which the woman did not cover her head but her husband wore a kufi cap and kanzu cotton dress. It was an accepted norm for ablution (or cleansing before praying) to be done with dirt or dust if water was not around.

The influence of fundamentalist groups has caused changes in how Islam is practiced, including an increase in the number of women who wear head covers. A head cover might signify religious affiliation, but it is also an indicator of socioeconomic class, since a nice headscarf worn in public is a sign of wealth. While older Muslim residents were more likely to attend mosque in the village, younger and wealthier men often chose to dedicate time to the larger, more fundamentalist mosque in town, where many of them go for work or are able to interact with men from other villages. The Tablique (also spelled Tabligh; Arabic for "to educate the people about religion") or Salafi are among the oldest of the fundamental sects, with leaders who have received training in Pakistan or other Muslim countries (see Kayunga 1994). Residents associate the Tablique with their appearance: the men have distinctive beards and shorter pants, and the women are fully covered except for their eyes. The common thought is that the Tablique also prohibit women from riding bicycles, to further restrict their physical mobility and access to sexual enticements, though I never had this confirmed by a religious leader. There is another wave of wealthier and younger Muslims in Iganga who do not identify with the Tablique sect but who, like the Tablique, claim to adhere more strictly to the Koran than the older African Sunni Muslims.

Like elsewhere in sub-Saharan Africa, the socially conservative Pentecostal movement is the fastest-growing religion in Uganda (Spear and Kimambo 1999; Gifford 1998; Englund 2011; Anderson 2004; Kalu 2008). According to the 2002 national census, the evangelical Pentecostals (*balokole*) made up around 5 percent of the population (UBOS 2006: 31).[9] I was told, however, that this is likely significantly less than the actual total because of inconsistencies in how the information was collected. Dating back to the early 1900s, the charismatic movement gained followers during specific moments in Uganda's recent history, and within the last couple of decades it has attracted many new members. Its leaders have aligned themselves with similar movements in donor countries, creating a global network of people, evangelical ideas, mission trips, and financial assistance. The church services and revivals include lively music, dancing, praise and worship, and public confessions from people about their journey of being "saved." People who consider themselves *balokole* with whom I spoke find the church and wider movement appealing because the sermons engage with people's everyday problems and offer hope and solutions. In addition to being able to connect with young adults while invoking the Bible, the movement appeals to young professionals through single adult ministries, community service groups, and education programs geared toward unmarried people. These faith-based activities and clubs provide a social space for young professionals to form civic and peer associations as a way of establishing their identities and their professional networks.

Sexuality and morality are popular topics for leaders in Uganda's evangelical movement. Pentecostal critiques about the corrupting influence of Western culture and the movement's belief that economic and social mobility are the reward for leading a moral life are delivered in charismatic sermons that weave together familiar local idioms, contemporary references, and references to the Bible. As *balokole* doctrine advocates monogamous relationships and sexual abstinence before marriage, many young professionals consider the churches an ideal place to meet potential socially mobile and "modern" partners.

While religion plays an important role in contemporary notions of sexuality, most youth in this study were not as active in religious institutions or fellowship groups as adults, and tended to identify with the religion of their parents. Young people are likely to be introduced to fundamentalist ideas through public revivals or services or through older relatives such as cousins or siblings, but during my research, very few identified themselves as formally belonging to one of the fundamentalist sects. By 2006, however, all of my then-young adult research assistants and initial research participants (who were considered youth at the beginning of this project) considered themselves *balokole*. Most became saved and *balokole* during points in their lives when they were struggling to piece together economic and educational opportunities; joining a moral movement offered hope and reassurance as well as new forms of civic affiliation. While Sam (see the beginning of this book) medicated his disappointment with alcohol and debauchery, other young people find hope in dedicating themselves to the evangelical movement. Particular evangelical leaders in Kampala have risen to great prominence in Uganda with support from foreign, often US-based, fundamentalist groups, leading to a great expansion of their congregations and their ministries. Their followers have become important constituencies in the movement's ability to influence politics in Uganda, such as in the drafting of. Uganda's Anti-Homosexuality Bill in 2009, which led to an extended legislative and global battle between antigay and gay rights advocates that had not been resolved as of this writing (Gettleman 2010; Kaoma 2009/2010). While initially thought to be organic and able to adapt to the needs of local communities, the Pentecostal movement has become increasingly socially conservative, as seen in the authority it has wielded in defining contemporary notions of morality and advocating morality both as the main protection from disease and as a route to economic prosperity.

Wealth

Socioeconomic status is a salient and visible distinction among Bulubandi residents.[10] In our mapping activities, residents developed four wealth categories, with the majority

TABLE 2.5. Wealth ranking of households in Bulubandi by sex of household heads, 1998

Wealth Ranking	Women		Men		Total	
	#	%	#	%	#	%
Very Poor	17	19%	30	9%	47	11%
Poor	47	52%	158	47%	205	48%
Average	18	20%	116	35%	134	32%
Rich	2	2%	24	7%	26	6%
Very Rich	1	1%	2	1%	3	1%
N/A	5	6%	3	1%	8	2%
Total	**90**	**100%**	**333**	**100%**	**423**	**100%**

of households (60 percent, or 252 households) falling into the "poor" or "very poor" categories, 34 percent into the "average" wealth category, and only 7 percent being considered wealthy (see Table 2.5). The wealth classification of a household was virtually isomorphic with the type of material used to construct the physical home, indicating that the physical appearance and construction of a house as an important social index for wealth (Figures 2.2 to 2.5). By 2015, there were visibly more households in the "average" and "wealthy" categories, reflecting the presence of newer residents who had purchased land and built homes, and the increased availability of wage jobs in town. Some of the households owned by elders and longer-term residents would have been categorized as poorer than newly constructed households, which points to some obvious limits of using household construction as a proxy for wealth.

In addition to the construction of one's house, a variety of other indicators provide constant reminders of a person's socioeconomic status, including the occupation of the head of household, the selection of schools for the children, the livestock and land ownership, the style of dress, the religious institutional affiliation (see below), and the consumption of luxury goods such as motorcycles, cars, and computers. While displays of consumption can bolster one's status and prestige, the goods also have to be properly managed within the village and exhibited only at appropriate times. People often try to conceal their wealth from their neighbors, fearing jealousy, theft, accusations of questionable acquisition, and unwanted requests. For example, Agnes told her neighbors that she was keeping the two cows in her backyard for someone else. I had heard that story so often that I had thought the cows belonged to someone else, although I did wonder why she would invest so much time into someone else's property. I discovered they were hers the morning one of the cows gave birth and an excited Agnes said, "Now we have three cows!" When I asked why she concealed her ownership, she explained that in the past jealous neighbors had bewitched her livestock, causing them to die.

While the conspicuous display of wealth has its social and cultural risks, higher economic status can serve to advance a person's social position in the community in the

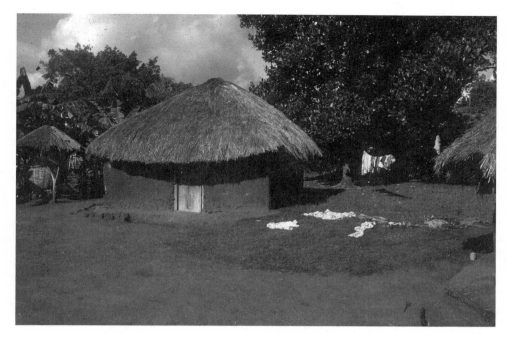

FIGURE 2.2. Very poor: Grass-thatched house with mud walls

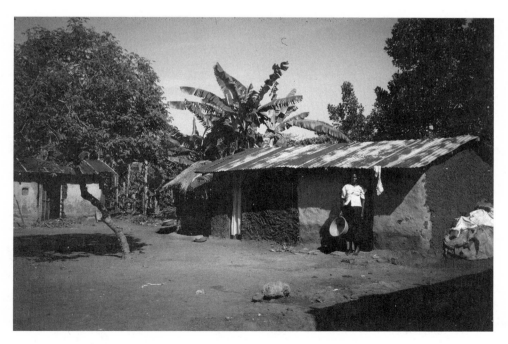

FIGURE 2.3. Poor: Temporary house with an iron roof and mud walls

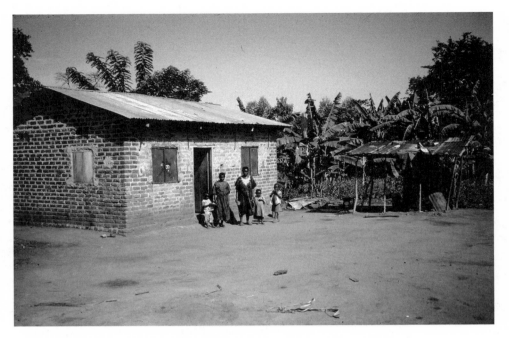

FIGURE 2.4. Average: Semi-permanent house with iron roof and brick walls

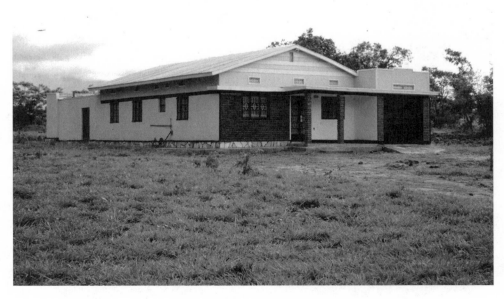

FIGURE 2.5. Wealthy to very wealthy: Permanent house with tile roof, painted exterior, and garage

form of patron-client ties (Vincent 1971). In such relationships, the patron maintains a superior position because of his or her greater capacity to give grants or services, and hence his or her ability to assemble loyal followers from whom intangible favors or debts can later be redeemed, such as votes for a local election, protection against petty thieves, or information that might not be easily available to village elites. Young people might subtly invoke their families' wealth status when negotiating a relationship with a peer. As seen in the story of the unemployed Sam and the nursing student Birungi, family status is an important criterion for parents as well. Since children are expected to serve as social security for the parents, parents have a vested interest in the socio-economic status of their future in-laws.

According to the World Bank, in 2012 19.5 percent of Uganda's population was below the relative poverty line. Fluctuating socioeconomic status is common and reflects the wider situation in the country, in which families that thrived during a particular economic context may feel economically worse in another period. According to economist Vali Jamal, in 1995 the average income in real terms was one-tenth that of the 1970s peak (1998:74). Even middle-class families have felt the pinch of rising inflation, unpredictable agricultural markets, and falling real wage incomes. By 2015, the growing middle class of residents in Iganga has significantly influenced social trends, the availability of consumer goods, and shifting systems of prestige, but as more luxury goods and greater educational opportunities become available in Uganda, people's inability to keep pace with their desires has exacerbated feelings of poverty and economic deprivation. Families in Bulubandi and Iganga often experience a further economic burden as they absorb AIDS orphans from deceased or sick relatives. For example, Agnes cared for two orphans on her husband's side in addition to six of her own children; a seventh child lived elsewhere.

Economic Livelihoods

In response to economic precarity and the demands of a monetized economy, people in Iganga are constantly engaged in multiple endeavors and creating new ways to generate income. As throughout Africa, households in Bulubandi perform a combination of farm and off-farm activities to diversify their income flow and hedge against seasonal trends. Most households (81 percent or 262), even those of white-collar professionals, participate in farming activities, and those who do not consist most commonly of either elders or people who migrate for work (see Table 2.6). Farming is generally still done manually with a hoe and, as such, is labor intensive and time consuming and the crop yield is highly unpredictable, even more so than in the past, according to elders as well as agricultural extension agents. Although the division of agricultural labor by sex has become blurred, labor in cash crops and home gardens is still commonly divided between husbands and wives, respectively, and among co-wives. Women are generally expected to plan and care for the home gardens that provide their households' daily starches (such as sweet potatoes) and vegetables. Men control what residents call the marketing or selling of cash crops, and hence the profits from women's labor. Women are acutely aware of this gender imbalance, commenting privately on how their labor

TABLE 2.6. **Main income-generating activities of households in Bulubandi, 1998**

Activity	#	%*
Farming	262	81%
Selling or trading	55	17%
Artisan work	44	14%
Grain mill work	40	12%
Shopkeeping	36	11%
Vocational work	31	10%
Service industry work	25	8%
Transport industry work	19	6%
Student	18	6%
Office work	16	5%
Teaching	9	3%
Renting property	6	2%
Other	5	2%

*The percentage is based on 323 households; for 100 households either no information was available or they were not involved with income-generating activities. Many households are engaged in more than one income-generating activity; therefore, the total percentage is greater than 100 percent.

is used to support their husbands' drinking or maintenance of outside lovers. Young people too are expected to contribute labor to their household's subsistence and cash crops, with larger contributions during school holidays and on the weekends. Academically promising offspring are excused from manual household labor—a privilege young men are more likely to exploit.

In 1998, nearly 80 percent of the households in Bulubandi engaged in off-farm income-generating activities. Men's participation in off-farm jobs increases women's and children's farm labor responsibilities. The most commonly cited off-farm activity (17 percent of the households) is the selling or trading of farm produce, foodstuffs, or goods in one of the market areas. A significant number of households also engaged in either artisan work (such as brick making, carpentry, tailoring, or construction) or vocational trades (such as auto repair, engineering, or welding) learned through apprenticeships or technical schools. Two extended family networks own grain mills in town, employing a large number of male kin. Owning or working in a shop, *ddukha*, or kiosk in Iganga provides income for some. Other people have office jobs with development agencies, government offices, or the hospital. The transportation industry and other service sectors (such as eating-houses, car washes, outlets for traditional medicine, religious institutions, photography studios, dry cleaners, and petrol stations) are other possible income sources. A defining characteristic of the informal economic sector is the ease of entry and exit, and people commonly switch between different income-generating activities. For example, for two seasons Charles was engaged in brick making in Bulubandi, after which he sold paraffin and ropes in town; currently he is training to be a photographer and is frequently sent to cover weddings.[11]

TABLE 2.7. Bulubandi households in extended family networks, 1998

Households	Female #	%	Male #	%	Total households #	%
Individual households (not in extended family network)	24	6%	68	16%	92	22%
Households in extended family networks	58	14%	251	59%	309	73%
Number of households in network						
2	7	2%	25	6%	32	8%
3	10	2%	23	5%	33	8%
4	7	2%	45	11%	52	12%
5	3	1%	22	5%	25	6%
6	4	1%	20	5%	24	6%
8	3	1%	5	1%	8	2%
10	4	1%	26	6%	30	7%
11	5	1%	17	4%	22	5%
13	1	0%	12	3%	13	3%
15	5	1%	10	2%	15	4%
20	4	1%	16	4%	20	5%
35	5	1%	30	7%	35	8%
Renting	8	2%	14	3%	22	5%
Total	**90**	**22%**	**333**	**78%**	**423**	**100%**

Households and Families

Extended families can play an important economic role in people's lives, in increasing one's economic opportunities or one's obligations to assist more people, as well as a key social role. Although *máka* is a cosmological term, as discussed earlier, residents also use it to refer to a compound whose inhabitants are bound together (through kinship, marriage, or other affiliations) in an intricate web of responsibility and reciprocity. Some *mákas* in Bulubandi are single-family homes (22 percent, or 92 households), but it is more common for a *máka* to contain the households of several related kin. In fact, 73 percent (309) of the households in Bulubandi belong to one of the 59 extended family networks in the village (see Table 2.7). On average, there are five households per extended family network. Most extended family networks contain only two generations of households (a father and several of his married sons, and perhaps a divorced or widowed daughter); however, three or even four generations is not uncommon. Within the context of Basoga patrilocality, in which a wife moves to her husband's land, a newly married

TABLE 2.8. Household membership in Bulubandi by sex of household heads, 1998

	Female-headed households		Male-headed households*		Total	
	#	%	#	%	#	%
1 member	18	4%	69	17%	87	21%
2–4 members	42	10%	97	24%	139	34%
5–7 members	22	5%	90	22%	112	27%
8–10 members	6	1%	41	10%	47	11%
11–13 members	2		20	5%	22	5%
>13 members			3	1%	3	1%
Total	**90**	**21%**	**320**	**79%**	**410**	**100%**

* These figures do not include the thirteen male-headed households that are vacant for most of the year.

woman may find herself removed from previous forms of social support, and residing on multigenerational compounds might further increase her dependence on and subordination to her in-laws. Although elders remark on the declining significance of the clan and extended family in the lives of young people, families still do have great influence over kin. An example of a three-generation network is the Bukampala family, which is the largest extended family in Bulubandi, with thirty-five households. According to elders, this family was given a large section of land by one of the original owners or headmen of the village. Over time, individual members have gradually sold off portions of their land, and relatives living elsewhere in Uganda have migrated to Bulubandi either to buy land or stay on a relative's plot. Today, the Bukampala households are settled in discontinuous areas scattered throughout the middle of Bulubandi, and some have started their own extended family networks. Most people associate the Bukampala family primarily with a cluster that contains the houses of the old man's widows, their adult children, and their adult grandchildren. Other extended families choose to live in separate compounds, which equally influences social and economic interrelationships among those households.

The average household size in Bulubandi is 4.7 members (see Table 2.8), but there is considerable variation in the composition, with some households, particularly households of older men, having just one resident, and others with as many as thirteen residents or more.[12] The actual members in a household are in constant flux. Angelique Haugerud's (1995) distinction between full-time and part-time household residents is a useful framework for conceptualizing the fluctuation. Full-time residents reside most of the year at the house and participate in the household's daily consumption and/or production. Part-time residents spend only part of the year in the household. Such residents include youth attending boarding schools or staying with relatives, heads of household who are temporarily absent for seasonal or long-term economic opportunities, and polygamous men who spend the majority of their time at other houses with other wives.

Gender and Status

People in Bulubandi believe that the public presentation of a homestead reflects the internal social health of a *máka*. In addition to reflecting the affective strength of residents of a *máka*, presentation is an important public marker of a family's status, aesthetic style, class, and social mobility; hence, residents take great care in maintaining their front yards and other areas that passers-by might see. Constructing and upgrading a house is an ongoing project that continues long after the family has moved in.

Domestic space is structured by gender and age. Women and children spend much of their time in the open areas and in buildings behind the main house that contain the sleeping quarters. In the open areas the women and children (and, on rare occasions, the men) tend to household chores, such as washing laundry, peeling food, ironing clothes, drying grain and beans, and cleaning dishes. Venturing here indicates a level of familiarity between a visitor and the residents of the home. The kitchen typically has a thatched roof over either wood stilts or mud walls and contains a wood or charcoal cooker constructed of three stones on the ground. As a person's income increases in a town where electricity and water are available, the auxiliary structures are incorporated into the main house. The man is thought to be responsible for building the main and auxiliary structures of the household, and the wife is responsible for making the paths among these structures. As I was told, the word for "woman," *mukazi*, is derived from "to dry" (*okúkazá*), as in drying out the grass by walking on it. The front yard is a place for entertaining visitors, and it is generally a woman's responsibility to keep it clean and well-groomed, although she might assign the task to a young person. Wives and adolescent girls are expected to welcome visitors upon little notice, offering them food, drink, and a comfortable place to sit. This can be a considerable task, as most households keep little by way of spare and easy-to-prepare food. Having visitors is considered a great honor and people believe it brings good fortune to the household, but it can also be a source of great tension if the wife does not meet the level of hospitality expected of the husband.

In most cases, husbands and wives both participate in the process of acquiring cash for the household; however, many women consider themselves nonworking "housewives." Married women are aware that their labor produces cash for the household, but they do not perceive themselves as actively participating in the cash economy except as consumers. For a woman, referring to herself as a housewife is also a strategy of social positioning that marks her as conforming to Basoga gender ideology, which links women's mobility to sexual permissiveness. Other women have complained that their husbands do not want them to work outside the home and off the farm because, as found in popular discourse, men fear that their wives will become sexually involved with other men. During a group discussion, one man explained, "Women *know* that their husbands cheat; husbands *suspect* that their wives cheat." While collecting a life history of a seventy-three-year-old woman, I asked her why her second husband in 1949 forbade her from teaching, which was her profession. She replied, "He felt if I worked he would not be able to fully control me as a wife. In the past men thought that letting a wife out of the home for any reason was giving her a chance to get other men or to do adultery." Fallers (1969) observed a similar suspicion between spouses and remarked that men felt insecure in marriage, leading some men to restrict not only the physical mobility of their wives (and hence their ability to work outside the homestead) but also their access to resources. Gender ideologies that formerly determined household chores and spaces have begun to fade, though both are still highly gendered. In the next chapter I take a closer look at marriage in Iganga.

Marriage is changing so kinship isn't as tightly bound

Gendered responses to this shift in marriage

↑ unmarried young people & sexual networking

Men often sleep w/ other women while on trips then return to their wives

overarching idea of weakening of kinship ties contributing to heightened risk

CHAPTER 3

Patriarchy, Marriage, and Gendered Respectability

As elsewhere in sub-Saharan Africa, marriage in Iganga marks an important transition in a person's life and social relationships, and is central to understanding how proper sexuality is locally conceptualized and achieved (Fortes 1962; Radcliffe-Brown and Forde 1950; Bledsoe 1990). Reflective of this social importance of and people's desire for marriage, 87 percent (366) of the household heads in Bulubandi have been or currently are married (see Table 3.1). The anthropology of marriage in Africa has a long history, having moved far beyond the original focus on its relationship to descent, alliance, and political and economic systems (Radcliffe-Brown and Forde 1950; Lévi-Strauss 1969; Mair 1969; Phillips 1953).[1] The analytic turn to the "processual" approach drew attention to, as Caroline Bledsoe and Gilles Pison explained, marriage "as a long, ambiguous process rather than a discrete event established by clear legal, ritual, and economic transactions" (1994:4).

In the study of marriage as a process, bridewealth exchanges have figured prominently as scholars highlighted strategies of elders and men in kinship groups who vied for power and status; in addition, insights from feminist and political economy approaches have showed how marriage transactions, including bridewealth, serve to establish and reinforce female oppression within societies and kinship groups (Rubin 1992; Goody 1973; Meillassoux 1981; Schlegel and Eloul 1988). More recent work has appreciated the role of bridewealth in reproducing gender inequalities while also examining how meanings and practices of bridewealth have changed over time, as have the ways women (as well as men) engage with the system according to their own motives and strategic ends, with varying outcomes (Wardlow 2006; Johnson-Hanks 2007; Feldman-Savelsberg 1999; Yan 2005). The study of marriage has also offered insight into how colonial and postcolonial states have attempted to impose particular ideological, moral, gender, and economic projects, and how these regulatory projects were neither hegemonic nor fully complete but were constantly challenged, complicated, and strategically adapted by communities (Berry 1993; Cooper 1997). Today, studies on marriage around the world include a broad set of concerns (some old, some new) such as gendered relations and inequalities, practices and desires of consumption, the nuclearization of the family, local reworkings of globalizing forms of intimacy (such as companionate marriage) and sexual identities (through gay rights movements, for example), and the way shifting notions of morality interact with wider economic, ideological, and social transformations.

TABLE 3.1. Marital status of household heads in Bulubandi, 1998*

	Female (N=90)		(N=333)		Male Total	
	#	%	#	%	#	%
Never married	2	0%	55	13%	57	13%
Previously married and now single	76	18%	25	6%	101	24%
Currently married	12	3%	253	60%	265	63%
Total	**90**	**21%**	**333**	**79%**	**423**	**100%**

*Data in this table and others in this chapter collected by the author and her research assistants, unless otherwise noted. All percentages have been rounded to the nearest whole number.

Absent from studies on conjugality is an appreciation of how marriage as experienced and evaluated by residents may feed into unmarried young people's imaginations about the possibilities and limitations of their own current and future partnerships. While many young people in Iganga with whom we spoke were critical of the gendered inequalities and difficulties they observed in the marriages of their parents and other relatives, they still desired to be married one day and believed that their unions would be more equitable—a place for mutual efforts to improve their economic and social standing. Adults as well as youth in Iganga recognize the complexities of marriage and understand that conjugal unions do not present themselves in a single form but rather, as Philip Burnham explains, in "a bundle of interactional possibilities" (1987:50). They are also aware of and engaged in debates about the fragile state of marriage today and the decline of formal marriage.

The "Letter" and the *Kwandhula* Ceremony: Legitimacy in Patriarchy

Two events mark the legitimacy of a Basoga marriage—a formal request from the prospective groom, made through the delivery of a "letter" to the father, and the *kwandhula* (or, introduction) ceremony that centers on the coming together of two kingroups. This solemnization process is practiced in ways that both reflects and reproduces the patrilineal kinship system and women's place in it. This does not mean that prospective brides (and female kin) are necessarily oppressed by and silenced in the premarital process or that prospective grooms (and male kin) are not burdened by it. However, the cultural legitimacy of a union is predicated on intergenerational and interclan male negotiations around the rights over the female body. The solemnization process is a series of rituals that symbolically transfer access to both the productive and reproductive labor of a woman from her father (and his clan) to her prospective husband (and his clan).

Marital histories we collected from the elders dating back to the 1930s indicate that for a long time there has been considerable variation in the solemnization process,

TABLE 3.2. Polygyny in Bulubandi by sex of household heads, 1998

	Female (N=88)		Male (N=278)		Total (N=366)	
	#	%	#	%	#	%
Polygynous*	6	7%	83	30%	89	24%
Wives in separate houses	6	100%	45	54%	51	57%
Wives in same house	0	0%	38	46%	38	43%

*Includes only individuals currently married.

although it was expected to follow a basic pattern. The delivery of an *ekibumbula mun-hwa* (literally "the opener of the mouth," figuratively a "letter") officially begins the process. Historically, the prospective groom sends a representative—such as the young man's father, another male relative, or a respectable age-mate—to deliver a "letter" to the father of the prospective bride. According to courtship narratives of the elders, the letter might simply be a verbal message of the young man's desire to marry the man's daughter, but it could also be an actual envelope containing money and a note. This letter "opens the mouth," initiating the negotiation process between the father and a representative of the prospective groom. In addition to the young woman's father, her mother and a *sônga* (Lusoga for "paternal aunt"; also *ssenga*, the more commonly recognized Luganda spelling) might also be present to receive the letter, and if it includes money, would expect to receive a share but might not know the entire amount sent in the envelope. The father and other (historically male) adult relatives then present their requirements to the man, negotiating for bridewealth and other gifts (such as clothing for particular relatives), as well as setting the date for the *kwandhula*. The bride's father has the upper hand in these negotiations, as a failed request for engagement would reflect poorly on the prospective groom's reputation; therefore, the young woman's male kin rarely accept the initial offer of the groom. Their deliberate display of shock and offense at the initial offer is a show of power that helps establish the social respect of the young woman's clan and is an acknowledgment of how well they had raised their daughters. "They give their daughters away easily" is an insult no man or clan wants to hear.

After an agreement is reached, the couple is considered betrothed. The young man promises to marry the young woman, relieving her father of any future economic burden in her upkeep; in turn, the father has to make sure she remains chaste and loyal until marriage. The young woman is sent to stay with her *sônga*, where she receives instruction on her sexual duties as a wife, such as "bedroom tricks" and other techniques for pleasing her husband (see Chapter 4). Given the frequency of polygyny among the Basoga (see Table 3.2), these bedroom techniques are particularly important strategies for wives, as they compete with co-wives and potential mistresses for their husband's economic and affective attention. This betrothal period gives the prospective groom time to gather the bridewealth, as well as necessary money and items for the staging of

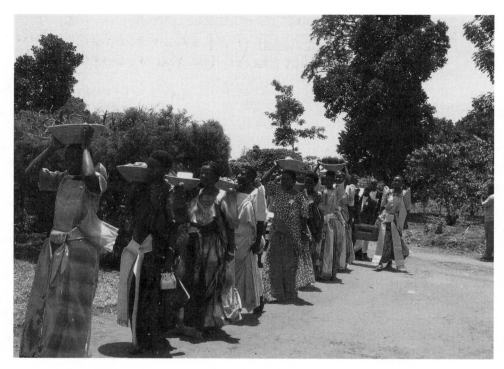

FIGURE 3.1. Bridewealth procession at a *kwandhula* ceremony

the *kwandhula*. If it is the man's first marriage, he is often assisted by his paternal male kin, but for subsequent marriages he would typically be expected to use his own wealth for much of the bridewealth and the *kwandhula*.

The *kwandhula* remains an important public performance, marking the entrance of a female as a wife into another clan, and symbolically culminates in the display of bridewealth as a demonstration of respect and prestige. The *kwandhula* can range from a small ceremony at the house of the bride's parents to a very elaborate production that includes a large feast and a grand presentation of gifts above the bridewealth (see Figure 3.1).[2] In some cases, a religious ceremony would follow—a practice that has been common among Muslims for some time and is becoming increasingly common and desirable among Christians. There are important distinctions in focus, social purpose, and significance among the *kwandhula* ceremony, the Christian wedding, and the Muslim ceremony. The central focus of the *kwandhula* is the performative coming together of two clans. The role of the bride and groom in the ceremony is minimal, and throughout much of the ceremony they are seated among their respective relatives instead of with each other.

Conversely, in Christian weddings in Iganga the focus is on the couple, who stand in front of the congregation with their respective attendants, who are often from their social network, and with their kingroup seated as audience members and witnesses (see Figure 3.2). The emphasis at Christian weddings is on the union of the husband and

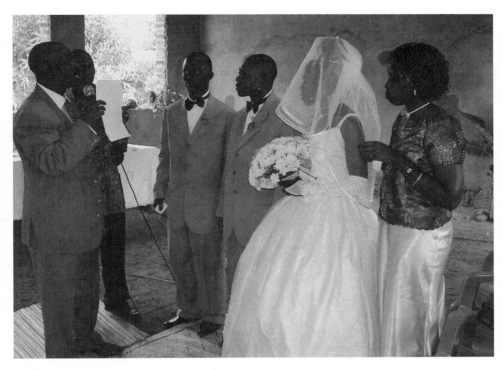

FIGURE 3.2. Christian exchange of wedding vows

wife through a representative of the church. At the center of Muslim ceremonies is the imam, who reads and interprets passages and tales from the Koran as he delivers lessons about the role, duties, and obligations of each party (the bride, groom, and the two families) in the life of the marriage.

There is an ongoing public debate in Uganda today about how the elaborate and expensive nature of the *kwandhula* and religious ceremonies (particularly Christian) has contributed to the increase in cohabitation, delays in marriage, and people's decisions not to marry at all. (There is a similar debate about bridewealth, but the Basoga do not have a practice of exorbitant bridewealth, except among the very wealthy). Even President Museveni has made public pleas to limit the cost of wedding ceremonies, arguing that in an attempt to show off to neighbors, some families are falling into tremendous debt. However, Museveni's pleas are in conflict with the glamorous images, goods, and services in Uganda's vibrant marriage ceremony industry, which fuel young men's and women's (as well as their families') dreams of elaborate *kwandhula* and wedding ceremonies that would include Ugandan and Western finery; a parade of flower girls, bridesmaids, and groomsmen; a fleet of rented Mercedes Benzes to carry the wedding party to the reception; and an abundance of food, drink, and entertainment at that grand reception.[3] These ceremonies are a deliberately conspicuous display of consumption and extravagance. Carrying social significance beyond the kinship groups, these performances are a public representation of the status, prestige, and future economic potential of the couple and of their arrival as a couple into a modern world. The culture of grand weddings is reproduced within social networks but also works as an obstacle to solemnizing a union.

A person can claim higher status over or speak disparagingly about a peer who is cohabitating but in a union that has not been publicly solemnized. The particular pressures and motivations for solemnization are different for men and women; conversely, there are gendered implications when a union is not formalized. For a man, the formal request and the public ceremonies are a demonstration of economic virility, masculine responsibility, and social status; if he does not celebrate the relationship formally, he often feels insecure about his wife's loyalty and his authority over her. For a woman, the solemnization process, like bridewealth, confers social respect and confirms her worth as a woman, wife, and mother; it is a public symbol that she has moved beyond her father's surveillance and home and has arrived into the world as an adult woman, albeit under the authority of another man. Having her family—and his, to some extent—invested and involved in the solemnization process helps ensure that the bride will be protected or looked after in case the marriage deteriorates or the husband is philandering and abusive. Some young women recognize that this protection comes at the cost of dependency: in accepting it, they open themselves up to having their actions as wives, in-laws, and mothers (to children who technically belong to the husband's clan) scrutinized by the invested parties. When older people complain about informal marriage and the decline of families' involvement in the marital process, they are expressing not only nostalgia for an idealized past but also anxiety about the loss of social and kinship protection and policing—particularly the protection and policing of young women—that they claim used to create the underlying moral economy of marriage and adult sexuality and gendered respectability.

Variations in Conjugality

Regardless of the perceived delay and decline of solemnization practices, the formal request and the *kwandhula* ceremony are still considered important steps in establishing the legitimacy of a union, particularly from the perspective of the woman's family and, as we will see later, in the eyes of the state. More often than not, however, marriage in Iganga does not follow the process described in the previous section, and marital histories of elders demonstrate that for at least the past fifty years or so there have been variations in the formation of marriages and the timing of *kwandhula* ceremonies. It is common for couples to cohabitate and have children before gathering enough money to stage a formal *kwandhula*—or, until the wife or her parents exert enough pressure on the young man in question. In 1998, 33 percent of the current marriages in Bulubandi were considered "customary," meaning that the couple had undergone some form of a *kwandhula* ceremony, or that the young man had at least gone through the formal process of getting approval from the bride's family and meeting her parents' demands, although the couple had not had a religious ceremony (see Table 3.3). The religious ceremonies are most frequently Islamic, with 25 percent of couples having

TABLE 3.3. Types of marriage of household heads in Bulubandi, 1998*

	Female		Male		Total	
	#	%	#	%	#	%
Customary (*kwandhula* only)	24	27%	95	34%	119	33%
Islamic	20	23%	73	26%	93	25%
Elopement	17	19%	66	24%	83	23%
Christian	9	10%	24	9%	33	9%
Unknown	18	20%	20	7%	38	10%
Total	**90**	**100%**	**278**	**100%**	**366**	**100%**

*Data are from only the 366 household heads who either are currently married or have been married in the past (but are now divorced or widowed). Data include only one (most often the first or most socially recognized) marriage of each household head, although many household heads have had more than one marriage.

gone through both the traditional process and an Islamic ceremony. In contrast, only 9 percent of heads of household in Bulubandi have had a Christian marriage ceremony as well as the traditional ceremony. The discrepancy between the number of Islamic and Christian weddings can be partially explained by the larger Muslim community in Bulubandi, but that alone does not account for the difference. It also reflects the role that the kinship groups and intergenerational interactions play in the life of younger Muslims and the difficulties in hosting the elaborate ceremony expected among many Christian congregations as described above.

For residents in Iganga, informal marriage (or elopement, as it translates in Lusoga) is a common and recognized marital form. These unions have not been formally approved by the young woman's parents, or the young man has not yet met the demands set by her parents, but the couple lives together and is socially recognized by residents as husband and wife. Nearly 25 percent of the households in Bulubandi were considered informal, but this figure is likely higher because in many cases we were able to collect information only on unions in Bulubandi. For instance, one man had wives in three different places—in Bulubandi, in another village, and in town—but we could reliably gather information only about the marriage in Bulubandi. While the man stated that his other two wives were "obtained through official routes," the wife and a couple of female neighbors in Bulubandi who had allegiance to the woman insisted that his other women were "temporary" wives.

Whereas residents, religious leaders, and politicians speak of informal marriage as a sign of moral decline and weakened Basoga patrilineage, in reality there is some ambivalence about it in everyday life in Bulubandi. Many elders had children and cohabited before a formal *kwandhula*, and residents are sympathetic to the difficulties involved in raising the money necessary to stage the increasingly elaborate and extravagant *kwandhula* (see also Hunter 2010:218). An informal marriage is more likely to be considered dishonorable when it is initially formed and especially if the parents and the community do not perceive the two people or the union as being "mature." But over time, if the couple remains together and particularly after children are born, the community might forget the status of the marriage. The woman's family might choose to ignore the fact that their demands were not met or might decide to consider some other gestures of the man (such as gift giving or service) to stand in the place of their demands or the introduction. For young professionals, though, cohabitating without a public *kwandhula* can be a source of great dissatisfaction and complaints among the wife and her family, for her reputation is at stake.

The act of eloping is a highly gendered concept. *Okúpáálá* is used to refer to the actions of a woman eloping and literally means "to run away without permission" from her father or parents. Holly Wardlow describes similar action among Huli passenger women in Papua New Guinea as a form of "negative agency . . . in which a woman severs from the social group that which should most be encompassed by it—her sexuality" (2006:15). Leaving one's parents' house without proper permission and a *kwandhula* is an act of disobedience and disrespect. Whereas a young woman's action of running away is seen as an indication of moral decline, this is less the case for the actions of the man who "stole" her. The term used to describe the man's action is *okupaaza*; that is, stealing a woman from another man without going through cultural conventions. It is a demonstration of masculine aggression. This concept is much less disparaging and stigmatizing than the one that describes the young woman. In fact, if a young man successfully steals a daughter without major repercussions (such as being publicly sued or physically confronted), his masculine prestige and reputation among his male peers may increase.

Older men complain that younger men today do not have the same respect for their elders as in the past—a lack of respect they see as being enabled by the state and the court system. As discussed in Chapter 6, during Fallers's research in the 1950s, a father of a young woman who had eloped could charge her partner with stealing his daughter, and the case could be resolved if the guilty man agreed either to pay *omutango* (a fine or compensation to the father) in addition to bridewealth or to return the daughter (Fallers 1969:108). While not obtaining proper permission from a young woman's father remains a source of considerable intergenerational conflict and tension among men, there are few cases today in which the father is awarded compensation in the courts. However, the cultural logic underlying *omutango* is deployed as a threat by parents who wish to end the romantic liaison of a daughter, as detailed further in Chapter 6. In short, the glue that historically held kinship groups together and gave legitimacy to social reproduction—the formal solemnization process that involved the official and public transfer of access to a young woman from her father to her husband—is perceived to be under threat by multiple forces, including the increased agency of young women, the economic difficulties in engaging in Uganda's globally influenced marriage industry, and the weakening of older men's power over young men and over their own daughters.

Dissolution of a Marriage and the Problematics of Legitimacy and Property

Lloyd Fallers (1957) once wrote that marriage is fragile and divorce is high among the Basoga as compared to other patrilineal Bantu groups. Finding that Max Gluckman's divorce hypothesis, in which he posits that patrilineal kinship leads to more stable marriages than bilateral kinship, did not fit the Basoga pattern, Fallers offered this revision: "Where a wife is not so absorbed [into the husband's lineage] and thus remains a member of the lineage into which she was born, patriliny tends to divide marriages by dividing the loyalties of spouses" (1957:114). This divided loyalty, he continued, is further facilitated by Basoga fathers who tend to be protective of and sympathetic to their daughters, both "jealously" guarding adolescent daughters from men's sexual advances and protecting them from abusive husbands. These reasons alone do not fully explain the rate of divorce in Bulubandi today, but provide interesting historical and cultural starting points from which to explore contemporary dissolutions of marriage.

In 1998, 55 percent of the heads of household in Bulubandi who had ever been married had also been divorced at least once, which represents only a slight increase over Fallers's 1950s data of 46 percent (see Table 3.4). Although residents tend to use the terms "divorce" and "separation" interchangeably in everyday conversations, the return of bridewealth differentiates the two terms. In general, divorce requires the return of the nongift portion of the bridewealth, while in a separation the couple is decidedly not living together but the refund has not (yet) been made. The refund of bridewealth to a husband is technically to be made by either the wife's father (or another male relative if the father is deceased or unable) or a prospective husband, the latter loosely defined. Bridewealth refund nullifies the initial marital contract and frees the woman from reproductive and productive labor obligations to the man and his family. Conversely, it also frees the man of obligations to her family and to her, except for child support.

Refunding the bridewealth is not always straightforward. Identifying the refundable portion can be a source of contention. The father or other male relative may not have the resources to enact the refund or want to use them in this way. The husband may not agree to accept a refund, to demonstrate his power, stubbornness, or even affection for his wife (which he may insist he still feels, despite actions that she finds no longer bearable, such as repeated extramarital philandering). When the bridewealth is not returned, the dissolution is considered incomplete, and the woman technically cannot marry another man, for polyandry is neither culturally nor legally permissible. It is not uncommon for a woman who is still attached to a husband through bridewealth to cohabit and have children with another man, but according to cultural convention her official husband can sue that man for damages and a refund in bridewealth. Fallers in the 1950s found cases of a husband suing another man for "harboring" (in the case of a father) or "stealing" (in the case of a lover) his wife if another man "kept" his wife (1969), but we found no such cases in the court system. Today bridewealth grievances are likely settled among kin groups or by village elected officials, or just dropped by the man.

Most people who have been divorced (or 58 percent of divorced people) report only one previous divorce, but based on conversations with residents we have reason to

TABLE 3.4. Divorce, separation, and widowhood histories of household heads in Bulubandi, 1998*

	Female (N=88)		Male (N=278)		Total (N=366)	
	#	%	#	%	#	%
Number of divorces reported	46	52%	156	56%	202	55%
1	32	70%	85	54%	117	58%
2	7	15%	32	21%	39	19%
3	4	9%	17	11%	21	10%
4	2	4%	10	6%	12	6%
5+	1	2%	12	8%	13	6%
Widowed	43	49%	39	14%	82	22%

*Includes only household heads either currently married or previously married but currently unmarried. Figures indicate whether the household head has been divorced or widowed.

believe that the actual number of divorces and separations is higher than reported. The underreporting of the number of divorces reveals gendered notions of sexual respectability. People begin to gossip and talk of sexual improprieties if a woman has had more than two marriages, so she may keep information about past conjugal relationships away from her neighbors. The practice of patrilocality (the wife's relocation to her husband's place) enables a woman to conceal a past marriage from current neighbors. On the contrary, it is more difficult for a man to hide previous unions, unless he has them in other places, which is not uncommon. Some men might try to downplay the nature of a past cohabitation relationship, making it seem more casual that it might have been, for a man who is seen as having a difficult time "keeping women" can develop a reputation of not being in control of his household and his women. For example, we collected information from a man who told us he had had five previous marriages (in addition to the one with his current wife). Over time, I found out it was common knowledge among his neighbors that he had had twelve previous marriages. The man was embarrassed and shocked when he discovered that his current wife and neighbors were aware of the number. While twelve marriages is an extreme case, it also highlights the blurred line between casual cohabitation and marriage. Furthermore, Jane Guyer (1994) notes that second and subsequent marriages tend to be more informal than first ones, and family involvement in these may not be as intimate as in the first marriage, particularly in the case of the man's family or if the couple is older. For Christian marriages, bridewealth is often not expected, unless it will be used as compensation to the first husband, as discussed above. While some observers argue that these second marriages are more likely love-marriages (the assumption being that first marriages are duty-marriages to satisfy a man's family), others argue that second and "outside" wives have less protection under state law and in local arbitration and kinship venues in cases of marital grievances or dissolution, as discussed below.

HIV has had a significant impact on the dissolution of unions. Not only has HIV increased cases of widowhood, but residents as well as researchers suggest that suspicions that a partner is HIV-positive or is engaging in HIV-risky behaviors (such as concurrent partnerships) have also motivated separation or divorce (see Porter et al. 2004). More females in Bulubandi than males report the death of a spouse (49 percent versus 14 percent, respectively), which reflects trends in other parts of Africa. According to health workers in Iganga, among serodiscordant couples (where one partner is HIV-positive and the other is HIV-negative) men are more likely than women to leave or separate from an HIV-positive spouse, which highlights the great stigmatization of HIV-infected women. There is also an expectation that a man will take another wife to look after him and his children should his wife die. However, the practice of levirate (a widow being "inherited" by a brother of the deceased man) has gradually faded among the Basoga, and because a woman is not fully absorbed into her husband's clan, a widow may not be able or want to remain in the matrimonial house after the death of her husband.

Widowhood, divorce, and separation are economically risky for women. Tales abound about widows being forced off the matrimonial property by in-laws who may stigmatize and ostracize the woman, claiming that she brought HIV into the compound and killed their son. In addition, the patrilineal system of inheritance alienates a woman from property in both her husband's clan and her father's clan. According to cultural convention, property is inherited by males through the male line and marital property is considered the husband's. Therefore, in cases of marital dissolution, the woman has limited, if any, claim over the property a man has inherited from his father's line and sometimes limited right over the property he acquired outside of his patrilineage. This practice is changing, and a family or other informal arbitrator may award a woman some portion of the "transportable" matrimonial property. The award, however, would likely not include the most valuable agrarian resource—land. Here, a distinction must be made between matrimonial property as *compensation*—that is, awarded by an arbitrator—and matrimonial property as a *right*, with the stronger claim being the latter. The loss of *rights* to matrimonial property may discourage some women from initiating a formal divorce, and women might instead choose to remain married so they can at least claim this status in social situations in which being married confers respect on a woman. On the other hand, the increasing practice of awarding women some compensation in cases of divorce may lead men to refuse to formally dissolve the marriages even when a woman leaves her matrimonial home. While in the past women often returned to their fathers' houses after divorces, the monetization of the economy has made it increasingly difficult for aging fathers to absorb adult daughters (and perhaps their children) into their already cash-strained households.

Women in Iganga have enacted a variety of strategies to protect their rights to matrimonial property. For instance, whereas most women leave their matrimonial house after a divorce, Kagoya, a woman in her late sixties, refused to do so. We discovered her situation while visiting a man's compound during our household surveys. When we inquired about a house in the back of the compound, the man replied, "My off-layer," a term used to refer to a chicken that can no longer lay eggs. In this case he was using the term to refer to his first wife, who is no longer able to produce children, unlike his current and younger wives. The man and Kagoya had separated some years before, but she refused to leave the land, claiming that years of her labor had helped build the houses and the farm. She added that her labor had also helped him "buy" the two wives with whom he was currently living. Kagoya was adamant about not leaving her matrimonial land, and her sons, two of whom also lived on the large plot of land, continued to support her decision and to tend to their mother's living needs. Although Kagoya's case was unique and a very bold act of defiance, many residents considered her justified in her decision to stay on the land she had helped develop. It created an awkward situation for all involved but, as some women suggested, it also provided a public reminder of persistent gender inequalities in marriage.

The strategy of remaining on the matrimonial property worked for Kagoya because her marriage was seen as legitimate in the eyes of the clans and the state. Conversely, the ambiguous legitimacy of informal marriages frequently undermines women's negotiating power and results in different strategies for women when conflicts arise. When marital conflicts arise, the two extended families are typically the first venue for arbitration, and if people are not satisfied with the families' resolution, they can take their grievances to outside arbitration venues, such as village elected officials or the Probate (Domestic Affairs) Office. Whereas sixty-some years ago, when Fallers conducted his research, women were prohibited from initiating cases in the colonial native court system, today women are more likely than men to seek arbitration for certain types of marital grievances outside the kinship route.

However, we found that in many of the cases we reviewed and witnessed in the Probate Office, the patriarchal view of gender and sexuality was often reproduced by state agents who had the authority to impose particular definitions of marriage and legitimacy that undermines women's marital rights. The case of twenty-five-year-old Mariam illustrates this point. Mariam went to the Probate Office with the hope of getting assistance for a reconciliation. She and her husband had lived together for over a year, but after she became pregnant, her husband stopped providing support and "abandoned" her at his house in the village. Unable to support herself and not receiving assistance from her in-laws, who were her neighbors, Mariam returned to her parents' house, where she delivered the baby. Her parents and her *ssenga* (paternal aunt) found the man and tried to encourage him to "take back" Mariam and their new baby. He "accepted" them back but eventually brought in another "wife." He asked Mariam to sleep in another room while the new wife took her bedroom and many of her household belongings. Mariam told the officer, "I took the case to the LC [local council official] and he told my co-wife and me to divide some items. Soon after, [my husband] stopped giving me and the baby assistance. Several times I have reported him to the LC, but he has failed to change, so the LC decided to send me to the Probate Office. I want to reconcile and for him to provide support for me and our child."

After listening to Mariam's grievance, the probate officer had one follow-up question: the type of her marriage. Mariam explained that she had not gone through the formal *kwandhula* ceremony but insisted that it was a marriage. The probate officer recorded the marriage as a "friendly relationship," however, which not only discursively stripped the union of legitimacy but also ideologically took away Mariam's ability to form a marriage without her father. The naming of the union as a "friendly relationship" reproduced patriarchal conceptions of marriage as an agreement between two men—the father and the husband—and called into question the legitimacy of Mariam's union with her child's father and hence her respectability as a woman. This ideological construction of women's sexuality had material implications as well. It transformed what Mariam had considered a marriage (with its bundle of responsibilities, duties, and obligations) into a casual union, effectively removing any marital economic obligations and responsibilities. Many state agents can and do claim that informal marriages do not fall under the legal jurisdiction of the state marriage laws, but this is slowly changing. In cases in which an informal marriage fails to meet the test of legitimacy in the eyes of the state or other official local arbitrators, we found that a domestic grievance is often recast in terms of paternity, child maintenance, or child custody. Hence, reproduction for a woman not only is a personal desire or an expression of an affective bond with a man, but can also be used as a strategy to strengthen the legitimacy of a union and her claims to matrimonial property and respectability. The strategy does not always produce the desired outcome. I spoke with Mariam as she walked away from the Probate Office with no legitimate claims for matrimonial support and with a young child for whom she expects to receive minimal economic support. Mariam told me that she knew of relatives and neighbors who had found themselves in similar situations, but had never imagined that she too would be in this position.

The Case of Nakagolo:
Networking, Reproduction, and Mobility

Life for many young adults and youth in Iganga can be transient, consisting of a series of temporary relocations to the houses of relatives and friends as they search for work, education, and other meaningful opportunities. This pattern of residence surfing (to borrow from the term "couch surfing," used to describe the transience of young people in the United States) is not only an accepted part of "searching for something to do" but also a way of distributing over a larger social landscape the economic and social responsibility of caring for un- or under-employed young people. Although some young people reside with their parents while suspended between schooling and employment, this option is not appealing or possible for all. Some parents retreat to rural areas with few opportunities for the young; others have urban accommodations too small to house their adult children; and many might provide surveillance and scrutiny, hoping to limit a young person's activities as well as to temper their imagination of grandiose future possibilities. Using Jennifer Johnson-Hanks's (2002) concept of "vital conjuncture" to capture the indeterminacy and innovation in young people's experiences, we can see how the story of Nakagolo illustrates the intersection of residence surfing patterns and emerging sexual, reproductive, and marital trajectories.

I met Nakagolo when she was thirty-nine-years old and very active in village affairs. She had eight children from relationships with five different men. She called two of these relationships "marriages," and during her relationships with four of the men, they were married to other women. She indicated that she was married during our household survey; however, over time I realized that her neighbors considered her the head of her household. Her fifty-eight-year-old husband, a charming former subcounty chief, was in declining health, provided her with minimal support, and lived with his first wife in a neighboring village; his second wife lived in yet another different village. Rumor was that he had fathered at least forty-seven children with various "wives" across the region over the course of his sexually active history. As his health deteriorated, his visits to Nakagalo became increasingly infrequent, but the three children they had had together, ranging in age from one to eight, provided evidence that the couple were performing their "marital duties," as sex between a husband and wife is politely coded. Nakogolo's story illuminates how the meanings of and motivations for sexual relationships are shaped by vital conjunctures that lie at the intersection of a person's progression through life stages, shifting residential locations, and gender- and class-related opportunities. Nakagolo explains:

> I began school in 1966 [age 6]. In 1977 [age 18], I completed secondary school and had nothing to do, so I was sent to stay with my half-sister in Kampala. While with my half-sister, I got pregnant by a man in her neighborhood. My half-sister sent me away from her place because she said that I was causing conflicts between her home and the wife of the man who had impregnated me. I came back to my mother in Bwanalira village with the pregnancy and gave birth from there.
>
> After the baby was a year old he was taken to my grandmother, and I went to Bugiri where my relatives found me a teaching job at a school. In 1979 [age 21], while at school in Bugiri, I fell in love with one of the teachers on staff. This man was a Mugisu [an ethnic category], and we got married in the same year. This man stopped teaching and took me to his home place in Bugisu. Our marriage was on a friendly basis. That man had given me a shop, but he used the money I made and spent it on other women. In 1981 [age 23], I left that man. I left two children; one was one year old and the other six months.
>
> The same year, my half-sister in Kampala again called for me to help around the house [as a housemaid]. I was impregnated by the young man who lived downstairs. He was a university student. He was not in a position to marry me, and I was sent away again. I came back to my mother and delivered from there.
>
> After I produced [a child], I fell in love with another man in the village. The man was a medical officer working at the subcounty offices. That was in 1983 [age 25]. The man rented for me a house and I stayed there. I produced one child with this man. The man was a Mugwere [an ethnic category]. Soon he was transferred to his home area where his wife lived. Our affair ended in that way in 1984.
>
> In 1988 [age 30], I was helped by one of my cousin's sisters to join the local administration as a clerical officer. I fell in love with the subcounty chief [Nakagolo's current husband]. This man took me to study as a cashier. In 1989, I was made the subcounty cashier and was transferred from Bulamogi Subcounty to Nakigo, but my husband remained in Bulamogi as subcounty chief.

In the same year, I produced a child with the subcounty chief. Between 1989 and 1994, I was in Nakigo as a subcounty cashier. In 1994, I produced the second child with the chief. The same year I was transferred from Nakigo to Namungalwe, and also my husband was laid off from his job in 1995.

In 1994, I bought a plot in Bulubandi and built a house there. In the same year I shifted from Namungalwe to my house in Bulubandi. In 1996 [age 38], I produced the third child with the former chief. Since that time I have been a housewife. In the most recent election, I was voted secretary for women on the Local Council 1 [the village level].

In Nakagolo's telling of her sexual narrative, she points to key vital conjunctures that tie her pattern of serial sexual relationships and reproduction to the geographic mobility and residence surfing set in motion by her limited economic and educational opportunities. Mobility facilitates sexual networking and allows people to conceal their sexual past and temporarily escape moral judgment in new locations. Combined with lack of access to resources, however, mobility leaves women such as Nakagolo particularly vulnerable. In Kampala, she found herself serving as a housemaid to her stepsister and greatly dependent on her. The men who impregnated her (the passive Lusoga verb she used suggesting lack of agency) were neither interested in a long-term relationship nor held responsibility for supporting the children produced from their sexual trysts. Much like Sam, whose story was recounted in the opening of this book, Nakagolo had in her youth imagined having a monogamous marriage, but her residence surfing landed her in places with few social ties and set off a series of relationships that were fragile and uncertain.

What also emerges in Nakagolo's history is a pattern of sexual relations with married men. Wambui Wa Karanja (1987) examines conjugal relationships of the elite in Nigeria and uses the term "outside wives" to describe mistresses of wealthy men (256).[4] While the term "informal wife" does not adequately account for the relationship among a man's "wives," Karanja's concept of "outside wife" foregrounds the legitimacy of the wives as well as their different status. She argues that for many young women there is a difference between "Mr. Right" and "Mr. Available." The former is their ideal, romantic, long-term mate, and the latter is often an older "married man of considerable means." From the vantage point of the younger "outside wife," the married man represents access to financial resources, and he often sets up a house for his mistress and their children. Although Nakagolo's relationships somewhat fit this framework, viewing her story solely through a transactional lens conceals the emotional, social, and reproductive motives underlying her sexual encounters and relations. Nakagolo was intolerant when her previous husband invested time and finances in his extramarital affairs, but later she was willing to be the "outside wife."

A thirty-something Nakagolo had had a string of failed relationships and five children by four different men. Tired of floating around as a *nakyewombekeire* and worried that she was past the age of marital eligibility, she felt anxious to ground herself somewhere and establish an identity as an adult (i.e., married) woman. The idea of being a first wife was not only unrealistic—for who would want to publicly "introduce" a woman with evidence of such a sordid sexual past?—but also socially limiting, for she would have to surrender the independence to which she had become accustomed. Hence, Nakagolo transformed herself from an illegitimate "outside" wife of the sub-county chief to one of his recognized official co-wives, becoming the youngest of his three wives. Living separately from his other wives, she remained socially independent while being able to conveniently call on the social respectability of being a married woman. The respectability bestowed on married women is more important to a woman's reputation in the rural setting in which Nakagolo resides than in an urban setting.

The birth of Nakagolo's second child with the former subcounty chief helped give her a measure of conjugal legitimacy, but without a formal *kwandhula* or letter of marital request, it was not sufficient, as she had learned from her past relationships. More significant in conferring conjugal legitimacy was the man's economic investment in helping her acquire a fixed asset (i.e., land) in Bulubandi and his visible presence and engagement as she established herself in her new community and during the early stages of the construction of their home. Whereas first wives are often afforded greater social recognition, respect, and status in the man's family and community, later wives often have to employ varying strategies to be recognized as wives; conversely, they have the chance to enjoy more social freedom if they can garner their own income from which to maintain the household and their children. After Nakagolo's husband's initial social and economic investment in their conjugal home, the industrious woman took over the management of the house construction, financing most of it with money from her various activities and connections. Her husband still came around and was helpful in connecting her to networks through which she advanced her involvement in various community-level projects, such as a participating in a village literary group and being elected as the village women's representative. However, her neighbors recognized that she was the household head and able to make decisions independent from her husband.

Like other married women living independently, Nakagolo's public visibility and autonomy positions her differently than other married women in the village, who may admire her ability to live without the restrictions that husbands impose. One woman commented, "Whenever a woman is leaving the home, she must seek permission from the husband first, even if it is an emergency. The woman must always wait for the husband and inform him first and see if he will accept her to go." The freedom of mobility and decision making that Nakagolo enjoys may be coveted by other married women; however, the knowledge that she is an "added on" wife (meaning, her husband's first obligation is to another wife) slightly diminishes her ranking as a respectable married woman. The fragile link she has to her husband means that her freedom and mobility become subject to wider surveillance and speculation among neighbors who see her as untethered to a particular patrilineage or man. Married women neighbors may view the independence of secondary wives with a bit of envy, but they also view those wives with a dose of suspicion, disapproval, and pity, since those women are left without a man (i.e., father or husband) to watch over them and their behaviors.

Ultimately, Nakagolo's story is not an example of the failure of patriarchy or patrilineage to work properly. Rather, patriarchy was working as it should. Nakagolo was born to an unwed mother. Her mother eventually became the fourth serial wife (not a concurrent or co-wife) of Kagoda, an older man with whom she had eight children. When Nakagolo's mother and stepfather separated, her mother moved back to her home area, which was about four hours away, and their children remained with the father. After Nakagolo completed her education in a poorly performing rural secondary school, her stepfather began to withdraw the little support he was providing her. While her eight older stepsiblings had attended fairly prestigious schools and were assisted by their father to secure salaried positions, they too provided Nakagolo with little emotional or economic support. Instead, their loyalties went to their biological mothers and full siblings. Nakagolo was for a time an "abandoned island," as she described, untethered from the protection as well as control of a patrilineage. Without the threat of an older male relative to make a claim against a suitor for damages or to demand a request for marriage, she was an ideal subject for sexual relationships, coerced or consensual. She learned to be entrepreneurial out of necessity, and her relationships with men became a strategy not only to survive but also to gain affection. Her marriage to the subcounty chief provided the patriarchal cover of respect she needed to pursue her activities in community development and local politics. Nakagolo's story is a familiar one among young and older people. Whereas for many residents in Iganga her story is evidence of moral decline and the weakening of the patrilineal system that had provided protection for its members, for women's rights groups these stories of women such as Nakagolo are a call to give women equal access to resources.

Marriage and Gender Equity Campaigns: Empowering Women or Undermining Men's Rights?

Since the British colonial period, there has been a long history of state and missionary interventions into marriage in Uganda (for instance, see Kalema Commission 1965). More recent legislative bills surrounding marriage—including the 2003 Domestic Relations Bill and the 2009 Marriage and Divorce Bill re-tabled for legislative discussion in 2013 and 2015—have been initiated by women's rights groups and women legislators as part of a broader and longer gender equity movement (as it is commonly called in Uganda) that began soon after independence but was interrupted and restarted at various times during Uganda's turbulent years of civil unrest (see Obbo 1980; Tamale 1999; Tripp 1994, 2000). Gender reforms have been a source of public debate, with reforms being criticized for intruding too far into cultural matters (Musiga and Okanya 2010; *New Vision* 2008; Mutunga 2012; Mugyenyi 1998). In response to the introduction and revisions of the Marriage and Divorce Bill, for instance, opponents have maintained that "marriage is a preserve of religious and cultural institutions and the state has no business meddling in the sacred union" (Akumu 2013). Key sticking points revolve around issues challenging the foundation of patriarchy and patrilineage, such as giving women rights to natal or matrimonial property, placing limitations on polygyny, recognizing marital rape, and making infidelity justifiable grounds for a woman to divorce a husband. Despite the flurry of criticisms about gender equality efforts and changes in the marriage laws, women activists have pursued their attempts to use the law to address gender inequality and women's disenfranchisement.

There are conflicting opinions and various interpretations in Iganga of the effects of gender equality, but a general consensus is that gender equality is not only about giving women greater access to resources but also about giving women greater social, sexual, and physical freedom. For some, these efforts have taken women further from the oversight of the patrilineage and husbands, contributing to the increase in *nakyewobekeire*, divorce, separation, and ultimately HIV and out-of-wedlock pregnancies. Men we interviewed frequently expressed feeling under attack by women's rights activists and legislators, the Museveni regime, and global discourses about women's rights. As fathers and as husbands, they may feel that their traditional and natural authority is being undermined and that the definition of and path to masculinity are slowly unraveling. Women, on the other hand, pointed to the protection provided by the state in cases where the kinship group failed. As one middle-aged woman remarked, compared to wives of the past, a young wife today does not hesitate to leave a husband if she is beaten or if a wealthier man approaches her.

Both men and women often agree that gender equity has led to greater cooperation between husbands and wives in "developing the home," a phrase residents use to reflect the economic projects as well as affective projects (such as raising children or marital intimacy) of the household. Some older men have had an ironic interpretation of this advancement: unlike in the past, when husbands had the burden of supporting the house and making all household decisions, wives today can and *should* contribute to the development of their matrimonial home. In 1997, Sefatiya, a seventy-five-year-old man who sat on an informal council of elders that settled local disputes, captured this sentiment while reflecting on earlier difficulties in gender equity efforts:

Now most women are obedient to their husbands. In the late 1980s when the current government began to give women responsibility, the first response of men was negative. We feared that if women were given responsibility they would rebel against us men. When women realized this, they knew that men were going to revoke the responsibilities given to them, so women began to be obedient to men again. Now even a woman Member of Parliament is obedient to her husband to the extent of taking him water for bathing. In the past women were not obedient and we used to beat them to get them to do what we wanted. . . .

Gender balance [equality] has improved the conditions for women. With an income, women can also contribute financially to the needs of the home. . . . But, before this, all women thought that the only person who could solve problems was the husband. . . . Women today are able to look after the children and still do business. A woman will leave home knowing that she has given food to her children.

This gender balance of Museveni's regime is really good. It refers to giving responsibility to the woman. But it should be the man who commands more respect in the home. Even if I am a small man, I rule over my wife.

Two elements in Sefatiya's interpretation of gender equality make the concept bearable to him and other men with whom I spoke. First, gender equity does not ultimately change the gender hierarchy in marriage, for a man is still the "ruler" of the home. Second, he casts gender equality not in terms of women's rights to resources but rather in terms of women's equal "responsibility" for the well-being of the household. In effect, the workload for women has doubled—taking care of the domestic chores as well as providing financial assistance. Women's increased economic responsibility and vocal assertions are beneficial only if they do not challenge the patriarchal order. This framing ameliorates the possible threat that the forces of equality and the realignment of the household economy could have on local gender hierarchies. Sefatiya's explanation reveals how men, and some women, in Iganga have transformed the effects of inevitable wider changes in ways that are palatable and fit within the framework of male authority and ideas of marriage. Changes for women are considered positive only if they do not disrupt a general pattern of male dominance over women. Otherwise, the women's movement and gender equality are still considered a threat to male authority and a feasible explanation for the decline of morality among young women.

Conclusion: Young People's Reflections on Marriage and the Burdens of Wives

I have detailed the processes and complexities of contemporary marriage in Iganga because conjugality, patrilineage, and bridewealth exchanges lie at the heart of Basoga understandings of sexuality. Furthermore, relationships among adult relatives and neighbors inform young people's ideas of marital and gender possibilities, even if they do so by providing them with a counterexample. I conclude this chapter with a brief discussion of how young people interpret the marriages of their parents and other adults with whom they are close and consider the configurations they imagine and desire for their own future marriages.

Young people with whom we spoke were highly critical of their parents' marriages and especially of the way their fathers mistreated their mothers or neglected to properly provide for the household's needs, including their own school fees. Virtually all the young people desired a marriage based on cooperation, communication, and mutual planning for needs of the household—what scholars call "companionate marriage"— something they did not think was fully realized in their parents' marriages. However, similar to Sefatiya's reflections above, their seemingly egalitarian notions kept intact basic Basoga and religious interpretations of gender ideologies—men rule and provide, and women follow and serve. For instance, young people described cooperation as occurring within specific gender roles in which the man is the "ruler," responsible for financial matters and giving advice, and the woman is responsible for cooking, cleaning, entertaining visitors, and caring for children and the husband.

Drawings and discussions by young people illustrated differences in boys' and girls' ideas of gender relations within marriage. There were notable distinctions in how boys and girls visually represented the physicality between a husband and wife. Adolescent males were more likely to draw this as a hierarchical relationship, often portraying the wife as kneeling in front of her husband—the customary Basoga way for a woman to greet a man. In their pictures, the "good" wife is frequently depicted as kneeling not

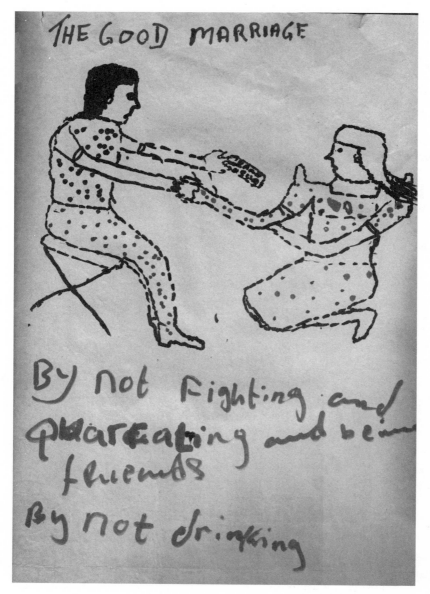

FIGURE 3.3. Drawing of a good marriage, by boys

only when greeting the husband but while either serving her husband food or receiving something from him such as money, as shown in a drawing by young people ages ten to fourteen years old (Figure 3.3). When I asked another group of young people if their parents' marriages were good, average, or bad, one boy wrote that his parents' marriage was good because "my mother does everything my father wants her to do." He expressed disappointment in his father's tardiness or absence in the evenings and his not paying the school fees on time, but overall he attributed his parents' success to his mother's coop-eration and hard work. Conversely, female participants emphasized the man's economic

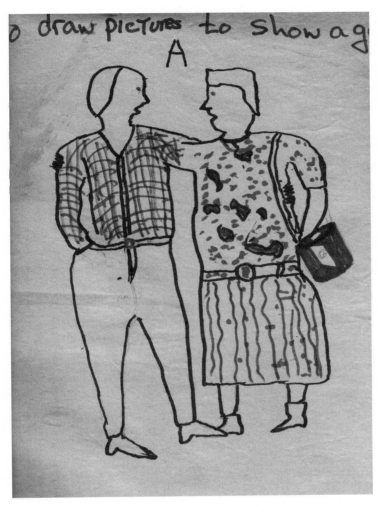

FIGURE 3.4. Drawing of a good marriage, by girls

role as the basis for a good marriage. A group of adolescent females wrote that in a good marriage, "the man loves his wife and he buys everything at home." Adolescent females believed that the husband is economically responsible for the home, but they also desired relationships in which the couple had mutual respect. They were more likely than their male counterparts to draw the husband and wife in an intimate relationship, often with the two figures touching, holding hands, and embracing (Figure 3.4).

There is materiality in young people's understandings of gender relations with a marriage, such as clothing style as an index of gender hierarchy. In pictures of women kneeling or serving, the woman is more likely to be dressed modestly in a *gomesi* (floor-length dress). In contrast, in drawings where the husband and wife are standing or sitting together, the woman is dressed in contemporary clothing and the man in a shirt and tie, both symbols of modernity and higher socioeconomic status. A key item in many adolescent females' pictures is a purse, which signifies freedom from village activities such as carrying firewood, water, or even babies, and full participation in the commercial economy. According to these girls, a woman's engagement with the modern consumer market is reflected in the contents of her purse, which would include money and her personal beauty products, such as lipstick, perfume, a cell phone, or a comb.

There were fewer differences and more similarities between adolescent boys' and girls' drawings of a "bad marriage." The most common theme was that of a drunken husband beating his wife (Figure 3.5). In bad marriage drawings, youth often used the word "fighting," which takes on gendered forms—a husband "beat" his wife, and a wife "quarreled" with her husband. Whereas older people in Iganga expressed the idea that "disciplining" a wife might be justified in certain situations, youth overwhelmingly saw it as harmful and were overwhelmingly sympathetic to the women in their drawings. One group of youth wrote under their picture, "The thing that makes a marriage bad is the man beating his wife every day. And another thing is he doesn't want to buy things at home, and he over drinks." This criticism of fathers and compassion for mothers might be a manifestation of the differences in children's emotional connections to their own mothers and fathers. In our interviews we found that adult men in general were much more sympathetic to their mothers than to their fathers, and most of the men I interviewed overtly disapproved of how their fathers had treated their mothers. Not only do mothers provide emotional support, but as scholars suggest, women often try to maintain positive ties with children, which is particularly critical given that children in Africa are the most reliable form of social security in old age for women who lack access to matrimonial property or inheritances from their fathers.

The youth we spoke with viewed extramarital affairs and polygyny as an unfortunate but integral and virtually inevitable aspect of marriage in Uganda. All the adolescent females and most of the adolescent males, both Christian and Muslim, wanted monogamous marriages in which they would socialize and make decisions together with their spouses. On the other hand, the youth were keenly aware that achieving such an ideal would be possible only through stable social and economic conditions, something many of them did not see in their parents' lives. Hence, the youth desired marriages different from their parents,' but they were aware that their parents' marital experiences have been shaped by wider conditions of poverty, mobility that is often unpredictable, lack of steady employment, and gender inequality. Having observed the relationships of older siblings, relatives, and peers, they are also aware that their own future relationship trajectories may be shaped by these conditions as well.

The structural constraints that surround conjugal as well as premarital relationships have been characteristic of the region for a long time, as examined in the previous chapter, and have been exacerbated by a history of demographic change, migration, and postcolonial political and social uncertainties in Uganda. These changes and constraints not only shape contemporary life and youth sexual culture, but in the *longue durée* have gradually uprooted young people from the *máka*, that sense of belonging that (at least ideally) ties an individual to a moral economy of protection and regulation. Among the patrilineal Basoga, the connection to a *máka* is highly gendered, and women, through bridewealth exchanges, exist somewhere between their father's lineage and their husband's. As the *kwandhula* and hence official marriages are delayed and as

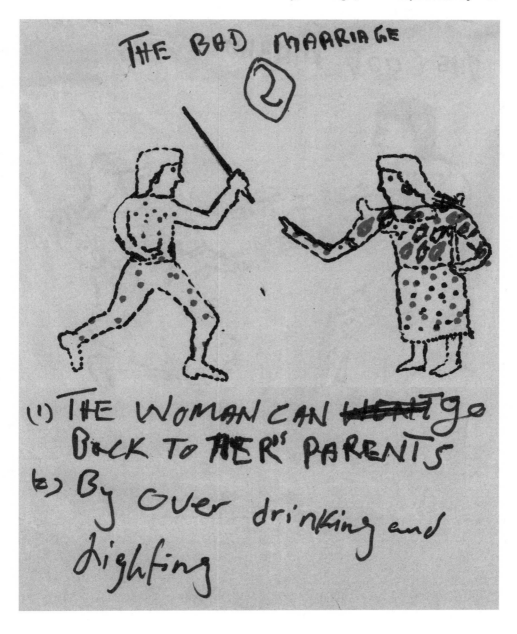

FIGURE 3.5. Youth drawing of a bad marriage

economic and demographic pressures propel young women, like their male counter-parts, into a pattern of residence surfing for survival and economic and educational opportunities, residents feel anxious about what they perceive as a visible and growing group of floating young *nakyewombekeire* who are unattached to, unprotected from, and unregulated by a *máka*. From the perspective of some residents, these morally un-attached young women are encouraged and empowered by the national interventions surrounding gender equality, and together they threaten to further disrupt an already weakened patriarchal moral order that would have offered these women (and, by exten-sion, their male lovers and society in general) protection against HIV, out-of-wedlock pregnancies, and other social depravities.

PART II

Publics

Interventions into Youth Sexuality

Yoweri Museveni and Nat'l Resistance Movement took over (power), standard story is he took action and boldly emphasized AIDS and prevention efforts

CHAPTER 4

The Social Evolution of HIV

Inequalities and Biomedical Citizenship

> Beyond the sheer weight of the numbers, what is perhaps most important about the shape of the HIV pandemic is the fact that the global distribution has been anything but equal. (Parker 2002:343)

> I first saw an AIDS patient in 1986. It was my brother who used to work in Kampala. He was brought back from Kampala when he was very sick, but we did not know that it was AIDS. We thought he had been bewitched from his place of work. He got sick and was bedridden for two years and then died. Then his wife also fell sick in the same way and also died, so we thought she was bewitched. We thought people were sending *juju*. Nobody suspected that it could be AIDS. And in the same village there was another person who died in a similar way. From there I also saw my husband having the same symptoms. He died in 1990. Then I knew it was AIDS doing all that. (Florence Kumunu, chair of Iganga's Buwolomera Development Association for HIV)

When the CDC first reported on what would later be known as AIDS in the June 5, 1981, issue of its *Morbidity and Mortality Weekly Report*, noting its appearance among five previously healthy "active homosexuals" in the United States, the virus had already made its way along the Uganda-Tanzania border in East Africa (Serwadda, Mugerwa, et al. 1985).[1] Health professionals working in the war-torn region at that time recall witnessing a dramatic increase in deaths from a new wasting disease that residents called *sslimu*, so named for its severe slimming effect on the body (see, for example, Garrett 1994:334–36; Thornton 2008; Epstein 2007:155–61; T. Barnett and Whiteside 2006:131–33). Evidence would later suggest that the epidemic took root and proliferated along the trade routes in the border region sometime in the 1970s, when fighting ensued between Idi Amin's army and opposition forces from Tanzania and Uganda. The armed conflict further exacerbated existing economic and social instability and fueled a network of soldiers, sex workers, and smugglers. It was "a risk environment *par excellence* and fertile ground for the development of an HIV epidemic" that would silently spread around the region during the next decade (T. Barnett and Whiteside 2002:133). By 1981, Amin's army had retreated from the border region, but the conflict had shifted into the Luwero Triangle, unfolding into a series of bloody guerilla struggles called the Ugandan Bush War, which lasted for five years. The virus followed the network of military, trade, and sexual exchanges.

As described earlier, the conflict ended in 1986 when Yoweri Museveni and his National Resistance Movement took control of the country, but left war orphans scattered throughout the Luwero Triangle. The HIV epidemic would soon take the lives of other adults, creating an even larger population of orphans as well as household and community instability. By the early 1990s, the epidemic had been comfortably traveling through the country via roadways, trade routes, and sexual networks. The HIV prevalence rate among pregnant women attending prenatal clinics in the conflict regions and in the capital reached as high as 30 percent, with a national average estimated at 18.3 percent (Serwadda, Wawer, et al. 1992; Wawer, Sewankambo, et al. 1994). The global media labeled Uganda's hardest-hit communities "AIDS villages," and journalists and scholars described hospitals overcrowded with withered bodies, along with a death rate among adults that was so high that households were being run by inexperienced children or overburdened grandparents (Konde-Lule and Sebina 1993). Uganda dominated the international news on HIV. Then, quite unexpectedly, in the early 1990s those hardest-hit regions began to show signs of declining HIV prevalence rates, dropping in some sites from 30 percent to 15 percent (UNAIDS 2008; Konde-Lule 1995; Kamali et al. 2000). Soon, other urban and rural surveillance sites experienced a similar decline in HIV prevalence (Hogle 2002; Stoneburner and Low-Beer 2004; Mbulaiteye et al. 2002).

Uganda's success story has received much media, scholarly, and policy attention (Kinsman 2010; Kuhanen 2008). The standard story is that Museveni initially heard of HIV over the radio while fighting in the bush (Museveni 1995). He later learned of the possible severity of the epidemic when he sent his troops halfway around the world to Cuba for training, where his soldiers were subjected to Cuba's mandatory HIV testing policy (Putzel 2004). The results were astonishing. About 40 percent of the soldiers tested positive for the HIV antibody. Museveni was shown a graph of the country's demographic and population trends if the epidemic were to continue unabated. The country's orphan population would explode, and the most economically productive sectors and age groups would be depleted.

The strategic and forward-thinking Museveni decided to take action. Within a few months of assuming the presidency, Museveni took the bold step of announcing to citizens of his country that they were facing a devastating sexually transmitted AIDS epidemic. He wove messages about HIV into every speech—advising people not to love recklessly, to be compassionate with those dying, that AIDS was not the result of *juju* (witchcraft), and, most importantly, to take AIDS seriously. Those speeches were broadcast over the radio and television. The government also initiated what was called a "multisectoral" approach to AIDS control by integrating HIV efforts into every ministry and at every level of government, from national to district to local. Uganda's AIDS Control Program (ACP) was established in 1987 within the Ministry of Health, and the Uganda AIDS Commission Act of 1992 established an independent body to coordinate the multisectoral approach to controlling the epidemic (UAC 1993, 1996).

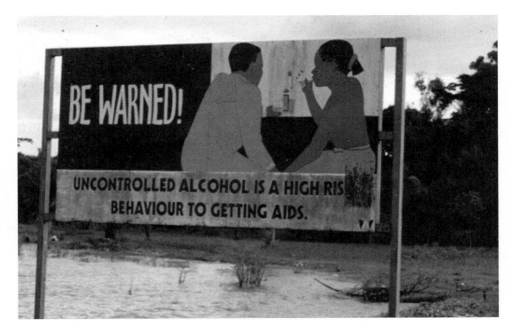

FIGURE 4.1. "Be warned!" billboard, built in the mid-1990s

This mainstreaming of the AIDS control plan at the national level was comple-
mented by an awareness campaign that was to be implemented through the new local
government structure. Museveni's government designed a five-tier local council (LC)
system—originally called "resistance councils" (RCs) for the work they provided during
the guerilla war—that began at the village level (LC1) to the subcounty and parish levels and eventually to the district level (LC5). Messages about HIV were to be disseminated through the LCs, dispelling myths and providing information about the spread
of the disease. The LC strategy was only partly successful. In Iganga, LC1 officials were
often busy settling disputes between neighbors or were too preoccupied with their own
political careers to dedicate themselves seriously to the task of delivering HIV messages.
One LC member in Iganga said that many feared that if you talked about AIDS, people
would think you had the disease, as reflected in the stories later in this chapter of Rev.
Jackson, Catherine, and Florence.

By all accounts, Museveni was strategic, pragmatic, and courageous in his approach
to HIV and nation-building (Kinsman 2010; Epstein 2007; Crane 2013; Thornton
2008). He knew that for the country to rebuild and grow, the cash-poor country needed
the assistance of international donors. Foreign development agencies, governments,
and research institutes had been driven out of Uganda during its previous periods of
insecurity, especially the Amin years, but were eager to return to the once-prosperous
country known as "the pearl of Africa." The social and political problems faced by the
new regime—the HIV epidemic, poverty, and an emerging capitalist democracy—
coincided with international development and research agendas. Museveni became the
darling of the international community of donors.

Likewise for foreign health researchers and scientists, Uganda was an ideal place to establish collaborations, laboratories, research projects, and clinical trials on the new global infectious disease. Prior to Amin's reign of terror, the country had been considered the intellectual hub of the East African colonial empire, serving as the home of foreign research institutes, but civil conflict had driven many away. Museveni's liberalization and opening-up policies welcomed back foreign researchers and international collaborations to help Uganda rebuild after the extended conflict. The Luwero Triangle and the border region in south-central Uganda that were ground zero for the epidemic became home to world-renowned HIV research projects and studies. Ugandan and foreign researchers and scientists collaborated to establish a premier longitudinal research center in 1988 in Rakai District (eventually known as the Rakai Health Sciences Program, or RHSP, and affiliated with Johns Hopkins Bloomberg School of Public Health) and another shortly thereafter in Masaka District (the Medical Research Council Programme on AIDS, MRC, affiliated with the London School of Hygiene and Tropical Medicine).

The sophisticated research infrastructure and collaborations in the region have resulted in a large number of highly respected and oft-cited epidemiological, medical, and longitudinal behavioral studies, and publications on trends related to the HIV epidemic. Investigative reporters also arrived in the region to unravel the extent of the epidemic and the toll it was having on communities. Influential science journalist Laurie Garrett, however, lamented about the increase of Western helicopter "safari" scientists who descended on Africa, extracting samples and information with sometimes questionable ethics and returning home to publish and advance their careers with their findings (1994:355–59). Uganda being under the global microscope drew heated criticism within the country as well. In Kampala, Uganda's *Monitor* newspaper celebrated Global AIDS Day on December 1, 1999, with an article entitled "Rakai like AIDS Laboratory, Its People like Laboratory Mice."

While this criticism of exploitation existed, so too did the awareness of economic stimulation from the AIDS industry. A young woman explained to me, "In some ways, AIDS was good for this country. Nowadays everyone has a job collecting data for HIV surveys, doing HIV prevention, caring for the sick . . . even carpenters have more work today by making caskets." She was not denying the suffering that HIV had caused, but she was acknowledging the reality that Uganda's epidemic had brought in billions of dollars from foreign donor countries and agencies, providing the funding and technical know-how to rebuild the public health system.

By the early 1990s, white Toyota Land Cruisers marked with names of AIDS-related agencies filled the streets of Kampala and the country's highway network; foreign aid workers brought equipment, supplies, and money; and an elaborate network of HIV surveillance, prevention, and care specialists emerged. According to surveillance reports, the efforts paid off. Knowledge about HIV and AIDS among people in Ugandan is high. People know that the disease spreads primarily through sexual intercourse, and can easily recite the now-famous ABCs—abstinence, be faithful, and condom use—of risk reduction (Konde-Lule, Musagara, and Musgrave 1993; Konde-Lule, Tumwesigye, and Lubanga 1997). Most people in Iganga also know the physical signs of someone dying of AIDS and the polite shorthand, "He is sick." By the 2000s, virtually everyone had heard of antiretrovirals (ARVs) and likely knows someone receiving the medicines. Some even know the biomedical terms for opportunistic infections and their symptoms. The campaign has done more than reduce HIV rates and increase awareness about the disease, its transmission, and risk-reduction strategies; it has also shaped local understandings of disease, infection, and forms of belonging.

AIDS Comes to Iganga: Cultures of Coping and Biomedical Citizenship

Nurse Catherine Njuba and I arrived at Florence Kumunu's house in the deep *kyalo* (village) after a bumpy forty-minute ride on the back of *boda-bodas* (bicycle or motorcycle taxis). The heavy downpour of the night before had turned the narrow path leading to the village into a muddy river. Instead of heading back to town and returning to get us a few hours later, the *boda-boda* drivers decided to wait for us, hoping that the sun would dry out the muddy path during our visit. Using every moment as a teaching opportunity, Florence signaled for them to join the meeting of the Buwolomera Development Association (BUDEA). She was dynamic; her energy and welcoming smile and bright eyes were captivating and reassuring. Two men played drums while women and children performed the Kisoga dance and sang an energetic welcome song:

> AIDS is among us.
> It lives here. [*first gesturing to themselves, then sweeping their hands outward*]
> It came to ruin our community, but we will not let it.
> We are BUDEA.
> We fight AIDS! We are not afraid!
> We are BUDEA.
> We fight AIDS! We are not afraid!

When I was first introduced to Florence in 1997, I did not know that she was considered a saint in her own and neighboring villages, but after almost two decades of knowing her I am not surprised. She has been talking publicly about HIV since she found out her positive status in 1990. It was unheard of at that time for a healthy-looking person to publicly declare a positive HIV status or even get tested. Speaking publicly was a risky move that came with high social, physical, and economic costs. But Florence felt it was her duty to educate others; according to her, "God would take care of me and protect me from possible harm from speaking out." After Museveni put HIV education on the top of his agenda, people in Iganga slowly began to learn about HIV through awareness posters, radio announcements, and billboards. But what Florence was doing was new in the village. It was common for residents to organize informal community networks to assist families and the already sick, but no one was speaking about his or her positive status or the fact that the virus might be lying dormant inside of any of them, and few spoke about how their own behaviors might be putting them at risk. I have met numerous people over the years who credit

Florence with inspiring them to get tested, join support groups, and "live positively," a slogan meaning to not excessively worry about the disease or death, to not overworking, to treat malaria and other ailments, and to not have sex or drink obsessively. For many people living with HIV, particularly women, these support groups have become their new *máka*.

Florence is not sure when she contracted HIV, but she is certain it was from her husband, so it was probably in the early or mid-1980s. She remembers first falling sick in 1988 with what she now believes were symptoms related to her HIV-weakened immune system or her period of seroconversion. The following year her husband developed a "terrible skin rash and fell seriously sick." At that time, she explains, "we were four women on one husband," but she and two other co-wives did not know about their last co-wife. Florence was the first wife. She and the second co-wife lived with their husband in the village; the third wife lived in another small trading town, which the husband used to frequent for trade, and the last one resided in Iganga Town, where his more recent trade activities were centered. His geographic distribution of wives (who provided homes to stay in, comfort, food, sex, and, as a result, children) mirrored his mobility and work patterns. It would be the last wife who would die first in 1989, but the husband "kept her death a secret and the other three of us did not know that the other co-wife in town had fallen sick. Even when she died, our husband went and buried her in Mabitende Village without our knowledge."

Then her husband became even more ill, and was bedridden for a period. Florence asked him if AIDS was still around. "He told me it is still in existence and that we are also going to die of the same." She cried for two days straight and decided to stay and care for him and their children. After he passed away in 1990, Florence decided that she wanted to know her status. She did not know of anyone who had gone for an HIV test. Iganga did not offer HIV testing at the government hospital, so she saved money to travel to the nearby town of Jinja, where she received counseling and a test at TASO (The AIDS Support Organization). Scared and feeling alone, she remembers, "When the results came out and I tested positive, I began telling my people, relatives, and friends that I had AIDS." Her co-wives were angry with Florence for speaking publicly about her status, and accused Florence of bringing *juju* into the family and of speaking publicly to receive aid from government programs. With the urging of Florence, however, the co-wives got tested and joined the support group. In early 1994, another co-wife died. Being the oldest wife, Florence knew she was next, but she remained active in the support group. When she did not die, she became even more active in the group and in doing HIV education.

Florence attributes her longevity and relatively good health to consistently "going for treatment," which in pre-antiretroviral therapy (ART) days included a combination of "social treatments" such as counseling and living positively with local medicinal treatments. Florence joined a group in a remote village that specialized in herbal medicines, organized by the son of a widely respected herbalist in her late eighties. The frail, elderly woman came from a long matrilineage of herbalists, and the community was concerned that the inherited local knowledge would die with her, as she had no surviving daughters. The group, therefore, focused on teaching its members and the

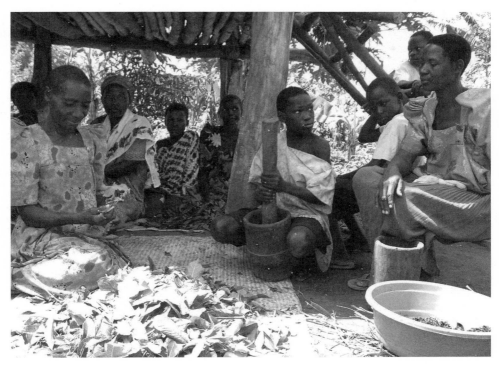

FIGURE 4.2. HIV support group making herbal medicine for HIV-related ailments

community about medicinal uses of local plants, including ones for boosting the immune system and for treating conditions commonly associated with an HIV-weakened system, such as sexually transmitted infections, herpes zoster (shingles), oral candidiasis (thrush), severe coughing (such as TB), and skin rashes. On the day Florence and I visited the group, the business meeting was being conducted as group members diligently tended to various stages of the two-day process of making a soap used for soothing skin rashes. Some members gathered leaves, others separated and pounded the leaves into a mixture, and yet others boiled the mixture in large *sufarias* (aluminum cooking pots) over a hot flame. A smaller group sat under a shade structure and divided a green powder mainly consisting of parts from the *moringa* tree (also locally known as the *mulinga* tree) into small plastic bags, adding to each a small piece of paper with directions for preparing the mixture. Though the aging and slightly built herbalist did not speak much (if at all) during the meeting, her presence was powerful and calming.

I visit with Florence each time I return to Iganga and have accompanied her to various meetings and community presentations. When we met in 2002, her last surviving co-wife had recently died, she believed in 2000 or 2001. Florence looked pained and worried when she discussed the passing of her co-wife, so I did not push her on the exact date. She said only that she had seen so many people die of AIDS over the years that she had begun to lose track of the exact dates. Watching her co-wife's agonizing death had proved quite difficult for Florence, as it brought into sharper relief the possibility that her own death might be near. She felt a greater sense of urgency

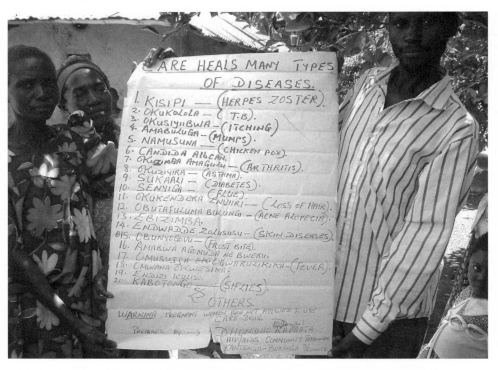

FIGURE 4.3. HIV support group's poster listing uses of the *moringa* medicinal plant

to prepare for the future of her six biological children and the orphaned relatives for whom she was caring. She was focused on finishing construction on her house, buying more chickens and goats for her livestock project, and making sure someone could help look after them when she was gone.

By the time I returned to Uganda in 2004, the antibiotic prophylaxis (cotrimoxazole) Florence had been receiving from TASO was no longer effective in warding off infections and illnesses. Florence had grown too frail and weak to travel with BUDEA on their educational tours to other villages. Her face was sunken and she spent most days in bed with a persistent cough that drained her energy and appetite. I wondered if her incoherence was partly a sign of AIDS dementia. Friends and neighbors were visibly worried about Florence's health, but no one spoke verbally about the imminence of her death. We arranged for her to visit the clinic in town to see about ARVs, but the sympathetic nurse regretfully told her that program was not accepting new patients.

A few months after I returned to the United States from that trip, I received the news that Florence had been accepted into the government ART program at the Iganga hospital. The members of BUDEA feared that she was too frail to make the journey to town and that her system was too weak for the drugs to have an effect. They dedicated a week to collecting the funds needed for renting a van to transport her to town and for other items necessary for her treatment. Florence began the common first-line ART treatment that combined into a single pill zidovudine (AZT), lamivudine (3TC), and nevirapine (NVP)—two nucleoside analog reverse-transcriptase inhibitors (NRTIs) and one nonnucleoside reverse transcriptase inhibitor (NNRTI), respectively. She did remarkably well on this fixed-dose combination. As her CD4 count (i.e., the number of helper T-cells, a type of white blood cell that fights infection) increased from below 70 mm to over 550 mm, she regained strength and put on some of the weight she had lost. She was able to resume farming and other income-generating activities and to perform again in the local HIV educational tours of her support group. As of my visit in 2015, Florence remains alive and receiving ARVs.

Some health professionals believe that it is only a matter of time before recipients of first-line drugs like Florence develop resistance to the limited options of first-line drugs, particularly since this regimen lacks a third class of drugs (namely, protease inhibitors) that is virtually always included in cocktail therapies in wealthier countries to provide additional protection against the replication of the virus in the body (MSF 2005). While critical of inferior treatments in poorer countries and of the high cost of second-line drugs, these health advocates argue that until second-line drug combinations are more easily accessible and affordable, the benefits of extending and improving the health quality of peoples' lives outweigh the risks of being on first-line drugs.

By chronicling Florence's experiences with HIV, I return to an issue central to this book. HIV is not simply a medical condition but also a socially constructed set of facts and a site for ideologically driven interventions. As the object of ideological and politi-cal intervening, HIV is absorbed into local landscapes in ways that reconfigure relationships, networks of affiliation, and meanings of life and morality. Specifically, Florence's history demonstrates how the emergence of new spaces for belonging, a concept so central to Basoga notions of personhood, has led to a shift for some residents from the kin-based *máka* to biomedical-based HIV support and education groups. Florence's and her community's history with HIV sheds light on how local understandings, responses, and strategies have greatly shifted over the course of the epidemic, being shaped by the creation and dissemination of information about the disease, wider advances in medicine, and global politics surrounding health policy and residents' access to health care.

These support groups are particularly appealing to women, given women's marginality from the patrilineal operations and property of the *máka* and given their increased role as the primary economic providers for children and other household dependents. Through Florence's story we see the creation of ways people can enter into emerging systems of rights, responsibilities, and obligations that gives them access to material and human resources. Specifically useful here is the concept of biological citizenship, or medical citizenship. In *Life Exposed: Biological Citizens after Chernobyl* (2002), Adriana Petryna uses the term "biological citizenship" to describe the "demand for, but limited access to, a form of social welfare based on medical, scientific, and legal criteria that recognize injury and compensate for it" during post-Chernobyl crises (261).

Scholars have used the term "biomedical citizenship" to describe the twin processes of entitlement and obligation through which people's participation in biomedical activities symbolizes not only the promises of medicine but also the process of complying with a health system's social and ideological expectations. For example, Joao Biehl describes those in Brazil who self-identify as AIDS patients and actively participate in the health-care system for continuous treatment as biomedical citizens. This requires one to adopt not only the state's definition of what it means to be an AIDS patient, but also the state's methods of treating AIDS (2004:120). Biomedical citizenship as enabled by donor programs and public health efforts allows residents such as Florence to increase their ability to access resources, services, and other entitlements, if they comply with biomedical expectations, knowledge, and practices as set forth by a cast of experts and professionals. While the nascent form of biomedical citizenship provides residents alternate forms of accessing resources, it is undergirded by a politics of exclusion in which those who are socially or medically noncompliant are denied access (Nguyen 2005; Petryna 2002; Rose and Novas 2005). In this sense, biomedical citizenship enables previously excluded persons to access entitlements, but also becomes a form of regulation, discipline, and control.

Reorganizations of Hope: IDAAC and the Globalization of the HIV Industry

As Florence spread the word in rural areas about the new disease that had come to the region, in Iganga Town a group of nurses among the district health-care providers were laying the ground for the town's first NGO dedicated to helping individuals and families affected by HIV. Rev. Jackson (a nurse who later became a Pentecostal preacher), Catherine Njuba (who had introduced me to Florence), and three other health-care providers were working in Iganga District Hospital when AIDS hit the town, sometime, they believe, in the late 1980s. Like medical personnel elsewhere, they recall patients in their late twenties and early thirties who had returned from other parts of Uganda being admitted to the hospital, suffering from ailments that were not responsive to usual antibiotic treatments. The extended hospital stays and intensive IV drips that usually worked on most infections made no difference, raising some concern among staff and hospital administrators. The number of young adult patients with similar conditions—excessive diarrhea, skin rashes, vomiting, weight loss, heavy coughing, and STIs—increased. Eventually these patients all died or were near death when they were released from the hospital. The hospital workers thought it was strange that so many young adults were wasting away so quickly. At first some of the hospital staff thought these patients (many of whom had been outside of Iganga for work) had contracted some bad disease from their distant places of work; others thought it was *juju*.

Rev. Jackson and Nurse Catherine wondered if this disease was related to news they had heard over the radio of a new, deadly disease in Rakai and Masaka called HIV, whose symptoms sounded similar to what they were seeing. After Museveni's government came to power, they both were invited to attend a government health seminar. Catherine remembers that the seminar presenters were not sure how extensively AIDS had spread through the country, but they had gotten reports from almost all reporting district hospitals indicating that the presence of the disease was far-reaching. The seminar leaders described how HIV patients in the hospital should be handled and told the providers that HIV could not be spread through casual contact or touching an AIDS patient. The facilitators advised them not to be afraid, since they could take precautionary measures, but seemed hesitant and tentative about the information. Participants in the seminar remained quiet. Rev. Jackson suspects some of the information was lost because people were in states of shock and fear. After the seminar, the health workers from Iganga concluded that those earlier, fatal illnesses were most likely this new disease called AIDS. Rev. Jackson and Catherine suspect that the silence around HIV among hospital staff was partly because of fear and also because many of them were uncertain if they or their coworkers were already infected.

Instead of increasing the healthcare providers' level of compassion and comfort, their new knowledge about the disease, combined with the incomplete medical information about transmission, led to greater stigmatization and fear of AIDS patients in the hospital. Rev. Jackson, Catherine, and others recounted stories about early AIDS patients being mistreated and ostracized in the hospital. As reported around the world, the fear of contracting HIV from sick patients led to the wearing of full-body protection and gloves among some hospital workers (see Parker and Aggleton 2003). Others refused to care for patients they suspected had AIDS. Not all hospital workers were as fearful, Rev. Jackson and Catherine reassured me, but the general tone among hospital staff was one of fear and anxiety, which fueled rumors and misconceptions. The disease and the infected were stigmatized in rural health-care settings, which were ill-equipped to administer confirmatory tests or take protective precautions.

Rose, a nurse at the district hospital, told me of a case that still haunts her. A very ill young mother of two was admitted to the hospital with profuse bleeding from a farming accident. After seeing the woman's wasting symptoms, hospital workers concluded that she had AIDS. Assuming the woman would soon die from AIDS, and being afraid to touch her, the staff moved her bed into the hallway to make room for other patients. The woman's young daughter was carrying her baby sister, crying for someone to help their mother. The woman's husband had left her a few months after the birth of their baby, when the woman kept getting sicker and weaker; her in-laws had abandoned her and her own relatives lived in another area. Her children were without adult assistance. Without money to transport herself back home, the woman died in the hallway later that evening with her two children by her side. Young Rose held the young woman's children, and housed them for a couple of days. After locating their relatives, she helped make sure they were taken to their new caregivers. Afterward, Rose visited the children every few months and provided clothes, rice, and other supplies.

After witnessing the lack of services and the helplessness of people infected and affected, Rev. Jackson, Catherine, and their colleagues decided to start an organization dedicated to alleviating some of the suffering and stigma. In 1991, they registered IDAAC (Integrated Development and AIDS Concern) as an NGO and worked closely with the hospital's STD and TB units to offer follow-up support to patients for psychosocial care and daily needs. In addition to counseling people with AIDS, they began to supply basic provisions such as rice, porridge, sugar, cooking oil, blankets, soap, and basins for bathing. Financial support for IDAAC came from the British Development Agency and Action AIDS, and with a grant from InterAID, the group expanded the food program. Being discharged from the hospital was what qualified the person for food services, but the team recognized two ripple effects of HIV infection: (1) an HIV infection of one adult affected the food production and needs of that person's entire household; and (2) providing nutrition during the latency period of the disease might help delay the onset of the illness. They opened up the food program to any household in need, even if no household member had been admitted into the hospital.

Rev. Jackson and Catherine are not sure if their efforts changed the community's understanding of HIV in Iganga, for people still found it hard to talk directly about the disease. However, providing food became a way of breaking down AIDS stigma in the health-care setting and hopefully in the community. The weekly food pantry offered a venue for speaking to people about HIV and recruiting them to attend seminars and other educational activities. Through the work of the pantry, Rev. Jackson and Catherine also began organizing groups of HIV widows and people who were regular patients at the TB clinic, since TB was an early sign of AIDS. Florence first became involved with the organization as a participant in one of these groups, and through people like her, IDAAC took its awareness program to villages, dispelling myths about people with AIDS and educating people about routes of transmission and ways to avoid HIV. This integrated approach that IDAAC and other early organic, community-based organizations took recognized that residents' immediate priority was economic survival and the well-being of household members. Hence, IDAAC next developed a program to train people in income generating activities. This program, Florence explained, keeps AIDS widows from having to "sell themselves" (i.e., engage in survival sex) or to marry another man, and in doing so to further spread HIV. At its height in the 1990s, IDAAC had twenty-two trained counseling volunteers who provided weekly one-on-one and group counseling at the hospital, in villages, and eventually at their office in town, and had organized numerous support and education groups in various villages around Iganga.

Even though IDAAC never became as well-known globally or nationally as TASO, older residents of Iganga recognize it as the first integrated HIV support and education agency in their area. In those early days, responses were organic and nimble but underfunded and not systematically measured. By the early 2000s, the increasingly bureaucratic nature of the global AIDS industry and particularly of the allocation of donor funding (such as PEPFAR's) began to have an impact on the operations of the local organizations that had played such a major role during the early days of the epidemic. IDAAC and other small community-based organizations (CBOs) were slowly squeezed out of the funding process. Without the financial resources required to develop systems to measure and track impact and to apply for donor assistance, IDAAC could not compete. When I returned in 2006, the oldest HIV agency in Iganga struggling to survive, and by 2015 more globally connected public health NGOs filled the landscape.

Shifting Etiologies of AIDS:
From *Juju* to Opportunistic Infection

In *AIDS and Accusations: Haiti and the Geography of Blame* (1992), Paul Farmer traces Do Kay Village residents' evolving etiologies of HIV. He argues that, as information became available and the patterns of disease emerged, residents' understanding of the new disease went from being a condition that was "sent" to wealthier people through sorcery as a result of jealousy to an infectious disease and eventually to a disease revealing

Haiti's historical place in global racial and economic inequalities. Farmer's analysis allows us to appreciate how local notions of illness causation are never stagnant but are intrinsically linked to concurrently occurring social processes. Furthermore, etiological models—in Farmer's case, *juju* and the biomedical model—are not mutually exclusive, but are more appropriately conceptualized as pluralistic systems (Ngokwey 1988). While etiological pluralism captures the complexities and contradictions of notions of illness causation, examining the etiological model that dominates at any particular moment offers insight into a community's deep-seated beliefs about causes of misfortune or their anxiety about the unknown.

In addition to the *juju* and biomedical causation models, two additional narrative trajectories in Iganga are worth mentioning, for they illuminate residents' understanding of their marginality and their lack of power in a changing world. First, when I arrived in Iganga in the mid-1990s, "AIDS-the-opportunistic-condition" that "just gets pleased with someone's body" was the most common understanding of HIV in Iganga. This was a shift from the stories of early HIV cases, which were associated either with the intricate web of trade, mobility, and transactional sex that emerged during Uganda's civil unrest period, or with rivalries between neighbors (see also Bond and Vincent 1991; Garrett 1994:334–36; Hooper 1999:37–43). After seeing ordinary people (such as rural farmers, poor women, and their babies) suffer from *sslimu*, the idea of rivalry and modernity-induced immorality as causes of infection no longer explained all cases. When residents began to see more cases that fell outside of the common narrative of HIV acquisition, such as the illness of someone whose sexual behavior wouldn't be deemed particularly hedonistic, residents became convinced that HIV selected its victims at random, even unjustly. This idea that HIV is not preventable because it opportunistically gets pleased with someone's body is precisely what Florence and other grassroots workers were and still are trying to combat. Florence found that this explanation allowed residents to avoid publicly discussing behaviors that were possibly fueling the epidemic—men having multiple outside lovers as a new form of prestige and modern masculinity, women having sex in exchange for money, young wives feeling the pressure to continually reproduce, and young people practicing "trial marriages." Blaming HIV on people's desire to find wealth by traveling outside of Iganga was no longer possible when the ailment began affecting families who had little connection with the world beyond the town. The sexual networking that was spreading HIV was located within Iganga, as Florence reminded people (see also Pickering et al. 1996, 1997; Obbo 1993; Thornton 2008).

As Museveni, Florence, and others spoke about the role of sexual networking in the spread of HIV, notions about HIV changed. Residents explain these new sexual cultures (including youth sexual culture) in terms of people adjusting to changing times: "These are not Basoga traditions, but people adopted them because of money, greed, and survival. Families began to move away from each other. They were unable to stop the new practices, so they continued," Florence stated. Florence and others talk about HIV as a disease produced by a breakdown of the moral order that had been provided by people's attachment and responsibility to a *máka*. This breakdown of morality reordered systems of greed and desire and led to excessive *obwenzi* (promiscuity). For the young people I met during my first research period, AIDS was already an integral part of the social landscape. They were born into a world in which HIV was already shaping social relations. To them, HIV's origin is not necessarily connected to events during a specific historical moment. Rather, it is a disease that has been in existence since they were old enough to understand death, sickness, and suffering. Many were able to tell me stories they had heard secondhand of wealthier relatives or neighbors returning from some distant place, often after doing "business." However, the fact that the spread of HIV was facilitated by the insecurity in southwestern Uganda is irrelevant to the young people with whom I spoke, for the AIDS they know has never been confined and has no geographic origin.

Like adults, young people conceptualize HIV as a foreign-introduced illness that is a consequence of modernity, urbanization, and globalization. Youth recall a common storyline of the earliest AIDS cases as follows: it was either a wealthy man who frequently traveled for trade and business or a *nakyewombekeire* who remained unmarried, making a living trading everything from clothes to her body (as a sex worker at a truck stop). The person came home to the village to die after contracting the disease from another place. Another common story has the young person caring for a dying relative—often an older (full or half-) sibling, a cousin, aunt or uncle, or even a parent. With vivid descriptions, in essays and dramas, youth detailed the progression of the condition, its symptoms, the reactions of the community and family, and the eventual withering and death of the body. Few, if any youth, attribute the main cause of HIV to *juju*. However, like adults, young people attribute the contracting of HIV to pluralistic causes: it is both a virus transmitted through blood and a misfortune that befalls a person either as retribution for past actions or as a demonstration of injustices in the modern world.

The Slow Development of Iganga's HIV Infrastructure

The medical advances in HIV treatment—from antibody testing to, more recently, ARVs—that have made their way to Iganga have not only abated suffering for some, but have also further exposed inequalities and facilitated new forms of secrecy about a person's access to resources. Medical advances have also been absorbed into the local landscape in ways that have altered residents' understandings of HIV, but that narrative needs to be explored as part of Iganga's historical interaction with national and global health systems. The organic beginning and demand for the services of IDAAC happened in large part because a formal public health infrastructure for HIV was relatively late in coming to Iganga as compared to other areas of Uganda. When I arrived in Iganga there were only minimal resources from the government and few international donors or foreign research-based university initiatives. These bodies were focusing on the harder-hit areas and larger towns. Iganga was not an epicenter of HIV like Rakai and Masaka, nor did it have the Luwero Triangle's concentration of orphans; it was not the capital city, with its problems of urban poverty and inadequate housing, nor did it garner global attention because of child soldiers or the unthinkable tyranny carried out by Joseph Kony's Lord Resistance Army in northern Uganda. There is nothing particularly extraordinary about Iganga to excite much attention from donors or NGOs. The

Basoga do not practice any of the behaviors that donor and public health reports had identified as contributing to HIV transmission, such as dry sex, forced child marriage, or extreme forms of widow inheritance. One health officer commented that Iganga is often in Phase 3 of the rollout of national or donor public health plans and is not a common pilot site for new interventions; hence, programs enter into Iganga much later than prioritized or globally connected sites.

The earliest AIDS biomedical control efforts in Iganga were ensuring the availability of clean needles and expanding STD testing and treatment services in the district hospital and in international clinics, such as those run by Marie Stopes International and Family Planning International. In terms of direct support for HIV and AIDS patients, however, services remained extremely limited at the local level, in the form of activities by groups such as IDAAC and people like Florence. It was not until almost a decade after the first testing centers opened in Uganda that Iganga District Hospital received funding to open what at the time was called a voluntary counseling and testing (VCT) center in 1998, and even then it was limited in its reach. Satellite testing centers were established in trading towns around Iganga to reach people who did not have easy access to town, such as women, youth, and poor framers. Because of the anonymity of town, many rural residents preferred to get tested in Iganga. Before the hospital acquired the necessary equipment and trained staff, people would typically discover their status when they were admitted to the hospital when already very ill. The hospital and other centers were able to draw blood, but their samples had to be taken to Kampala or Jinja for testing. Or, like Florence, people traveled to Jinja but had to go back weeks later to collect the results, which was difficult for many rural and poor residents. Someone at TASO suspected that less than 40 percent of the people from outside Jinja returned for their tests. Based on the patient registry for Iganga District Hospital. 1,786 people received HIV counseling and testing during the eighteen months between January 2005 and June 2006. Of those people, almost 28 percent tested positive for the HIV antibody, with women having a higher HIV-positive rate than men and children (30 percent, 25 percent, and 27 percent, respectively). Compared to the estimated overall prevalence rate of 5.5 percent that same year, this percentage indicates that testing efforts were reaching those infected. Consistent with findings throughout much of sub-Saharan Africa, adult women make up the largest number of people going for VCT services in Iganga, representing 55 percent of all patients, compared to 37 percent for men and 8 percent for children.

But to health-care workers, promoting the new testing center presented a new dilemma: how to pursue the national strategy of encouraging people to get tested while knowing that there was no formal support, care, or hope that they could provide for these newly diagnosed people. They grappled with the reality that the global scale-up for VCT greatly outpaced the development of the necessary health-care infrastructure, systems, and medicines needed throughout Uganda to care for people diagnosed with HIV. This imbalance in the need for services versus capacity was known and severely experienced on the ground.

In 2004, the health-care workers' dilemma and disparity in services was exacerbated by the arrival of Iganga's ART, offered through Iganga District Hospital by the

Joint Clinical Research Center (JCRC), a nongovernmental HIV research and clinical organization. JCRC was the first UNAIDS-accredited organization in Uganda and, at the time, the largest provider of ARVs in the country. The JCRC program provided drugs that were subsidized but not free, which excluded many rural and poor patients. The following year, the Ministry of Health rolled out the government's free ART program in Iganga, a program that previously had been offered in higher-priority areas.

As reflected in Florence's story above, "care" for people with HIV had previously existed only as treatment of opportunistic infections (OIs) and STDs, counseling, and supplies of the antibacterial medicine cotrimoxazole as a prophylaxis for OIs.[2] The introduction of ARTs into Iganga gave hope to many for whom the traditional "care" model was failing.

But most Iganga residents would not have access to the life-extending medicines. The initial roll-out guaranteed only three hundred slots in the free medicine program, with many of these slots reserved for patients who had demonstrated "success" in the subsidized program. In 2005, the government rolled out the national ART program in Iganga. The scale-up was slowly implemented in health centers around the district, expanding ART coverage in 2009 to an estimated 15 percent of those meeting the criteria for "need" with retention in care estimated at 8.1 percent. By 2015, a supervisor at the hospital ART program estimated that there were 2,700 "active" patients, but believed many have fallen out of care. The uneven introduction of ARTs also changed the face of HIV-related death. As people continued to die, but in ways that did not resemble the familiar wasting-away of AIDS patients, rumors of bewitching and foul play began to resurface.

Despair, Suicide, and Gender

Within the context of new ways of experiencing AIDS deaths, politics of triage, and tensions between residents' knowledge about biomedical advances and their lack of access to them, the increased visibility of AIDS-related suicides that I encountered during later research stints becomes intriguing. While I am not making claims about whether the aforementioned factors can be directly correlated to these suicides, a general conclusion can be made that the suicides were motivated by despair, shame, and fear occasioned by HIV infection. During my seven-month research trip in 2004, three men whom I knew in Iganga took their lives for AIDS-related reasons, and one woman killed herself shortly after I returned to the United States. The body of a man who delivered the morning newspaper to my house was found hanging from a rafter in his rented room in Iganga Town. On a nearby table was a jar of money and a note written on tattered paper with instructions to use the money to transport his body back home and to pay his burial expenses. He did not want to be a burden to his already financially taxed family. Residents believed he killed himself not only because he was distraught about the HIV infection but also because his fiancée had recently left him for another man. Apparently she could not bear the stigma of being with someone who was known to have HIV. Residents believed, however, that the fiancée had brought HIV into their relationship, since one of her past lovers was thought to have died of AIDS.

Another suicide victim was a laid-off accountant who had amassed an enormous amount of debt in trying to receive care and treatment for his HIV-related illnesses. His numerous attempts to enroll in the district ART programs had failed, as had his attempts to be retained in one of the programs in Jinja Town. When his financial situation allowed it, he had purchased medicines from various types of pharmacies and through other avenues and informal markets, but the inconsistent supply and quality had led to a variety of other ailments, conditions, and stress. Once considered a member of Iganga's professional class, his socioeconomic status had rapidly declined over two years, leading his neighbors (who likely did not know his HIV status) to speculate that he had gone mad. As his debt grew and his spirit and body weakened, he became so desperate and worried that he decided to end his life. But in ending his own suffering, he transferred the burden of the disease to his poorly educated widow, who had never had formal employment or a source of income. At the funeral, the thin woman stood stoic and emotionless, clutching the shoulders of her two young children in obvious shock and dismay. Marrying right after completing secondary school, she had gone directly from the house of her protective father to her equally watchful husband, and had never navigated the complicated maze of social and institutional structures that would soon greet her. Being known as an AIDS widow with the additional social stigma of her husband's suicide meant that it was highly unlikely she would marry again, bringing into sharper relief the fact that for the rest of her life, she would be the household head. As I offered her some condolence money, her eyes were glazed over and she stared blankly into space. I am uncertain what became of her, but neighbors suspect she stayed for a while with her ailing parents.

The third man who committed suicide during this period was a wealthy government official and former diplomat from a village near Iganga who was living in Kampala. It was said that, after losing his six-year-old son to HIV two years earlier, he frequently stated that he had no reason to live. His wife had died a few years before the death of his son, and with the two people he loved most gone, the man was often heard questioning the meaning of life. Suffering from a combination of survivor's guilt (over being the only family member not yet dead from the disease), loneliness, and alcohol-exacerbated depression, he decided to expedite his own death rather than remaining alone and isolated. After being off ARVs for a period of time, he ingested a large dose of poison and told his brother and sister to take him to the hospital. His timing was impeccable. His siblings suspect that, not wanting to die alone at home but certain that he wanted to die, he likely waited until it was too late for the doctors to treat him for the poison. The general reaction to his act was, "How could a rich man commit suicide?"

Iganga residents believe that suicide is more common among men (see also Fallers and Fallers 1960), which is consistent with data from much of the world, as well as data from Uganda in general. For instance, mortuary data from 375 suicide cases over a thirty-year period, from 1975 to 2004, in Kampala found that 77 percent were males and 23 percent were females, with feelings of shame being reported as the most common stressor (16.1 percent); hanging was the most frequently used method (63 percent) and ingesting poison (25.8 percent) the second most common method (Kinyanda et al. 2011).

I end this chapter with suicide stories to underscore the ways in which HIV—as an infection of inequality, a social fact, and a site for uneven and mediated intervention—has penetrated the lived realities and performative actions of residents. My telling of these stories is also intended to highlight how interventions and responses to the epidemic have been highly gendered. Specifically, the gendered nature of HIV-related suicides might reveal something about the distinct ways in which the laying of blame on men for the epidemic in Africa deflects attention to the wider structures of inequality that are ripe for HIV to thrive. Suicide as a gendered coping strategy also suggests that local gender expectations and obligations might conflict with the way interventions and resources are packaged and accessible to differently situated residents, such that some men may see ending their lives as the only way to escape despair, shame, and failed masculinity.

A functional explanation for this gender imbalance in suicides that resonates with residents is that no matter how desperate a woman feels, her culturally inflected sense of duty to care for her children keeps her alive. In fact, "planning for my children's future" was the top priority expressed by women with HIV whom I knew. Fear of what would happen to their children in their absence became a motivating factor, as it was for Florence, to "live positively" with HIV, giving them a deep sense of urgency and responsibility to survive despite difficult times. This explanation, however, is inadequate, for the privileging of survival and resiliency obscures the emotional, physical, and material suffering of women. A functional explanation also fails to account for the limited nondestructive options for achieving masculine ideals and the fragility of masculinity in a patriarchal and capitalist context in which downward social mobility is highly probable. To complicate the narrative of gender, despair, and suicide, I end this section with a story of Jovena, a young woman who killed herself shortly after I returned to the United States from that same 2004 trip.

Jovena married her husband, Mugabi, when they were in their early twenties and as he was quickly moving up the ranks in a local branch of a foreign NGO, rising from driver to project manager. For a rural man with only a secondary education, Mugabi had done well for himself, providing the couple with a nice house in town full of luxury items and a maid, and taking yearly trips to Europe for training. His luck with the NGO quickly changed after the branch received a new director. He lost his job, and he began selling off their luxury items to pay bills and past debts and to retain the public appearance of wealth. Unable to find a comparable salaried position, yet used to the social prestige he once enjoyed, Mugabi began seeking attention from girls attending neighboring schools, while Jovena took up various domestic tasks for wealthier people in town. By the time I met Jovena, she had grown frustrated and deeply embarrassed by her husband's repeated affairs with schoolgirls. The penalties and bribes to avoid prosecution for having sex with underage girls were putting a tremendous financial strain on their household. Jovena also worried that in her husband's years of philandering, he might have given her HIV, along with the other STIs that she had contracted from him. A few months after I last spoke to her, she ended her life.

These tragic suicide stories in the time of ARVs show the extent to which residents are keenly aware of their alienation from resources for controlling the epidemic. For young people, death from sex is more than just an abstract warning; it is a reality that they regularly witness in their communities and among older relatives and neighbors. These paths to death provide the young people who witness them from the sidelines with a set of possible outcomes of their future relationships and with options for how to cope with a future of uncertainties while still pursuing socially expected life projects such as love, romance, and reproduction.

- songa = auntie explains sex and marriage to neice
AIDS marketing → sexuality discourse became more
public, but sex talk changed
"pleasure talk" → "risk talk"
- senga = advice column

CHAPTER 5

From Auntie to Disco

Risk and Pleasure in Sexuality Education

James Kyagaba and Esther Nakilanda were married in 2003. Although they had both been students at the prestigious Makerere University in Kampala, overlapping by a couple of years, they did not know each other. They met instead through mutual friends after they graduated. They were both beginning their professional careers in Kampala—he as a banker, she as a research nurse for reproductive health projects. After a two-year courtship, they decided to enroll in their Pentecostal church's required premarital counseling. After their union was declared godly, they publicly announced their engagement. They were considered the model Christian couple among their church friends—active in the church and waiting patiently until marriage to engage in sexual intercourse. They had a much-talked-about, extravagant *kwandhula* ceremony and feast in Esther's home village, near Iganga Town. A week later, they had an even grander and costlier wedding at their church in Kampala. James was offered a promotion and transfer to Iganga later that year, and the couple decided it was best to be closer to their families as they began planning to have children. To residents in Iganga, their marriage represented the ideal modern relationship—they had had Christian and Basoga ceremonies and were well traveled, university educated, salaried, members of a well-known and globally connected megachurch in Kampala, and owners of a car.

Despite public appearances, James was becoming increasingly frustrated with his wife's *tamumatiza mubululi* (inability to satisfy him in bed). He found Esther detached and unresponsive during sex, as if she was having sex to fulfill her marital obligation rather than out of desire. She never came close to uttering the Basoga bedroom noises (*kusikina*) James had learned about in his youth as signs of a woman receiving sexual pleasure. Following Basoga cultural convention, James enlisted the assistance of Esther's mother and designated *sôngá* (paternal aunt), requesting that they take their daughter home to "talk to her" about marriage and how to achieve *kusikina*. Such a request is more than just a complaint about his wife's sexual frigidity. It is also an indictment of the mother's and *sôngá*'s failure to perform their Basoga cultural duty of preparing the young woman for marriage. Unsure of how to proceed, Esther's mother and *sôngá* contacted Mpoyenda, an *ababulidho* (a "commoner" or peasant woman). The woman lived in a village only a few kilometers from the two women seeking assistance, but in a vastly different world. The depth of her cultural knowledge and the number of years that had passed since she was betrothed (she estimates around twenty), however, temporarily reversed the socioeconomic and age hierarchy that would have typically structured her interactions with the two much wealthier women, who were more than a decade her senior.

My first extended conversation with Mpoyenda was in collecting her life and sexual history. She appeared wiser and older than her thirty-four years would suggest. Her face appeared young but she had the gracefully reserved mannerisms and comportment of a more mature, even wealthy, person. Mpoyenda was a woman of few words, but when she did speak, her gift for storytelling and advising became apparent.

As we packed up from our interview and Mpoyenda escorted me along the path heading to town, she called on the story of Esther as a way of illustrating points she had made earlier about the state of marriage and intimacy today. To Mpoyenda, Esther represented a young woman caught amid a confusing array of alternative and competing moralities, finding that no one single moral universe provided complete guidance through the complex and shifting realities shaping her intimate life and desires.

Although people commonly identify sexual problems as a source of marital tension, I begin this chapter with Esther's story not as an entry into a discussion about marital intimacy but rather to complicate the tendency to privilege health communication interventions that are designed and evaluated by often Western or Western-trained professionalized health experts. In many such cases what is ignored is a serious consideration of local ways of defining and transmitting information about sexuality and sexual health. Yet these existing structures, which have often endured and transformed through many generations, might serve as a productive foundation for disseminating information about newer ailments or treatments (the community health worker [CHW] model promoted by the WHO is one such use of existing local systems). Rather than building on local systems and customs, culture, particularly of the poor or socially marginalized, is frequently portrayed as an obstacle that needs to be overcome or changed in the quest for "good health," as defined by the experts. This chapter uses coming-of-age stories of elders, stories that date back to the 1930s, to examine the Basoga sexual learning system and ideology as well as transformations in the system that have been occasioned by some of the demographic shifts discussed in Chapter 2, such as geographic dispersal of clans, globalization, formal education, and interventions concerning the body and sexuality since colonial days.[1] As Esther's story highlights, there is not a unilinear and predictable transition in which "new" practices replace and are uncritically assumed to be better than "old" ones. Instead, what has emerged is a variety of moral alternatives, each possessing different cultural currency and significance depending on the specific contexts or prestige structures.[2]

Second, building on this book's larger interest in unintended consequences of interventions around sexuality, this chapter argues that HIV campaigns have contributed to the gradual bifurcation of ideologies of sexual risk and sexual pleasure that, according to my interviews with elders in Iganga, ideally are intertwined in Basoga notions of sexual morality.[3] I am not arguing that the HIV campaigns *caused* the bifurcation, but rather that they further exacerbated and gave new biomedical authority a process that was already in motion. For adolescent girls, Basoga coming-of-age conventions involve two key aspects, as explored in this chapter: (1) "visiting the bush" (meaning, going to a private place) with other adolescent girls, during which a girl is instructed on how to elongate her labia minora and receives information about her body and sexuality; and (2) learning Basoga marital "bedroom tricks" after betrothal through indirect instruction from her designated *sôngá*. Without undergoing this learning process, elders argue, the next generation of women lack full knowledge about the intertwining of sexual danger and pleasure and ways of carefully balancing and deploying them.

The Disconnect: Notions of Risk and Pleasure Today

This bifurcation of risk and pleasure is reflected in survey results from 260 young people in Iganga, ages thirteen to twenty.[4] I asked respondents to identify their greatest fear about or the greatest risk of sex. Eighty-seven percent stated that their greatest fear was contracting HIV or another STI, and 10 percent, mainly girls, listed pregnancy. These fears reflect the main two messages in public health campaigns at the time, indicating that the campaigns were indeed working.[5] Conversely, in response to questions about where they first learned and still learn about sex, none of the respondents listed reproductive and sexual health campaigns and programs, though in follow-up discussions some stated that *Straight Talk* was a good source for information about sex. (Their definitions of sex included what I would call sexuality and sexual intimacy, ranging from gendered ways of flirting and holding hands to initiating sexual activity and ultimately engaging in sexual intercourse). Respondents perceived public health messages as moral admonitions against sex rather than as a source of knowledge about intimacy, sex, and sexuality. Most reported that they learned about sex from discussions with friends, watching sexual interactions of older people in social places such as discos and other evening spaces, and popular culture and the mass media. The same youth said that they would prefer to learn about sex from relatives (aunts or uncles), parents, or knowledgeable adults, such as health professionals or teachers.

Policy makers and health communication experts are aware of this discrepancy. Whereas in the late 1990s and early 2000s policy makers and planners were proud of their success in reducing Uganda's HIV prevalence rate, they were also drawn into public debates about a new dilemma: "Who should teach our youth about sex?"[6] They were grappling with the fact that the 1986-initiated AIDS campaigns had thrust sex into the public domain by educating people about sexual risk and ways to reduce risk, but without directly addressing sex acts, sexual pleasure, and alternative sexualities. The public, for instance, learned about the risk-reduction benefits of using a condom without being offered from the same source specifics about when and how to incorporate the device in an intimate or sexual encounter. This absence of discussion about pleasure and sex acts in prevention messages allowed for the entry of other sources of information. The variety of alternative moralities served to heighten anxiety around young people's experiences with sexuality, particularly during a time when adults in Iganga felt that youth were not being properly educated in Basoga sexuality customs and regulations. But these same adults were themselves unsure of how best to transmit the information and how relevant those lessons are today.

Basoga Ideologies of Sex: Gendering Bodies and Pleasures

Elders in Iganga provide similar accounts of the Basoga kin-based system of sexual learning and of the proper presentation of gendered sexual selves, and most also bemoan the fact that these past ways and ideas differ greatly from those of today.[7] In elders' historical narratives, sexual learning involved the gradual development of a sexual self that elaborated expected gendered roles in the family and society, and expressions of a sexualized self was to be fully actualized in marriage, where it was appropriately nested within marital intimacy, reproduction, family reputation, and marital obligation. These Basoga notions of sexual maturation were highly gendered. Boys naturally and gradually transitioned into sexualized adult men, their sexual selves and desires emerging as a natural progression from boyhood to manhood that needed little more than them observing older relatives and neighbors and overhearing men's conversations and joking about the role of sexual encounters, performance, and sexuality in masculine prestige and identity. Men's sexuality was not only natural but also healthy and necessary for the survival and reproduction of the patriclan, the primary social and economic unit. Unlike some ethnic groups in sub-Saharan Africa, Basoga boys do not undergo a formal initiation process into manhood, such as the formal recognition of coming of age that culminates into a public ceremony, as is often the purpose of circumcision ceremonies.[8]

The natural and socially unmarked development of male sexuality and desires stood in stark contrast to young women's sexuality and bodies, which needed direct and supervised shaping, controlling, and grooming. While boys naturally emerged into men, girls required careful and continuous sexual nurturing, socialization, and disciplining. The grooming of the sexuality and bodies of adolescent girls, in particular the vaginal area, was in part an attempt to assuage the kinship and social anxiety caused by women's unregulated reproductive and sexual powers. Fallers observed in the 1950s that "the ideology of male dominance . . . centers about the sexual and child-bearing potentialities of women" (Fallers 1965:78), and hence much attention was given to the proper bodily discipline of girls. Elder women spoke about being prohibited from leaving the family compound without permission and being closely supervised, as their families feared that young females would be seduced away or "stolen" by men.[9] For men, women's sexual powers extended beyond their reproductive capacities. Women's bodies, particularly in the hip and thigh areas, were a source of great sexual power over men—a threat to patriarchy in their ability to generate intoxicating desire in and jealousy-based violence between competing men.

At an early age both young girls and young boys gradually learned about Basoga gendered notions of sexuality at village gatherings and ceremonies through watching older relatives and neighbors. Given the culture of sexual discretion, the temporary suspension of propriety stood out as key learning moments to elders with whom I spoke. Elders frequently mentioned burial ceremonies as a social space where they learned about gendered ways of adult interactions. Burial ceremonies involved extended overnight stays at the host compound during which an outdoor shelter was made, and men, women, and children who traveled from other places would camp out to show support and grieve with the family. An elder who came of age in the 1950s when

African ceremonies were restricted to village settings recalled that "young people used to learn about sex through burial ceremonies. These ceremonies used to take more than one month. During this time older people used to do a lot of *obwenzi* [unauthorized sexual liaisons; often translated as "promiscuity"], and the young people used to watch this. That is how they came to know about sex." Elders talk about burial ceremonies as a time when people returned to the village of their youth and became reunited with childhood playmates and sweethearts. The darkness of the evening provided an opportunity for former playmates to find a secluded place to share stories or rekindle an old romance.

Both young and older residents commonly cite twin-naming ceremonies (a culturally required festivity to satisfy the spirits after the birth of twins) as the one intergenerational and coed cultural space in which topics of sexuality, desire, and transgression are explicitly performed, providing an opportunity for young people to acquire knowledge about issues otherwise considered taboo and obscene. Marked by their temporary suspension of cultural propriety and gendered respectability, vulgar speech is permitted and encouraged by reactions from the audience. Men and women participate in transgender performances, songs, and dances, during which they dramatize various sex roles of the opposite sex and exaggerated ways of being sexually enticing. During the two ceremonies I attended, the level of applause and encouragement a performer received was directly related to their ability to enact transgender gestures and displays of sexuality. Men performing an exaggerated femininity and sexual seduction were by far the most entertaining to the audience, suggesting both that women's sexuality is considered more provocative and objectified for public gaze and that men's transgressions are more alluring and voyeuristically pleasurable.

In addition to gender and sexual transgressions, the suspension of propriety at twin-naming ceremonies allows for the use of sexual language and the direct naming of sexualized body parts. Hence, whereas genitalia and sex were typically talked about in highly coded ways, the pleasure of twin-naming ceremonies is precisely the publicness of taboo terms and simulated sex acts. As performers used terms that were otherwise considered vulgar and simulated sex acts that were typically inappropriate for public show, young people learned about sex and the body. These performances not only allow youth to learn Basoga ideas about sexualized acts and bodies but also serve as a counterexample for what was appropriate for everyday life. One older man who recalled learning about the gendered roles in sex in a twin-naming ceremony described a performance by his uncle and a female neighbor in which they simulated a sex act. The male character (played by the woman) aggressively "conquered" the woman (played by his uncle) and forced her into sexual submission. After struggling to get away, eventually the "woman" submitted to sex, screaming with joy and excitement during the act. The crowd, he remembered, burst out in laughter, appreciating the familiar portrayal.[10] Such highly theatrical performances of acts of sexual domination and aggression shaped the ideas of sexually maturing and curious youth. According to elders, these rituals are less common today, a situation that partly reflects the emergence of other outlets for entertainment, as well as a bend in moral sensibility among middle-class and religious fundamental groups, for whom these performances represent the immorality of the past.

Less affected by moral interpretations of middle-class bourgeoisie sensibilities is the more visible and common Basoga dancing. Basoga dancing provided and still provides public opportunities for young people not only to observe culturally attractive movements of the hips and also to practice and perfect them. Done by both men and women, dancing featured a cloth, a grass skirt, or other material tied below the waist to accentuate the hips. While keeping their shoulders and torsos still, the dancers use their lower-hip muscles to create a rapid, controlled, and rhythmic movement that alternates between side to side and front to back, or circular motions (Figure 5.1). In homes, mothers instruct girls in this dancing technique, and at certain events skilled young female dancers are the center of attention. In the context of an observing crowd, dancing is a celebration of skilled movement, demonstrating an attention to the labor and precision of movement. Similarly, there is a competitive element to this cultural production of body performance. The dancer is the object of the gaze, and hence it is common for a man to say that he would not allow his wife to engage in Basoga dancing publicly, implying that he does not want her sexuality on public display for fear that she might attract the attention of other men.

Elders also recall childhood games as places for learning about and experimenting with gendered sexual identity. An elder in Balikabona Village remembers a game called "house" that was played by village children when he was young:

> We used to play together with girls. And we used to divide ourselves into a father, a mother, and children. Those who acted as the father and mother were always the eldest in the group, and they used to be of the opposite sex. In the process there would come a time when those acting as parents would tell the children to go and play and that they would call them if they wanted them, or the "parents" would say that it's time to sleep. The two people—the father and mother—would sleep together and sometimes we used to pretend to play sex at an early age.

Young people today play similar games and also cite such games as being early sources of sexual learning and spaces for the playful but instructive enactment of adult gender roles. A game called "war" more explicitly enacted gendered norms around sexual conquest, as boys from two competing villages battled with each other over who could "steal" the largest number of girls from their opponent's village. Elders readily remember that intergenerational village gatherings provided their earliest learnings about sexuality. Their critique that young people today learn about sex from town settings that are more age-segregated and contain strangers from unfamiliar families and places reflects their larger anxiety about the loss of control and about the outside influence on younger generations.

The *Sôngá* and the Grooming of Female Sexuality

According to Basoga ideologies of sexuality, young females requires more specific knowledge than is learned through informal activities and conversations with peers. A girl's sexual education and bodily preparation are the joint responsibility of her mother and her designated *sôngá*. The mother oversees the transition of a girl's body by stressing the importance

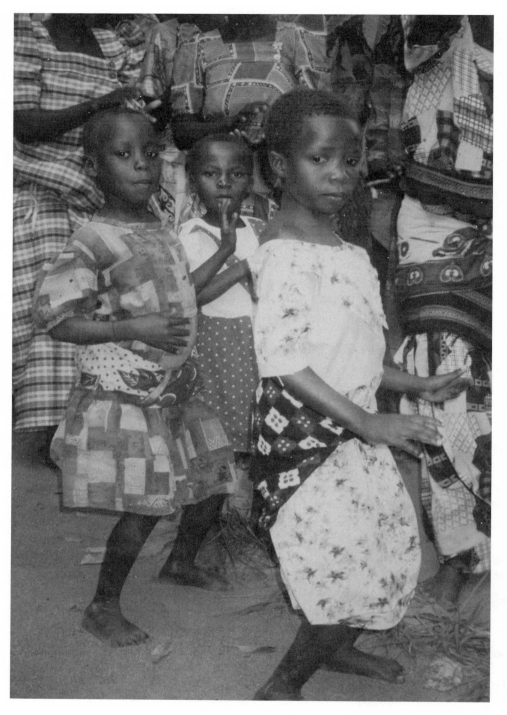

FIGURE 5.1. Basoga dancing

of physical attractiveness, feminine hygiene, and modesty, which, as discussed above, centered on the waist, hip, and thigh area. The mother's gaze and instruction ideally began at a young age and intensified after a girl began menstruating, to prevent pregnancy in her father's house and the possible reduction in her marriageability or bridewealth. Whereas the mother's persistent surveillance was intended to ensure the proper embodiment of adult female modesty, the girl's *sôngá* directly guided her sexual development and later served as her sexual advisor. In the Basoga moral economy of fair exchange, the father's lineage, from which the *sôngá* came, had an economic interest in the sexual abilities of its younger female kin. There was the possibility that their son-in-law's marital satisfaction might translate into a flow of gifts to show appreciation for their preparation of his wife for marriage (for a description of a similar pattern in Southern Africa, see Jeater 1993).

Premenarche: Elongating the Labia Minora

The common Basoga practice of child lending (which was less formal and for shorter periods than fostering), during which a girl resided with and assisted her *sôngá* and the matrimonial family of the *sôngá*, created opportunities for the girl's early sexual instruction under the watch of her father's clan. Instruction from the *sôngá* began before menarche, continued during puberty, and became more focused and intense after the girl was betrothed. A major role of the *sôngá* was to ensure that her niece learned and participated in stretching or pulling her labia minora (*okusika enfuli*).[11] The *sôngá* either described the details directly to the girl and provided the necessary items, or indirectly provided instruction by arranging an opportunity for the girl to learn the practice, such as connecting her to a group of girls to "fetch firewood," "collect firewood," or "visit the bush" at night. Mpoyenda, the cultural sex expert described earlier in this chapter, explained to me that the older girls would then tell the new member that "it wasn't the real firewood that they meant, it was something else." The *sôngá* or older girls would show her how to numb the area with a sticky substance—most likely sap from a tree—and how to roll the inner vaginal lip around a twig. This instruction began when the girl was around eight or nine years old, and she would continue the pulling continued until her labia reached a few centimeters long or she began menstruating, for after menarche it was believed that the lips became too tough to pull. Often girls were not told why the practice was important, but simply that if they did not do it they would encounter misfortune. When Mpoyenda complained to her mother that the pulling was painful, her mother invoked the common Kisoga threat I heard from other women: "If you don't, they [your in-laws] will bring two stale eggs and pour sorghum in your 'things' [vagina] and then a chicken will pick [eat] it." Even today, although men know of the act, pulling is still considered a part of female knowledge, and with cultural revival in some circles, its importance is reemerging.

Many elder women said that they did not know the reasons for pulling while participating in the custom, but as they matured and assisted their older sisters and aunts with childbirth or overheard women discussing marital problems, they came to know the significance of the practice. Norah, an elderly birth attendant in her late sixties, provided a common explanation about the role of pulling in childbirth: "Long ago they used to say that if you do not visit the bush to pull you would not give birth. In reality," she continued, "pulling is useful because if you never pulled, during the time of delivery a baby will fear to come, seeing that she is coming in a very open place. And even the men did not like to have sex with women who never pulled. To men, a woman who never pulled looked to them like entering a house that has no door." Like Norah, elder women commonly invoked the idea of a vagina needing a cover and the image of a door, associating both with a sense of modesty. Similarly, elder men were not circumcised (unless they were Muslim) because it was believed that exposing their uncovered genitalia was, as one anthropological observer put it, "an act of indecent exposure" (Orley 1970:13). As Norah suggested, pulling was closely associated with ideas of fertility as well, linking a female's external genital transformation with her reproductive capacities (see also Jeater 1993:24). A girl received a stern warning that if she did not pull she would either be unable to give birth or would experience complications during delivery.

On a more social level, "visiting the bush" provided a girl a forum for sharing information and gossip with her age-mates, helping to establish a homosocial network. One woman with whom I spoke laughed as she remembered visiting the bush with other girls. Although pulling was painful, she said, girls would take longer than necessary just so they could temporarily escape the drudgery of housework and constant supervision. According to my discussions with a group of young women, the bonding that occurs among young women while "visiting the bush" remains an important aspect of the practice, motivating their desires to continue the practice.

In addition to providing protection by covering the vaginal introitus (or opening), pulling was believed to increase a man's sexual satisfaction by elongating the passage through which the penis passed. When a woman was sexually aroused, the increased blood flow to her labia would cause them to swell; the longer labia engorged with blood extended the canal for the penis. The erotic appeal of an elongated labia minora was considered one of the most effective ways to win the favor of a husband. For instance, Faridah, an affable and almost blind widow in her seventies, was the third of five co-wives and was jealously known by the other wives as the favored one. Faridah attributes her favored status to her good sexual grooming: "If a woman who never pulled was in a polygynous family, her husband would give her less [sexual] attention than her cowives who had pulled. She could be disliked." She chuckled and stated that she had a *sôngá bulungi* (a very good aunt). The *sôngá* received credit or blame for a young woman's sexual conduct and moral behavior. A sexually well-groomed young wife would be a source of pride for her *sôngá*—an extension of the aunt's own sexual-social self. Likewise, a sexually lackluster young bride (much like Esther in the opening vignette) reflected the sexual inadequacies of her *sôngá*. In the latter cases, the flow of gifts from the young woman's disappointed husband to his in-laws, including the *sôngá*, would diminish over time. The practice of pulling reinforced the connection between risk (a vagina not having a cover) and bodily pleasures.

Betrothal: Bedroom Tricks

After a girl pulled, her body was prepared and she was ready for sexual instruction by her *sôngá*, which she would receive when she was either considered ready for marriage or already betrothed, intensifying during the period between the formal engagement ceremony (*okwandhula*) and the wedding ceremony. Sexual instruction was facilitated by another period of child lending, during which the girl returned to her *sôngá*'s house.[12] Mainly through observation, rather than verbal instruction, the girl would gather cultural tips on intimacy and sexual performance, or what elder women called "bedroom tricks" (*okulamba obukodyo bwomubulili*, literally "advice about techniques of the bed"). I was told several stories by elder and adult females about *sôngás* who discreetly arranged for them to hide under their aunt's bed or directly outside the bedroom while the aunt and her husband had sexual intercourse. It was there that the niece would learn the bedroom tricks. One of these was bedroom dancing, similar to Kisoga dancing, a movement used during both foreplay and coitus. The proper wearing or use of waist beads (*obutiti*) was important to bedroom dancing, and beads were given to a betrothed girl by her *sôngá*.[13] Imbued with sexual significance, waist beads were guaranteed to cause great sexual arousal in men. The *sôngá* also gave her betrothed niece a cotton *kitambaa* (cloth) to use for cleaning the man after sexual intercourse.[14] Along with instructions on its proper use, the girl would receive the stern warning that if her husband ever found her carrying the *kitambaa* when she was not in the bedroom with him, he would have sufficient evidence to accuse her of adultery. Another important lesson involved proper bodily hygiene, including how to cleanse the body and rid it of foul odors by using herbs and other vegetation (see also Burke 1996:23–31).

A betrothed woman was encouraged to enjoy intimacy and sex and was taught to play the subtle seductress role with her bedroom dancing and waist beads; however, she also learned that the man should believe he is the sexual initiator. His pleasure, she learned, should be seen to supersede hers. To achieve this, girls were coached in managing expressions of sexuality, such as bedroom sounds (*kusikina*). One older woman aged sixty-four remembered being "told that during the real act of sex, sexual intercourse, I should not keep quiet but I must make some sounds [*kusikina*] showing the man that I am enjoying what he is doing to me and it will also encourage the man so much." *Kusikina* was thought to further arouse the man, making him more eager to please the woman. Mastery of sexual intimacy also entailed risks for women—if not managed carefully, a woman could be accused of having engaged in pre- or extramarital sex, which was often collapsed into the moral term *obwenzi* (promiscuity), and the woman would run the risk of being called a *malaya* (prostitute).[15] Here lies the tension between sexual risk and sexual pleasure in Basoga ideologies regarding female sexuality—the balance between orchestrating pleasure for herself and her husband against the risk of being considered too sexually knowledgeable. Although most married women (as well as men) agreed that sexual intercourse should satisfy both the man and the woman, social validation of sexual pleasure did not mean that *all* sexual encounters were consensual and pleasurable for both. Many women talked about their first sexual experience with a lover or their husband as being coerced or forced, and many used Lusoga terms meaning "conquered," "violent," or "rape" (see also Fritz 1998:153).

Consummation of marriage on the wedding night marked both the official transfer of the rights over the bride's sexuality from her father to her husband and the first official test of a young woman's sexual abilities. "On the wedding night," Fallers documented (1957:112), "the bride is accompanied to the bridegroom's house by her brother and her father's sister, who remain for one night to assure themselves of the bridegroom's potency and who, on the following day, must be given a token gift 'to drive them away.'" According to elders I spoke with, the *sôngá* was also interested in assessing the effectiveness of the girl's education or, as I was told, "if she was able to play sex as accepted." If the girl was a virgin, as indicated by blood on the bedding (often banana fibers), the *sôngá* was rewarded with a goat. If the girl was not a virgin, however, no action was taken against the girl or *sôngá*. I also heard stories about *sôngás* who would be in the bedroom to give instruction to the couple, and though at first I thought this seemed odd, given Basoga notions of sexual privacy, I heard it too often to not believe there was some truth in it.

The Basoga sexualization process for women must be understood in the moral economy of marriage that is structured around the exchange of bridewealth and polygyny, which inspires competition among co-wives and competing clans; in this context a young woman's sexual competency was one way of securing greater resources and attention for her as well as her family. This required a young woman to be sexually skilled in the bedroom and an attractive object of gaze at public events, while simultaneously remaining modest and controlled. A woman was believed to have more sexual powers than a man, further fueling her family's and the community's motivation for strict regulation and supervision. A woman such as Mpoyenda was awarded great respect for her ability to manage her public reputation as a sexually well-groomed and knowledgeable woman ("sexually" here meaning more than just the act of sex and more like "sensual") while remaining sexually unavailable to men other than her husband. Successfully maintaining this balance publicly worked to advance the prestige of the husband as the "owner" of the woman, and wives often used this power in helping shape a man's reputation to their advantage and to the advantage of their children and natal family.

Alternative Moralities

Changes such as greater mobility and the dispersion of kin groups, religious movements, urbanization, and newer forms of sexual information have facilitated transformations in the Basoga sexual learning system and the role of the *sôngá*. Uganda's postcolonial turmoil and insecurity partly caused the situation in which many women I interviewed who came of age in the 1960s and 1970s did not reside near their *sôngá*; others were not assigned an official one until they were securely betrothed and perhaps already sexually experienced. Although many of the now middle-aged women lived with a *sôngá* for short periods during their youth, few recalled their *sôngá* providing them with the extensive sexual training described above, and only some said their *sôngá* was the one who instructed them on pulling. When I asked these same women if they had discussed issues of sexuality with their nieces, very few said that they did. Others explained that strained relationships between their sisters-in-law because of jealousy over children, wealth, or differences in ideologies or religious beliefs also contributed to their reluctance to perform the role of the *sôngá*. Many women wanted to talk to their own daughters about sex, as opposed to leaving it to the *sôngá*, but because of deeply embedded cultural norms and anxieties surrounding direct parent-child sexual discussions, few of them actually did. These same adults are critical of how young people today learn about sex, yet they feel ill-equipped and reluctant to act as sexual advisors to their children.

There has also been a shift in the instruction about and the practice of pulling. It has changed from a practice overseen by the *sôngá* and often reinforced in peer groups to one that is frequently missing a direct adult presence and in which the female peer group is central. Older adolescent girls teach younger ones, in schools or around the village, the practice of pulling, and in the process sexual information is transmitted, but it lacks the authority of an older relative. Hence, the practice of pulling does not exist as older women remember it, but adolescent girls at the time of my initial research were still "visiting the bush" with their peers.[16] The dispersal of the clan contributed to the decline in the practice of pulling. In addition, birth attendants, who initially encountered the practice while delivering babies, and Christian missionaries believed that pulling was masturbation or body mutilation, hence uncivilized and immoral. Women missionaries stationed at schools and health wards asserted that pulling promoted promiscuity by introducing girls at an early age to their genitalia and sexual sensation.

Nabirye, an elderly woman who had an unusually high level of education for a female of her time, attended a Catholic boarding school in the 1940s. The sisters and the health official forbade the practice of pulling and performed random screenings of the girls to ensure that girls did not continue the practice. Although Nabirye never underwent a random screening, she often heard rumors of girls who were suspected or reported to be involved in pulling being called into the nurse's office for a "check on their vagina for signs of pulling." After a mass screening that led to the expulsion of girls from one dormitory, her *sôngá* advised Nabirye's parents to transfer the girl to another school. The *sôngá* feared that the twin liability of being educated (and hence, culturally subversive and expensive in terms of bridewealth) and not pulling (and hence, culturally less sexually desirable and prepared) would jeopardize her niece's chances of marrying and reproducing. Nabirye never finished pulling and, as an adult, had a string of miscarriages, divorces, and episodes of barrenness. Nabirye attributes her series of misfortunes to not pulling and to bewitching by a jealous stepmother.

Nabirye's story represents how, since the late nineteenth century, foreign religions, mainly Christianity, have interacted in complex and multiple ways with local ideas about sexual learning and morality through the colonial project aimed at "civilizing" African sexuality (see articles in K. T. Hansen 1992). During the early part of the twentieth century, these competing ideas led to a long debate among missionaries and between colonial officials and missionaries about how to achieve the goal of ideal African subjects who would serve the larger economic and political interests of the colonial government and companies. As the process progressed, Christian marriages emerged as the ideal model through which to domesticate and create a group of African elites (Giblin 1999; Morris 1967; Kalema Commission 1965). It was believed that Christian families should consider "churches and hospitals as the proper places for sex education and care of reproductive health" (Giblin 1999:313). As a result, the church and public health institutions became important sites of reformulating African bodies and sexuality, and notions of premarital abstinence and sin became significant discourses. Such notions were easily appropriated into local moralities because they relied on moral and practical criteria that had been part of Basoga ideologies of sexuality long before the penetration of Christianity. Many women also resisted such constructions and continued the practice that had been central to Basoga conceptions of female sensuality and female bonding.

Furthermore, as hospital maternity wards became sites for monitoring and attempting to halt the practice of pulling, some women chose to avoid hospital maternity wards and opted instead to deliver in village settings. While older women recall attending health meetings in the village about maternal health and hospital delivery and visits from representatives of Mothers Unions, they have little memory of receiving information similar to what they received from their *sôngá* about sexuality and sex. An alternative morality had emerged that privileged a pedantic learning style in which experts disseminated knowledge that was a shift from the sharing of women's knowledge across generations. Women with whom I spoke did not consider the messages received through churches, clinics, or schools as containing messages about what they would consider intimate matters of marriage, or sexuality.

Apart from messages of sexual abstinence, churches and mosques in Iganga today have remained virtually absent from the sexual education of young people, maintaining that unmarried people should not engage in sex and that learning about sex should correspond with pre-wedding arrangements.[17] Sexual learning finds its way into some premarital counseling required by religious institutions, which (as seen in Esther's case at the beginning of this chapter) focuses on gendered sexual obligations, the role of reproduction, and the importance of fidelity. More commonly, however, sex becomes an object for invoking moral projects (see Adams and Pigg 2005). When I asked a reverend from the Church Mission Society (CMS) in Iganga about Uganda's HIV education campaigns, he applauded them but was highly critical of what he saw as the overemphasis on condoms. He argued that "if we encourage the young people to use them [condoms], it means that we are encouraging prostitution and adultery, which is against the biblical teaching." For him, as for others, teaching about condoms is equivalent to encouraging people to engage in unrestrained sexual activity. To illustrate his point, he recalled a dance at the teacher's college that bordered his church compound. The day of the dance, an NGO held an HIV awareness event during which they distributed condoms and demonstrated how to use them. The day after the dance, according to the reverend, used condoms and wrappers were scattered everywhere. He assumed that without access to condoms the young people would not have engaged in sexual intercourse, an assumption commonly made by people who argue against the distribution of condoms (for example, Pfeiffer 2004).

Another church leader complained that young people today are learning "incorrect ideas about sex" from videos, books, and discos and argued that, although the role of the *sôngá* has significantly declined, she was the ideal person to educate young females about sex. When I asked if his church had tried to replace the teachings of the *sôngá* or encouraged the congregation to reinstitute the practice, he replied: "In fact the church has tried to incorporate that in its teachings. For example, that's why we have opened up counseling clinics and we send people especially from the Mother's Union groups to these clinics to go and teach the young people. So, these have taken up the role of the *sôngá* after realizing its importance." For the reverend, as in the past, sexuality education, and hence the problematic of morality, is associated with women—a woman's responsibility. According to the chair of the Mother's Union, however, the Union does not offer sexual advice to unmarried or childless females. Instead, she explained, the Union assists poor rural women with pre- and post-natal health advice, showing them "proper" techniques for running a household and caring for new babies and toddlers, akin to the domesticity projects of the same organizations during the colonial era (Allman and Tashjian 2000; Hunt 1999). A common perception is that being married or already having reproduced are criteria for accessing reproductive health programs such as the Mother's Union. This perception further alienates young people from sexuality programs and arises from the idea that educating about sex promotes sex.

Religion is invoked to explain the decline of historical practices that regulated youth sexuality and is simultaneously woven into commentaries about today's sexually misbehaving youth. While in elders' narratives, Christianity helped erode Basoga notions of morality and regulation, their critiques of contemporary impropriety are infused with Christian and Islamic discourses and logics. Although religion provides a rhetorical and moral framework in promoting premarital sexual abstinence, I almost never heard anyone in Iganga say that religious institutions or leaders are the ideal sexual educators of young people. Hence, in addition to sexual risk and pleasure being bifurcated in the sexuality learning process, recent constructions of morality have placed it in the domain of religion and dislocated it from the workings of clan reproduction and bridewealth. This newer alternative moral order, which has been emerging gradually since colonial missionary interventions, often privileges an obligation or contract that a person has with god or more recently with public health, as opposed to an obligation that the person has to his or her clan; however, that same religious teaching falls short in transmitting knowledge about intimacy and the sexual body that were so central in the Basoga sexual/morality learning system. Morality and sexuality learning are viewed increasingly as projects of the individual, focused on creating an autonomous individual rather than on creating an individual grounded in a *máka* and situated within kin and social networks.

The Commercialization of Pleasure: From the Personal Sôngá to the Public Ssenga

Uganda's active public culture producers, the bentu (see Chapter 1), have found that the repackaging of past practices of sexual pleasure and intimacy makes ideal material for entrepreneurial enterprises. In Uganda's current cultural renaissance—or, the "reinvention of tradition," as Terence Ranger (1983) reminds us—the figure of the sexually wise auntie has risen to public prominence as the expert on sexuality. In the process, the Basoga *sôngá* has become commodified and commercialized and repackaged as the national *ssenga*, which is the Luganda term for a paternal aunt who played a similar role in the sexual development and grooming of her niece (as mentioned in Chapter 2, Luganda is the language of the more dominant group, the Baganda). Techno-savvy

Nowadays they are made with fastening hooks
The sacred loin beads!

By Keturah Kamugasa Akiiki

LOIN beads, that is the latest fashion craze in town. Increasingly, women are going for strands of small beads worn around the loins. Go anywhere in town and you will find these sacred beads hanging in the shop displays.

A lady in a Kampala Road shop told me that many women were buying the beads. So why the sudden interest in the beads? I asked her.

"Some women buy them because they want to rekindle the passion in their marriages. Others because they want to be fashionable. There are women who buy them at the recommendation of their husbands."

"I wear them because I want to give my husband everything at home so that he does not go for other women, especially prostitutes. I hear many prostitutes now wear them," she said.

Angela, in her late twenties has always worn beads around her loins. In her culture, women have traditionally worn beads for centuries. "Besides, my boyfriend loves them to bits. He wants to keep them hanging on a nail in his bedroom so that I only wear them when I am with him," she says.

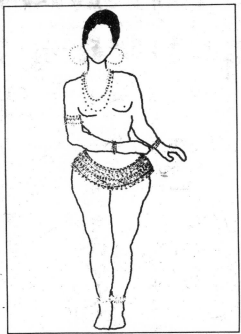

An art piece showing how beads are worn by women in many of the African cultures. Loin beads are becoming more popular these days. File Photo.

Do men love them? "Oh yes," says one man. I went home one evening and my wife surprised me when she walked into our bedroom from the bathroom wearing nothing but the beads around her loins. I felt good that she'd gone out of her way to surprise me. They certainly have added 'spice' to our marriage," he chuckles mischievously.

Some women are, however, embarrassed by the whole ideal of wearing these beads. When some women suggested to buy them for a friend's wedding anniversary, she was scandalised. "I will not wear them," she vowed much to their amusement.

Loin beads are not a new phenomena in Africa. Our fore-mothers wore them and they were part of a woman's beauty and sexuality. Even the most pious of women's groups in Uganda, Mothers' Union recommended them highly to a friend who got married recently. They make theirs in the union's colours of white and blue.

She declined at the time but she is interested now. So come her wedding anniversary, I will be there with two sets of beads. In the past, women wore them permanently around the loins. This has changed ever since a woman was embarrassed when the string snapped and the beads went flying everywhere.

Nowadays, they are made with fastening hooks so that they can be adjusted whenever the need arises.

In town, they come in various colours. The choice is yours. You need to measure your loin area before you buy them just to ensure that they fit comfortably. Go on, be adventurous, recapture your Africanness.

FIGURE 5.2. Waist beads article and picture, *New Vision*, May 6, 1997

bentu bring into one medium, whether radio, magazine, or TV, a constant interplay between a reinvented Ugandan past and contemporary constructions of a modern global morality and sexuality based on freedom, pleasure, and autonomy. As discourses of pleasure and desire get sanitized by religious institutions, schools, and medical institutions and constructed as a sign of depravity, these commercial venues fill the gap by bringing to the public sphere of sexual pleasure repackaged and reinvented as African traditions. Hence, while public culture discourses about pleasure and desire are frequently in English and adapt African customs, many community-based HIV awareness campaigns are conducted in local languages and use foreign constructions of medical risk and risk reduction. Using English provides a license for discussions that would be considered too vulgar or inappropriate for public consumption if uttered in local languages.[18]

I turn to an example to illustrate this point about popular culture and the transmission of African sexual (reinvented) traditions. During my initial research stint, two excited girls ran into my office in Iganga Town waving an issue of *Chic*, a soft-sex/leisure magazine that uses scantily dressed cover girls to attract attention. The title of the issue's feature article boldly occupied the glossy cover of the magazine: "Ladies: To Pull or Not to Pull Is the Question." During a discussion about sexual learning with students at their school the previous week, some of the girls told me about a "good article" on the practice of pulling in a new magazine. "The article was accurate," they assured me, and would tell me everything I wanted to know about pulling. The magazine article recast the purpose of pulling from a practice to please the man into a practice that increased the woman's sexual pleasure. This privileging of female sexual pleasure was woven throughout the article, with testimonials from informants:

> The results are usually pleasurable, some women admitted. "Every time I shower with warm water I feel great down there," Joy confessed. By increasing the sensitive surface area, pulling is believed to enhance sexual desire and masturbatory pleasure. "Ever since I carried out that function I have found jogging more enjoyable. I don't need a man to get an orgasm; all I do is jog!" Mary, an athlete, said. (*Chic* 1997).

The article concluded with a brief description of an expensive Western surgical procedure that cost 2,300 British pounds and provided what the article described as the same "effect as the traditional African" practice. The author challenged the reader to consider the irony: "What Europeans today pay top dollar for, we have been doing for years and for free." In the magazine's creatively refashioned version of the practice and moral sensibilities, pulling was removed from the context of marriage, reproduction, and patrilineal ties to one in which the young woman pursued her own sexual desires.

Yet that same year, on October 11, another story about the purpose of pulling appeared in a sex advice column in the *Monitor* (Kampala). This one more closely resembled reasons offered by older women. A perplexed, perhaps fictitious, reader asked: "At the tender age of 11, I was made to extend the outer [*sic*] labia of the genitals. . . . What is the purpose of extending the outer labia?" The advisor responded, "You are one of the few lucky modern ladies who had the opportunity to perform this ritual at such a tender age, and didn't shun it. . . . The purpose of extending the outer labia of the female genitalia, dear Sandra, is plainly to increase your partner's satisfaction during sex. . . . That is why women are advised to perform it, because it keeps their men satisfied and limits their wandering." According to the advisor of the column, the outer labia, not the inner ones as described by elders, are the parts of the genitalia that are pulled. Pulling, the girl and the public are informed, increases a man's sexual pleasure and discourages him from "wandering" to other women. In both articles, pulling is framed in the context of individual pleasures. For many young men and women, such popularized versions of past sex practices that are generated by the unseen yet

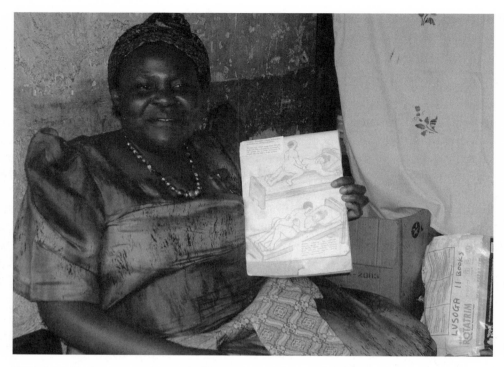

FIGURE 5.3. Contemporary *ssenga* holding sex manual for married people

omniscient sexperts inform their knowledge about sex, the old days, and their own bodies. Ironically, these frequently male advisors have become the experts on what was formerly known as women's knowledge and have recast versions of tradition based on clan reproduction through a modernist lens of the individual pursuit of pleasure.

As the sexpert trend was taking hold, the *ssenga* emerged as one of the most profitable mass-produced sexual icons (see also Scheier 2003). She became a cultural reference to the old days—a time without AIDS. The commercialized *ssenga* draws on the authority of the roles, duties, and sexual wisdom attributed to the kin-based *sôngá* and is conveniently packaged into a powerful symbol of cultural heritage and modern knowledge. Starting in the mid-1990s and flourishing by the end of the decade, various media and commercial outlets began to run serial advice pieces bearing the name *ssenga*, including advice columns, radio shows, counseling centers, education seminars, and TV programs. People in Iganga easily associate this emerging public counselor as a familiar and trusted person. Leading the way in the public commodification of the *ssenga* was the *Monitor*, with an advice column called "Agony Column with Ssenga Nambwere." Another "Agony Column" appears in a competing newspaper in the women's section. In both columns the *ssenga* consoles broken hearts, advises on modern romance and love, and offers solutions to sex problems (such as impotence or genital warts) and anxieties (such as first sex experiences and intercourse during menstruation). The columns encourage the modern reader to seek help from the expert: "Want to share your problems or seek help? Write to Ssenga Nambwere, c/o the *Monitor*."

The troubled modern sex citizens could also fax or e-mail their questions. Titles of the columns include "He Loves His Ex," "Is It Okay to Use a Vibrator?" and "How Do I Tell If My Wife Reached an Orgasm?" The once-private conversations with the *sônga* are now shared with a wider audience that is blended along gender, class, and age lines.

In the process of commercial packaging, the *ssenga* that has emerged is removed from the private lessons of girls and is now targeting an audience of adults who are interested in improving their sex lives and getting answers to questions about their bodies that the AIDS campaigns do not address. Once associated with the instruction of prepubescent and betrothed girls, the *ssenga* has been transformed into a counselor for "mature" men and women, married couples, and sexually precocious young people, according to local perceptions. The *ssenga* as a modern-day cultural icon has been seamlessly woven into an invisible and expert voice in affairs of love, romance, and other more banal aspects of relationships between adults. Partly because of the faceless nature of the media, the *ssenga* is able to creatively push and merge the distinctions between traditional and modern and unapologetically defy the boundary between illicit and acceptable. Whereas the public *ssenga* has risen to national prominence, in Iganga the role of the *sônga* in teaching pubescent girls about sexuality has been greatly weakened. Today, the *sônga* who acts as the bride's representative is selected more for her social status in civic society than for her role in the girl's sexual development. The construction of modern sexuality as an individualistic pursuit removed from the moral economy of the clan provides another moral alternative through which sexually curious youth and adults understand sexuality.

The Sex Education Debate

A question that frequently reemerges in Uganda is: If the historical role of the *sônga* has declined and religious leaders do not feel comfortable talking with youth about sex, who should teach youth? Two common answers I received from Iganga residents were "parents" and "schools." It remains culturally inappropriate for parents to talk directly to their children about sex, although indirect communication through riddles or strategically situated gossip exchanges has long been accepted and normal. An elder woman in Iganga expressed another perspective on the parent-as-sex-educator idea. She stated that it was the current adult generation and their promiscuity that had caused the rampant spread of AIDS. Since adults cannot control themselves sexually, she explained, how could they possibly teach young people about sex and sexual morality? In her opinion, adults *should* be embarrassed, because their unregulated sexual behavior has caused the spread of HIV and the dissolution of marriage. Although many parents do not discuss sexuality with their children, it is no longer the *sônga* who is blamed for a young woman's sexual deficiencies or excesses but her parents (and particularly the mother, who is criticized when her child's behavior goes beyond the boundaries of propriety).

Most young people believe that school is the ideal place to learn about sex, asserting that teachers are socially respectable and knowledgeable. Compared to magazines and videos, students feel that schools "would give correct information on sex." While young people enjoy the sexual images and counseling programs, they are often confused about the accuracy of the information. However, in the schools around Iganga, sex education contains a unit on the biology of reproduction, and another on anatomy, and today increasingly focuses on scientific lessons about HIV. One fifteen-year-old girl remembered: "When I was in primary five [equivalent to fifth grade] a teacher talked about sex one day. She did not want to talk too much about it, but the children kept on asking her so many questions, and we came to realize that sex has been there since our great-grandfathers' time. But she wouldn't talk more." What is revealed in this quote is that by the age of ten or eleven these students knew vaguely about what has recently become lumped under the term "sex" through the AIDS campaigns, radio programs, local gossip, or observing older siblings.

Teachers are reluctant to discuss sexuality with students for fear of being accused of "seducing" students or of encouraging premarital sex among students. Hence, within this context, the risk of getting a bad reputation from speaking to young people about sex is greater than the public health risk of negative sexual health outcomes among youth. Despite young people's access to sexualized images in the media, teachers and other adult authority figures in Iganga expressed hesitation in educating young people about sexuality, beyond warning about HIV, STIs, and unplanned pregnancy. When I asked the headmaster of a secondary school if his school had instituted the sexual education curriculum as presented in the Ministry of Education's Moral Education module, he responded:

> At the moment, no. I remember having tried to introduce sex education here, but when the parents had a general meeting, they stopped it. They thought that when you talk about sex you are telling people to do it or you are describing the real act of sex. Yet we wanted to reflect what the *sôngá* used to teach. But the parents had a misconception about it. . . . We first should educate the parents about the need to educate the children and have the sex education at hand. So there is no sex education in the school although we sent someone to train and she came back, but we are reluctant to teach because of the parents' attitude towards it.

The headmaster was open to introducing sex education in his school. Like parents, however, the school needed first to learn how to teach it. Although the sex education curriculum had not been implemented in Iganga schools when I conducted my initial research, it is revealing that the curriculum was included in the section on marriage and moral education. The module treats sexual intercourse solely as a marital *obligation*, not as one of desire or love. Therefore, since people only need to know about it when they are preparing to wed, schools as well as other adults are excused from teaching about sexual activity and sexuality. The embedded moral message suggests that sexual pleasure leads to dangerous consequences such as unplanned pregnancy or HIV.

Sources that people identify as ideal sex educators, such as parents, religious institutions, and schools, do not feel comfortable or able to discuss sex with a group of people who, according to moral doctrine, should not be sexually active. The *sôngá*, on the other hand, has been transformed from a sex educator for girls into a broader

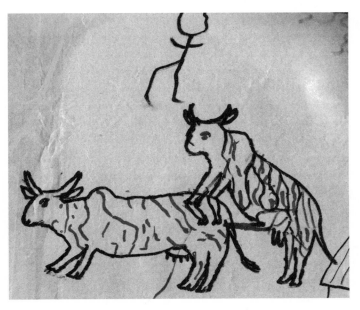

FIGURE 5.4. Learning about sex: Youth drawing of cows mating

educator for both males and females, often neglecting the biological and sociological questions of youth. Furthermore, public health and HIV campaign workers view their role as educating people about risk reduction, not sexual pleasure. People in Iganga and Uganda in general acknowledge that sexuality education for young people is needed, but they remain uncertain about how to institutionalize it in a way that accommodates the concerns of adults and the needs of youth.

Learning about Sexuality beyond the Sôngá: Discos, Bars, and Video Halls

Learning how to be a sexual being is important to young people today, as it was to elders and as well as to James (the dissatisfied husband introduced at the opening of this chapter). As the kin-based system declines and age-segregated social events become more prominent than cross-generational ones (displacing occasions such as twin-naming ceremonies), young people turn to other sources for information on how to enact and embody sexuality. Most youth learn about sexual intercourse from routine village living, such as watching animals mate (see Figure 5.4). However, for youth, being a sexual being is not just about intercourse or risk. Rather, sex is performed through a range of practices, such as gendered ways of flirting, persuading, negotiating, courting, engaging in foreplay, and seeking pleasure. Same-sex and coed peer groups allow youth to discuss sexual issues and learn from each other. As seen in the practice of pulling, older youth become the experts and younger ones eagerly listen to their experiences and notions of sexual relations. In peer groups, youth also make sense of the cultural scripts of sexuality and morality that they observe when

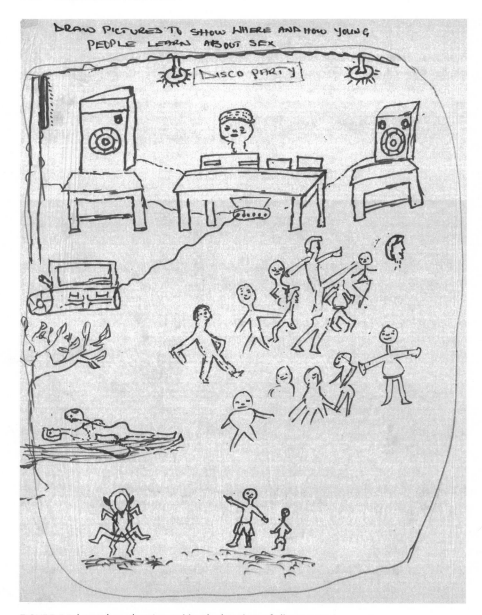

FIGURE 5.5. Learning about sex: Youth drawing of disco party

watching young adults interact in discos, bars, marketplaces, the village, and in Western pornography.[19]

Watching older youth and young adults is central to a young person's first lessons on intimacy, and often these same venues eventually provide that person's first experiences with enactments of sexuality and romance. School holidays similarly offer young people an opportunity to explore town life, meeting with schoolmates who live in neighboring villages (Kinsman, Nyanzi, and Pool 2000; Konde-Lule, Sewankambo, and Morris

1997). "Transnight" discos that last all night stir excitement during school breaks. Announcing transnight discos, pickup trucks carrying a group of young men in urban wear slowly cruise through busy market areas. Young and old stop their activities, descending from offices, homes, and informal selling shacks to watch the colorful truck and listen to the fast-talking DJ and the loud dance music blaring from large speakers. Some frown in disapproval and turn away; others wave and cheer at the sign that Iganga is part of a global urban network. For youth, the display announces another opportunity for them to see adults at play, and they may indulge in a little adult play themselves.

The dress code at discos is "modern, sexy casual," defined in part by the particular location but also clearly informed by regional and global aesthetics as seen in music videos, television shows, and advertisements. For adolescent boys this could include jeans, baggy pants, T-shirts, colorful satiny shirts, and brimmed hats or baseball caps. Like elsewhere in the world, the definition of sexually hip for young women changes more frequently and can include miniskirts, half tops or sheer blouses, skinny jeans or pants, and strappy, dressy high heels. Youth select from a variety of aesthetic options, depending on their financial resources and how they desire to create a public identity. The atmosphere of discos and bars is created by modern stereo systems, disco lights, a mixture of Western and African dance music (the latter mostly from Uganda and Zaire, but more recently from South Africa), bottled beer, and energetic disc jockeys. Early in the night, men dance in groups with other men and women with other women. As the night wears on and libations flow, social mixing of the sexes increases; the songs, dancing, mingling of sexes, and flowing beer are common images that guide sexual narratives of youth. As one secondary student offered, "young children today easily learn about sex in discos. In slow songs men and women hold each other while the young ones watch. At times from such moments of close contact men and women end up playing sex in dark corners or in the bush while the young children see them." For this youth, and others as well, the excitement is not with whom people go but with whom people leave. He continues, "After seeing, the young people go and practice what they have seen."

Watching intently, youth learn secrets of adult sexualized interactions and then share their disco narratives with their friends, until the narratives become well-known sexual scripts among youth. When youth lack the financial means to enter the disco, congregating outside presents a form of entertainment and a social scene that they can share with classmates. One adolescent female recounted a story of a man trying to convince a woman to leave with him. After the man bought the woman drinks and danced closely with her, the couple meandered to a dark corridor behind the dance hall. Another young male said, "The disco is the best place to learn sex from. This is because you are able to see how a boy begins to approach a girl—how the affair develops until you see them playing sex." Bush discos held in the village to celebrate political victories, housewarming parties, or marital engagements offer youth other chances to observe adult play and flirting.

For older people, these discos and bars that play a major role in the sexualization of young people symbolize a myriad of conflicting changes in society—changes such as the fading of tradition, assimilation into modernity, the blending of local and foreign, youth gone wild, and new opportunities for youth (Parikh 2005). Although these recreational venues are not new, for many have been in Uganda for decades, they continue to serve as targets for accusations of social and moral decay. Western videos provide young people (as well as adults) with an up-close look at sex acts. US action movies, kung fu films, Indian melodrama-romance musicals, and sports tapes are screened during the day and early evening in Iganga's video halls. At night, "blue movies" (pornographic and X-rated movies) from the United States and Europe replace these films, providing youth with images of interpersonal sexual scripts that emphasize sexual positions, noises, foreplay, and visual plots within which youth can imaginatively insert themselves, though the settings of these movies are often far removed from Ugandan youth's lives (Figure 5.6). Adolescent males secretly flock to these video halls, either peeping through windows or paying the admission to go inside and watch foreign men and women indulge in sexual intercourse. Girls, often too embarrassed to watch intently, catch glimpses as they pass by slowly with their friends on detours from evening market trips. One secondary schoolboy commented that from blue movies "you learn best styles of playing sex." Another student added, "Young people like to attend video shows concerning sex most. This is because they want to improve on their sexual abilities. . . . Boys especially need to know how to balance [on top of a girl]. And also young people are interested in sex films so as to learn many skills and styles and to know which one is the best." Even if young people do not view these films, the details are eagerly retold and embellished by friends, offering the visual imagery and sexual scripts through which they can imagine sexual possibilities outside or despite local realities. Same-sex and mixed peer groups allow youth to further discuss and explore issues of sexuality, with older youth acting as experts and younger ones eagerly listening. Through these networks, youth make sense of sexual behaviors and begin to understand their own sexuality. Youth, however, are very critical and mistrust what their peers say about sex, but many do not feel that they have a trusted adult with whom they can speak openly without fear of reprimand (see also Dilger 2003).

The venues through which youth gather sexual scripts have specific gendered constructions of sexuality. Women who frequent bars and discos are often referred to as promiscuous and are perceived as defying sexual propriety. This often sends mixed messages to young girls. For them, discos and bars are places where men and women *perform* gendered sexuality, but girls are not sure how to enact these roles without jeopardizing their own reputations. One girl said, "The women in the bars are beautiful, but they are not good women." Girls and some boys must grapple with this tension between risking their reputations and negotiating their way through alternative moralities.

Reconciling Risk and Pleasure in the Age of Public Sex

Given the array of competing sexual moralities in contemporary Uganda, Esther's sexual paralysis (presented at the beginning of this chapter) makes sense. Her desire to embody evangelical Christian values of female sexual naïveté and restraint, combined with her professional work at the medical research clinic, which sanitized affection and pleasure from the act of intimacy, led to her uncertainty about the most appropriate way to pursue pleasure with her new husband. In addition, the Sunday sermons

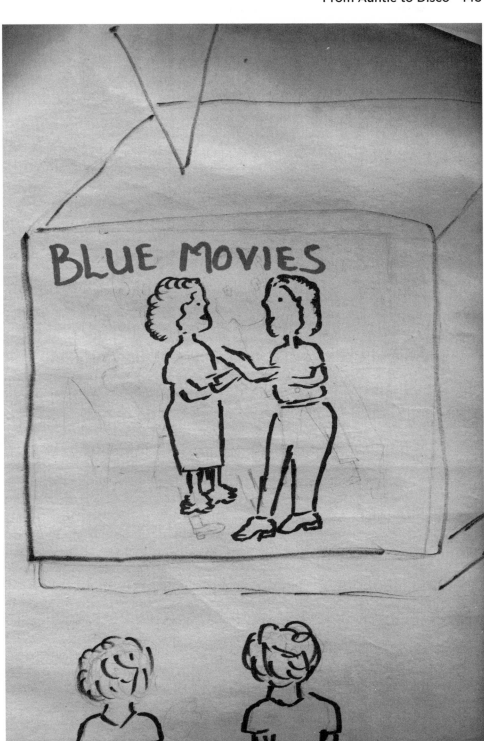

FIGURE 5.6. Learning about sex: Youth drawing of blue movies (pornography)

attacking the sexually explicit images and messages in popular culture, and the increasingly conservative public commentary about the growing number of *nakyewombekeire* and other sexual reprobates, left her fearful that performances of desire would call into question her respectability and premarital chastity. The entry into the Basoga moral landscape by her husband, her mother, and her *sôngá*, to seek advice from a respected person—a person of lower socioeconomic status with whom they likely would not otherwise have engaged—reveals the lingering nostalgia for a perceived uncomplicated past in which moral judgment and punishment were more localized affairs. The trio's quest for appropriate pleasure highlights what many see as a main problem with the moral alternatives of today—the breakdown of women's intergenerational sharing and regulation of sexual knowledge. An elder woman, Egulansi, offered this commentary about generational tensions in sexuality education:

> The relationship is very poor between the young and old. Today young people hardly listen to any advice from old people. Whatever they are told, they will always say, "That's of the past and it can't work now." Young women believe that they have a generation with everything new. . . . Today people who get educated see it as a shame to ask or be told by a *sôngá* things to do with marriage or sex. At the same time young people today claim to know everything. Worse still, young people today do not give elders the chance to teach them, especially about sex. For instance, so many young people today, especially the girls, get into sex before they reach the age at which we used to teach about sex. So today they find out the bad and the good by themselves.

Many adults and elders share Egulansi's sentiments about feeling marginalized and irrelevant in the sexual development of young people (see also Stewart 2000). Yet they are constantly reminded of the complexities of life that youth face—uncertain futures, limited jobs, the desire for foreign goods and ideas, an increased policing of sexuality, and HIV. Older people are resigned to the notion of young people "finding out things by themselves," recognizing that sexual learning and knowledge tied to kinship and the familiar village setting has firmly shifted toward newer "technologies of sex and self" generated by national and global cultural brokers, including public health, religion, commercial entertainment, and the media. This public convergence rearranges vocabularies of sexual morality that include new standards of bodily hygiene and grooming, medico-moral notions of reproductive health and risk reduction, and religion-infused rhetorics that privilege women's sexual purity and equate it with sexual ignorance. This represents a departure from Basoga morality, in which a woman's knowledge of sex was necessary for her and her patrilineage to keep its powers safely located within the patriarchal system of the clan. This is the precise reason that the *nakyewombekeire* has received so much criticism—she has taken her sexuality out of the patrilineage, in what Holly Wardlow calls acts of "negative agency" (2006).

Removing oneself from the patrilineage, whether intentionally or not, is shaped by the declining role of the *sôngá*, for this relationship provided a maturing girl with her moral connection to her father's lineage—a *máka* of sorts. The transformation of the *sôngá* from an intimate and personal educator of girls to a public icon speaking about "healthy" relationships within national projects of modernity symbolizes an era of sexual bifurcation in which meanings of pleasure have shifted from a reflection of a harmonious marriage and proper functioning of the kin group to individual projects of desire and risk as an avoidable moral issue with serious health and social consequences. However, as Iganga residents are constantly reminded, the risk that they are told can be avoided if one behaves in medico-moral ways finds its way into the lived realities of adolescent girls who experience a high rate of pregnancy and have higher rates of HIV and STDs than their male counterparts. Anxiety about this reality engenders, as it has in the past, intense policing of the young female body—a policing that occurs at various levels. Recent legislative attempts to protect adolescent girls have been creatively deployed locally as a technology to police the sexuality of daughters while demonizing their youthful lovers with the ultimate aim of protecting the respectability and health of their patriclan and community, as explored in the next chapter.

CHAPTER 6

"They arrested me for loving a schoolgirl"

Controlling Delinquent Daughters and Punishing Defiant Boyfriends

I met twenty-four-year-old Yahaya Waigongolo in 2002. The thin, soft-spoken man was working as a manual laborer, loading and unloading trucks for a beverage depot in Iganga Town. He recently had been released from federal prison after serving a thirty-two-month sentence for defilement, the crime of having sexual intercourse with a female who was under eighteen years old. At the time of his arrest, Yahaya was twenty years old, and the alleged victim, Lydia, was a few months shy of her seventeenth birthday. By all the accounts that I collected, the relationship had been consensual, though Lydia's protective father was known for strictly prohibiting his daughter from engaging in a romantic relationship. Lydia's display of interest in Yahaya made this relationship particularly problematic for the man. In the ninth month of the relationship Lydia started showing signs commonly associated with pregnancy—withdrawing from social activities, nausea, general lethargy, and wearing loosely fitted clothing. Lydia's angry father threatened to throw his despoiled daughter out of the house unless she disclosed the name of her lover. When the father found out that the girl's mother had received sixty-five thousand shillings (about 35 USD) to help with medical expenses—and hence collaborated in keeping the secret—the even more enraged man went to the police station to charge Yahaya with defilement. With evidence of paternity (the evidence being Yahaya's financial assistance), and with Yahaya's lack of sufficient economic or social capital to settle out of court, the case easily sped through the justice system, and Yahaya was sent to prison. During our initial interview, his eyes cast downward, Yahaya said, "They arrested me for loving a schoolgirl."

The intervention around youth sexuality I examine in this chapter is a legal one, specifically the defilement law that sent Yahaya to prison. An analysis of local uses of the defilement law demonstrates that it is used in communities to address the existing anxiety around adolescent female sexual agency and youth sexual liaisons in general by bringing daughters back under the control of their patrilineage. As argued in this book, most people and agencies in Uganda agreed that there was a crisis of youth sexuality, but they diverged in their understanding of the causes and how best to deal the crisis. On one side, conservative social critics were bemoaning the moral decline of young people and expressed public outrage over the proliferation of sexualized images in the media, the thriving coed commercial social spaces for unmarried people, young women's independent quest for material gain, and seemingly endless sexual possibilities (such as same-sex desire). On the other side, policy makers and public health experts were warning about the impact of gender inequality on health as revealed in the grim picture painted by

TABLE 6.1. Defilement charges, Chief Magistrate Court, 1990–2001

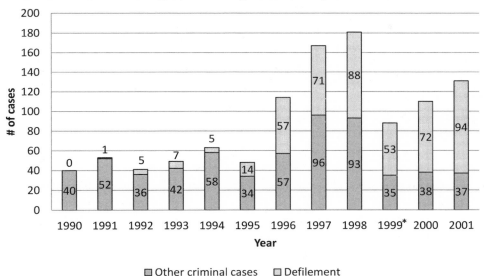

☐ Other criminal cases   ☐ Defilement

*In 1999, the Iganga Chief Magistrate was divided into two jurisdictions serving different parts of the region, resulting in an overall decline in cases sent to the Iganga Chief Magistrate.

population surveys and reports about the state of young women and girls in Uganda. While the former preached about the moral dangers of *nakyewombekeire* and their unrestrained sexual agency, progressive policy makers depicted these same young women as victims of patriarchal culture and systemic gender inequality. Within communities such as Iganga, the real effects of youth sexuality had practical consequences in the form of pregnant daughters, a disproportionately high rate of HIV, and abandonment. The divergent conceptualizations of the problem and intervention efforts led to a perfect storm for Yahaya and other poor young men who became easy and dispensable collateral damage amid conflicting attempts to protect young girls from lives of poverty and destruction.

Communities throughout Uganda found that the newly amended and highly publicized defilement law provided a legal mechanism for dealing with the youth crisis. But that was not the intention of the law's designers and advocates. In 1990, women's and children's rights advocates won a legislative battle to increase the age of consent from fourteen to eighteen years old and to elevate the categorization of the offence from civil to criminal, with the maximum penalty of death by hanging (section 123 of the Ugandan penal code [1950], cap. 106).[1] A main aim of the law was to address the sexual exploitation of adolescent and young girls from older men, which was thought to be a major factor in the gender disparities in health and social outcomes. The aggressive anti-defilement campaign that immediately followed the passing of the law led to a rapid increase in reported defilement cases throughout Uganda. Data my research assistants and I compiled from the chief magistrate's court in Iganga confirms this. For instance, there were zero reported cases of defilement in 1990, but they accounted for 50 percent of all criminal cases in 1996 and over 70 percent in 2001 (see Table 6.1).

Despite the demonstrated success in promoting the law, and the dramatic increase in reported cases, the law had unintended consequences locally. This sentiment was shared by other stakeholders. The Iganga chief magistrate felt the rapid increase of defilement cases was causing a "severe backlog of cases," many of which fell into a "gray area," where criminality and consent were unclear. Women's advocates in Kampala also expressed concern about the law. They worried that the intended offenders—sugar daddies and pedophiles—were evading the law while the law was being used to settle other sorts of community and household conflicts. Our data confirms both the magistrate's and women's rights advocates' concerns. Specifically, the average age of the males accused of defilement in the Iganga legal system was 21.5 years old, and further investigation reveals that many of these young men were charged with having sex with an adolescent girl.

A look at how cases of youth sexual liaisons were being arbitrated before the defilement amendment brings things into sharper focus. Before the amendment and aggressive campaigns, such cases found their way into state arbitration venues as child support cases. They were commonly referred to the Probate (Domestic Affairs) Office when village-level approaches failed to offer an adequate outcome. Yahaya's case represented what had been an ongoing anxiety over pregnant teenage daughters, but the defilement law allowed parents to stop a relationship before it resulted in a conception. At the heart of the issue in many of the teen pregnancy and child support cases were parents' concerns about having to provide extended economic support for their pregnant daughters to help raise a child that technically belonged to a different patrilineage. Hence, the predominance of teen pregnancy and child support cases in the Probate Office demonstrated that there had already been a growing concern about legitimacy, belonging, and the economy.

The large number of cases involving young lovers—and, conversely, the frequency with which the intended perpetrators, sugar daddies, evade the law—demonstrates how, when refracted through local anxieties and hierarchies, the deployment of the age of consent law has had unintended uses and consequences. Specifically, despite their stated efforts to *protect* adolescent females from sugar daddies and pedophiles and the subsequent burdens of HIV and single motherhood that these men bring, legal reformers and community residents have inadvertently bolstered patriarchal *control* over the female body—what feminist legal scholar Michelle Oberman calls "the twin themes of protection and patriarchal control over a girl's sexuality" (2001:803). An analysis of defilement cases in Iganga reveals that what is "defiled" in many instances is not necessarily the girl's sexual rights (as intended by the law's advocates), but rather her father's patriarchal rights over his daughter's sexuality, honor, and potential economic gain from bridewealth and other gifts from future husbands, in-laws, and grandchildren. This conception of the female body as the property of a male guardian is precisely what helped facilitate the public acceptance of the defilement law nationally and in Iganga. As Oberman argues (in discussing the case of the United States), the notion of age of consent is a reflection of the long-standing assumption that "virginity was so highly prized that a man who took a girl's virginity without her father's permission was considered to have committed a theft against the father" (2001:802).

Much of the existing scholarship on the evolution and use of age of consent and statutory rape laws is based on those of the United States and northern Europe and primarily focuses on either fathers' rights or progressive female reformers' efforts to domesticate and lift up lower-class young females.[2] In Uganda the law is as much about the patriarchal regulation of young (poor) men's sexual access to young females as it is about fathers' rights and notions of modern girlhood.[3] Hence, the law has reinstated two important features of patriarchy. First, the law provides a way for fathers to reassert their *traditional* authority over their daughters' sexuality—an authority that residents believe has been fading over the last few decades as freely floating young women with weakened ties to patrilineal groups assert their sexual autonomy (as discussed in the previous chapter). Second, the law becomes a tool for reinstating or sustaining age and class hierarchies among men. Importantly, I argue that patriarchy is not simply about men's dominance over women, but also about hierarchies among men. In short, against the backdrop of moral anxieties and shifting economic relationships, the defilement law provides senior men a way to restore some of their historical but weakened authority over the sexual and reproductive affairs of unmarried young women within their kin group as well as addressing junior men's blatant disrespect for obtaining proper permission from senior males. My main analytic aim of this chapter is not to document discourses and legal logic used within the legal system—what is often called a case approach to legal reasoning—but rather to see how legal tools and ideas surrounding the age of consent are reworked and folded into everyday understandings of and anxieties surrounding sexuality, the female body, and rights.[4]

Debating Access and Rights to Young Female Bodies

The debates about Uganda's defilement law in Uganda hearken back to the early 1900s, when the British colonial government instituted throughout many of its colonies "Offenses against Morality" statutes, setting the age of consent at fourteen years old. This was part of the larger colonial morality project aimed at spreading British Christian ideologies around issues of sexuality and gender by defining and classifying acts such as rape, elopement, indecent assault, defilement, prostitution, bestiality, incest, and sodomy. While cases of and debates about prostitution, incest, "offences against nature" (such as same-sex acts), and elopement are found in colonial records and likely reflected contemporary concerns in Britain at the time, I found no evidence that age of consent violations had risen to the same level of concern. Many of the colonial laws governing sexual matters in Africa focused on marriage and adult sexuality, often with the purpose of ensuring a labor supply through the regulation of adult female sexuality and settling disputes among men about rights over a woman and her labor (see, for example, Allman and Tashjian 2000; Jeater 1993; Thomas 2003; White 1990; Schmidt 1990). During the same period in Britain, the socioeconomic status of the girl played a large role in determining if sexual activity with a girl under the age of consent was considered a crime, with the sexuality of lower-class girls seen as already soiled and available to wealthier men (a situation that moral reformers hoped to change).

Oral histories I collected in Iganga suggest that sexual violations involving young females were typically handled between the girl's family (which was seen as the victim) and the offending party or adjudicated by local elders or chief's councils. An important aspect of understanding contemporary uses of the defilement law is that consent violations were not tied to a girl's ability to consent but rather whether consent had been obtained from the father. There was no standard biological age that established a girl's sexual availability; rather, this determination was based on several interconnected factors, such as menarche, socioeconomic class, and bodily appearance. Consent to obtain sexual access to a female among the Basoga, as in other groups in Africa, was established by gaining permission from the father (often through the negotiation of bridewealth) or through the payment of a fine (*omutango*) to the father if the man had engaged with sex before obtaining permission. A father's leverage to negotiate for either bridewealth or *omutango* largely depended on his socioeconomic position within the community and the public reputation or purity of his daughter, leading in some cases to strict supervision of daughters, as seen in Lydia's case.

The age of consent began to receive national attention after Museveni took power in the late 1980s. Women advocates found Museveni's initial platform conducive for tackling the gender violence and inequality that they believed had escalated and gone unchecked during Uganda's previous twenty-five years of internal insecurity. They believed that the abuses of gender violence enacted by the military and state police had helped to create a general ambivalence toward gender violence and exploitation. The age of consent bill was part of a series of strategies that sought to call attention to and abate this social acceptability and frequency of gender violence and sexual violations against women and girls. Of specific concern were (1) data that showed Uganda had the highest teenage pregnancy rate in sub-Saharan Africa, at 31 percent for females ages 15–19 (or 203 per 1,000), and (2) serosurveys that revealed girls were disproportionately infected with HIV (at a rate of 5:1) compared to their male counterparts (Population Reference Bureau 2007). Studies had shown that the sugar daddy phenomenon was a major factor in fueling the poor outcomes, and providing girls legal protection seemed to offer punishment with the most teeth. The law's advocates wanted not only to provide young females legal protection against preying men but, equally important, to publicly challenge what had become the social acceptability of older men's pursuit of adolescent and younger women, a practice that had become not only a common occurrence among the military and other men of power but also a survival strategy for young women during the previous decades of unrest. The early years of President Museveni's regime offered a political environment suitable for gender-progressive policies.

The initial response among some policy makers was to trivialize the measure, for it was seen as an unnecessary distraction from more serious problems. The general sentiment among many male policy makers was that rebuilding the economy, controlling the conflict in the northern and western parts of the country, and revitalizing a decaying public infrastructure should take precedent over domestic issues such as gender and sexuality. However, the foundation of President Museveni's national restructuring plan, as laid out in a ten-point plan, explicitly included investigations into human rights violations, specifically by the police and soldiers, and women advocates leaned on this policy emphasis for legitimacy (Khiddu-Makubuya 1991; Mutibwa 1992; Pirouet 1991). While women's rights were not listed as a specific aspect of human rights protection, Museveni publicly stated his commitment to women's issues and gender equality to Parliament, the media, and to international and national women's rights organizations (Mbire-Barungi 1999). Some claimed that Museveni's speeches about gender equality were more about rhetoric than conviction and were designed to gain favor and attract funding from international donors, governments, and bodies (Boyd 1989). Regardless of Museveni's intention, women's advocates seized on his desire to present his regime as forward- thinking to an international audience eager to return to Uganda.

Although Uganda began receiving positive international publicity, the notion of the rights of the girl child met resistance and trivializing during early discussions about the Children's Bill, the initial legislation that proposed to extend the protected category of "child" from fourteen to eighteen and therefore provided the legal basis for the amended defilement law. The new definition of a child being a person under the age of eighteen drew great ridicule, particularly when it came to defining a girl child. Sylvia Tamale reports that "during the [1990] debate on the children's bill . . . a Muslim MP stood up and said, 'Increasing the age of minority to eighteen years is unrealistic and unscientific; the prophet Mohammed married Aisha when she was nine years old.' Loud laughter ensued" (1999:122). Such opposition followed the discussion of the amended defilement law. Many MPs and political observers believed that age of consent violations were part of the private realm and thus more appropriately handled at the community level (Tamale 2001).

Even more powerful was how critics spun the debates into evidence of a Museveni-backed feminist campaign against men. Miria Matembe, a member of Parliament and a well-known women's rights advocate, became a favorite target. In an article entitled "Women Demand Castration for Men over Sex Abuse," Matembe's soon-to-be-famous quote first appeared: "Men are in possession of a potentially dangerous instrument which should be cut off unless it is properly used" (Muhangi 1991). Critics of the age of consent crusade repeatedly invoked Matembe's call to castrate men as a way of drawing attention to the social terror being promoted by radical female social reformers, viewing it as yet another attack on the already crumbling patrilineal kinship system that historically offered communities local stability and cohesion through reinforcing male power.

A satirical cartoon appearing in the *New Vision* newspaper a few days after the Matembe story visually reinforced the idea that the defilement law was unnecessarily barbaric and damaging to community cohesion. The 1991 cartoon showed a scared and vulnerable man with bound hands at the entrance of a "Castration Center," being greeted by two robust women, one holding a large pair of scissors and the other wielding a machete. His prepubescent accuser stands next to him, displaying equal fear and confusion as the man prepares for his impending emasculation. Directly below the fear-invoking cartoon was a separate editorial about the seductive strategies of adolescent girls entitled "School girls provoke." Together, the cartoon and the editorial provide an example of the daily images and discourses that fed the public perception of the anti-defilement campaign as a misdirected war against men. According

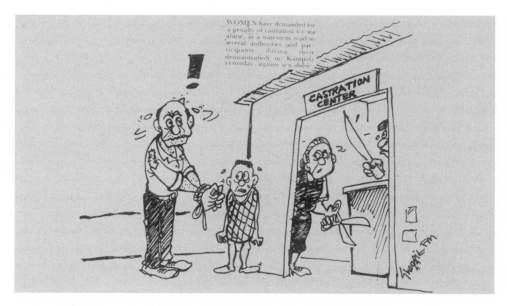

FIGURE 6.1. "Castration Center" cartoon, *New Vision*, December 18, 1991

to this narrative, men are not the perpetrators of sexual exploitation but rather the victims of adolescent girls' sexual seduction and the helpless targets of feminist attacks. Women activists were portrayed as emotional, irrational, and jealous of nubile, sexually attractive young women—a segment of the population recast as Uganda's new breed of self-interested *femmes fatales*. Other earlier critiques of the defilement law portrayed women reformers as anti-modern by highlighting how the bill curtailed young women's free will and their ability to select sexual partners for themselves. Beneath the surface of popular debates about the proper role of government in protecting girls and young women from older men, an even more revealing sub-conversation was taking place, showing how the category of "adolescence"—that is, deserving of protection—is intricately tied to class, education, and family status. The debates revealed how players with ideologically different agendas construct visions of the health of the nation in the context of HIV and teenage pregnancy based on particular conceptions of young women's sexual agency and men's sexual privilege.

The ongoing conflicts about women's and girls' rights and the role of the state in private matters reflects the construction of women activists as a threat to the natural patriarchal order that had historically allowed for the reproduction of African societies. Matembe became a symbol of the anti-man and hence anti-African movement, with opponents periodically invoking her castration threat to serve both as a warning to men to be vigilant about their rights and as a fear tactic to discourage other women from following her lead. However, instead of discouraging the support of women, the idea of Matembe as the leader of the "castration brigade" was appropriated by women reformers to mobilize for causes and was embraced by younger and older women in Iganga with whom I interacted. Matembe was seen as a mother of the women's movement, with an increasing following and admirers. In a newspaper commentary entitled

"Matembe: 'Castration brigade' takes charge," author and politician Mary Karooro Okurut proclaimed, "Thank God the gender-quake is rocking Uganda in a positive direction" (1998).

Each gender and sexual rights law that has passed since has been done after careful recrafting of the initial public message, making the intent and spirit behind the specific proposed law less about dismantling African traditions, a discourse used in this instance to invoke safety and security, and more about allowing citizens to live with both protections and freedoms. In the case of the anti-defilement campaigns, amid public scrutiny of the intention, advocates of the law formulated new arguments in favor of increasing the age of consent, eventually finding widespread and less controversial appeal in the image of the innocent girl child. By shifting the issue away from the prosecution of men and calling attention to data that showed the vulnerability of girl children, reformers were able to deflect allegations that the law was an attack on men and men's historical (and hence, natural) gender role and rights. Invoking the need to protect the innocent girl child is an indirect and unthreatening strategy used by women reformers—a strategy called "maternalism" in scholarship on the United States and Northern Europe (Gordon 1990, 1995; Koven and Michel 1993; Gordon 1995). Scholars note that maternalist strategies have been effectively used in highly patriarchal legislatures and in contexts where structural gender inequalities and gender violence are central to the construction of hegemonic masculinity. The maternalist strategy produces successful results because women are not seen as asking for their own rights; rather, they call on male legislators (as well as men in general) to stand by them to protect innocent daughters, sisters, and nieces. By drawing on the idea of the innocent child, feminist reformers in Uganda ended up with a greater voice and more power in political debates without seeming to request rights or equality for themselves. Ironically, the maternalist strategy that produced such results had the unintended consequence of reinforcing the patriarchal notion that young women and adolescent girls need to be protected not only from exploitation by others but also from their own potentially self-destructive choices.

Advocates' deployment of the rights of children emerged within a global context of growing humanitarian attention around the 1989 International Convention on the Rights of the Child (ICRC) and related international reports, declarations, and conferences.[5] Global media and donor interest in children's rights (particularly in the Third World) offered Uganda's anti-defilement campaign legitimacy, strength, discursive framing, and, importantly, ample financial and technical resources. The language of children's rights allowed women reformers to justify legally extending childhood until the age of eighteen on the grounds that the nation needed to catch up to a modern world. By positioning females under the age of eighteen as under the protected status of children, advocates sought to recast gendered health and social inequalities not as natural occurrences, but rather as the consequence of illegal and coercive male sexual behavior toward underage girls who lacked the mental, emotional, or physical ability to resist. Defilement thus was woven into various seduction narratives in which girls were depicted as innocent victims trying to overcome great odds at home, in the community, and at school. If a girl went astray, it was not of her own free will, but because her innocence was violated. She was defiled—either by being married off, seduced by a man, or impregnated—and heartlessly left to suffer. Raising and enforcing the age of consent, according to advocates of the law, would shield young women from sexual predators by legally lengthening their childhood, thereby providing them with a protected environment in which to mature physically and emotionally and allowing them to develop skills that would lead to greater economic and social independence from men.

However, the application of a universalist notion of rights, as scholars have demonstrated in other places and times, is often fraught with unintended contradictions, paradoxes, and miscalculations (see Goodale 2006a, 2006b; Merry 2001; Messer 1997; Cowan 2006; Adams 1998; Stoeltje 2002). In this particular instance, the sugar daddy who evades legal consequences, and his nemesis, the poor younger boyfriend, represent such contradictions. While the amended law expressly targeted cases involving sugar daddies and pedophiles, such cases were in reality largely settled out of court and were commonly dealt with as they had been in the past, either by negotiations between the offending man and the girl's family or by ignoring the incident because the economic benefit accrued to the family outweighed any moral dilemma. On the other hand, relationships such as that of Yahaya and Lydia made up the bulk of prosecuted cases. Understanding how this paradox was generated and sustained requires a look at historically and socially produced sexual economies within a specific setting.

Local Uses and Abuses of the Defilement Law: Age, Gender, and Class

When I began ethnographic research in Iganga in 1996, the defilement law was fairly common knowledge among younger and older residents. Posters depicting adolescent girls being preyed on by older men were regularly seen in government buildings and in health clinics around the dusty agrarian town. Slogans such as "Support Your Friends" and "Report Defilers" attempted to shift the culture of silence into a collective obligation to speak about sexual abuse and vigilantly protect girls from sexual predators and the transmission of HIV (Figure 6.2). Another set of posters featured a prepubescent girl being enticed by a friendly-looking man holding out a piece of candy. Gossip about local cases spread easily through gathering places, and rarely did I hear great shock over the numerous defilement stories reported in the media. The idea of men having (and taking advantage of their) sexual privilege over younger females was not new. The defilement campaign was at the heart of a social marketing campaign that attempted to consolidate the wide range of configurations of these liaisons into one shared concept. The social marketing campaign was designed to bring what had been general public silence about these relationships into the public sphere of discussion, debate, and outrage, transforming how communities thought about male sexual privilege and access to girls' sexuality. Given its relatively recent insertion into public discourse and the initial heated debates, I was struck by how easily the defilement law fit into local ideology, talk, and practice in Iganga. This was especially surprising given that men's sexual advances toward much younger women were a historical social reality (though they often defied cultural rules, as discussed below), and had not previously been conceptualized locally as defilement. However, the ease with which the concept of sexual violations of

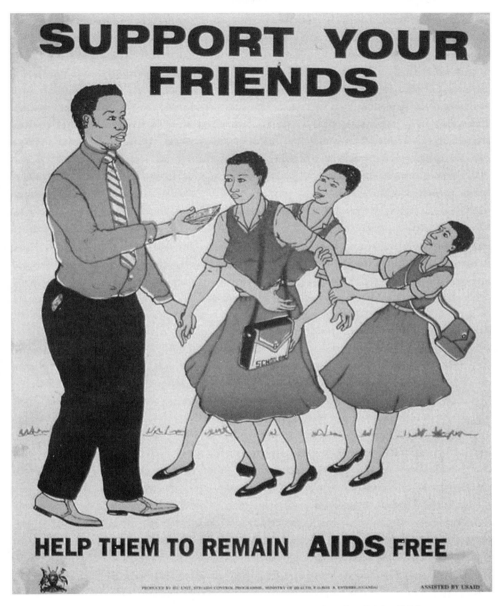

FIGURE 6.2. Defilement campaign: Poster of sugar daddy with schoolgirls, 1990s

girls was absorbed into local discourse reflected fears about the state of youth sexuality, and particularly adolescent female sexuality.

Whereas residents of Iganga are generally aware that Uganda's 1990 law and public discourse extended childhood to the age of eighteen, they hold complex views about the age categorization and sexual agency of adolescent girls. Historically, the transition from child to adult depended less on chronological age and more on biological, economic, and social factors, such as a girl's physical body, reproductive history, family's economic status, and educational prospects. The economic status of a girl and her family inevitably underwrites perceptions about a girl's maturation and sexual responsibility. A girl from a poor family not attending school is perceived as transitioning out of innocent childhood and into a sexually available woman sooner than a school-going girl—say, from a middle-class family. Likewise, a girl under the age of consent who reproduces is considered adult enough to take on adult responsibilities and duties, and subsequent cases of older men having sexual relations with her might not be seen as defilement. Hence, the status of innocence and the legal protection that accompanies the international category of "child"—two central aspects of the defilement law as reformers conceived it—are more accessible to adolescent girls who are perceived by communities and law enforcement as future productive (read: middle- and upper-class) members of society. Their poorer counterparts, on the other hand, are often perceived as sexually knowing or, as elders say, "despoiled" because they are assumed either to have knowledge about sex or to have engaged in sexual liaisons (see Patton 1996). These sexually "knowing" young people fall outside of the protection of the state, which is reserved for the "innocent" girl child for whom adulthood is properly delayed. Given their low economic and education status, poorer girls are instead perceived as potential burdens to society because their out-of-wedlock pregnancies drain resources from the natal family and the community or because they might be lured into dubious economic activities, such as commercial sex work or selling local brew and hence pleasures to (married) men. This flexible social classification of the teenage girl—as either innocent child or sexually knowing adult—has complicated local uses of the defilement law.

The anti-defilement campaigns attempted to broaden the range of punishable male sexual pursuits to include not only acts that were historically considered egregious (such as pedophilia) but also liaisons that had not previously been considered improper (such as relationships between adolescent girls and older men).[6] In narratives of elders, it is clear that liaisons between pubescent girls and older, middle-class men represent a historical privilege of wealthy men within a context of economic desperation. These were not conceptualized as abuses of power, but rather privileges of power. Yet there were increasingly vocal opinions, especially among older women, that these liaisons were unacceptable, for they left the adolescent girl with limited social mobility and options.

This vocal opinion of women, however, does not necessarily translate into their use of the defilement law in prosecuting sugar daddies. While women are critical of men's abuses of power over adolescent girls and young women, mothers are much less likely than fathers to initiate defilement cases. This gender difference in the use of the state court system has a long historical trajectory that began during the British colonial regime, when women were considered dependents of their fathers or husbands. As a result, women were unable to bring cases themselves to the colonial state court and often were not able to offer an official testimony (Fallers 1969). Instead, a woman would enlist the assistance of a male representative to present her case. The intertwining of this colonial court history and contemporary gender equalities in formal institutions has had a tremendous impact on the gendered use of the state legal system. This is not to say that women do not air their grievances; rather, they are more likely to go to one of the more recent and accessible arbitration venues, such as the Probate Office, local councils, or NGO legal services. These alternative offices, however, cannot convict offenders and are focused on negotiation and arbitration. Similar to the past, today most of the defilement cases brought through the legal system in Iganga are initiated by the father of the girl. "Father" here can refer to a girl's biological father, another male in her patrilineage, or at times the brother of her mother working on behalf of the mother. There is also a gender difference in how mothers and fathers choose to settle cases. Women are less likely to use the threat of defilement against boyfriends but are more likely to make public cases involving sugar daddies, though they do not necessarily take them to the legal system. Sugar daddy cases remain a significantly smaller portion of prosecution and trial registries. The case of Musa, a fifty-something serial sugar daddy, demonstrates why these cases continue to evade the judicial system.

Senior Men: Sugar Daddies, Fathers, and *Omutango*

Musa is an affable and charming wealthy businessman and is respected among residents not for his morality but for having the cleverness and drive to rise from a poor background to become one of the elites in town. I met Musa in 2004, shortly after the youngest of his four co-wives, Aisha, had posted bail for him. I developed a friendly relationship with both of them, though I rarely engaged with them together. Aisha was frustrated with his repeated affairs with schoolgirls and the money his family wasted on getting him out of trouble, but she did not easily recognize that her own marriage had begun in the same manner some six years earlier. She appeared to be more upset that his most recent relationship was with her younger sister than she was with the latest defilement charges against him. Aisha was conflicted but heavily jealous about her husband's liaisons with her sister. In one interview she declared that her husband's affair with her sister was almost over, while in the next she revealed that he had built her a house in town. To Aisha, the relationship between her sister and husband posed the greatest threat to her marriage, in addition to being an inexcusable betrayal of sororal loyalty. Aisha managed to dismiss the public humiliation she might have felt from Musa's reputation as a serial sugar daddy with a weakness for adolescent schoolgirls.

Many of Musa's liaisons with schoolgirls did not result in formal legal cases, but were settled when Musa, through an emissary, offered money or other compensatory arrangements to the girls' parents, such as paying off debts or helping a family member obtain employment. The case that was being resolved when I met the couple had been reported to the police by a local official; I heard conflicting rumors about why this particular local leader decided to file a report. One rumor was that he had a personal feud with Musa; another was that the official's female counterparts pressured him to follow official procedures for sexual abuse cases; and yet another version places the dissatisfied and angry father of the schoolgirl at the center of Musa's arrest. This particular case landed Musa in jail overnight and led Aisha on a frantic hunt to secure the large cash bond of two-and-a-half-million shillings (about 1,400 USD) for his release. Soon after, though, the case was dropped. According to rumor, part of the bail money was a bribe to get the case dropped; it was supposedly split among the relevant police officers, the schoolgirl's parents, and the reporting local official. The parents expressed concern about the relationship but eventually decided to resolve the case outside the formal judicial system in exchange for financial compensation.

The cases involving Musa demonstrate how some parents are willing to ignore a man's illegal liaisons with their daughters in exchange for material gain. In attempting to account for this tendency, many people I spoke with pointed to the widespread corruption among local law enforcement officials and the ability of middle-class men to meet the financial demands of the girls' parents. The Iganga chief magistrate commented on sugar daddies' abilities to avoid the law by remarking, "It's hard to charge that one" in court if "the man is a source of income for the parents." The income from the man may be direct, as in the form of a cash payment, or indirect, as in the form of paying for school fees, clothing, or other future needs of the family. Given Uganda's widespread poverty and high unemployment, the patron-client ties this dynamic revolves around remain crucial to the lives of the majority of people in the country. Jeopardizing such ties by prosecuting the wealthy man could mean risking future economic or social benefits from a local "big-man" (Vincent 1971) or alienating oneself from neighbors who also reap or hope to reap benefits from the man. "A rich criminal is greater use to a community out of jail than in jail," an older woman commented. Thus, the economic gain from a settlement is transferred from the girl—who likely reaped some gain in the transactional liaison—to her parents, who use the threat of the defilement law to secure a financial reward for themselves.

This economic rationalization, however, fails to take into account an important cultural dimension of sexual relationships between older men and adolescent girls in Uganda. This same liaison that is a continual source of frustration for women reformers and HIV agencies, paradoxically, comprises powerful signs of modernity—the wealthy, suit-wearing older male and the neatly uniformed and disciplined schoolgirl. This symbolic pairing not only draws from images of Uganda's future progress but can also be understood as part of a historical trajectory during which elite landholding men were given sexual access to the daughters of commoners, through marriage, temporary domestic servitude, or some other arrangement, to pay off debts or in return for continual favors—an extension of the big-man phenomena. The sugar daddy/schoolgirl pairing is a modern-day, repackaged version of a historically occurring and sometimes sanctioned relationship (Parikh 2004). This pairing not only provided a way for poorer families to pay off debt, but formed part of a social network that assisted in solidifying ties within areas, serving to mediate relations between potentially warring groups, avoid social conflicts, and secure new territories for leaders.

There is yet another way that cases such as Musa's fit into the local sexual economy. The historical use of young women and girls as sexual pawns in social and economic negotiations had its own set of moral rules that tied it to the patrilineage system. Basoga tradition offered a father or another guardian two options if he were dissatisfied about his daughter's entering into a sexual union or cohabitation without his consent. He could sue for her return, which Fallers (1969) found common in Busoga local courts in the 1950s, he could claim *omutango* (compensation) for unauthorized sexual access to his daughter, or he could at times try both options. Over time, both practices have gradually become a less significant part of the local social system as the influence of poorer fathers over daughters has weakened. The defilement law has become a recent, state-sponsored way to initiate the historical process of obtaining *omutango* from unauthorized sexual partners of daughters. Wealthier men such as Musa have the economic resources to pay *omutango* and the social capital to evade the law. Normally, the prosecution of younger men stems from having limited access to both. What emerges is a vulnerable masculinity among younger men, as in the case of Yahaya.

Generational Tensions: Delinquent Daughters, Defiant Boys

Early on the day of his arrest, two police officers met Yahaya. After a brief exchange, the officers hauled the young man to the police station, where they handcuffed him to a metal table. He remained in the darkened room for a few hours until more law enforcement agents appeared with a man and his pregnant teenaged daughter. The pregnant girl stood behind her father as three police officers began their interrogation. After a series of routine questions, they asked the young man if he knew the girl in the room. Yahaya said yes, explaining that she was the daughter of the middle-aged man in the room, a neighbor who lived across the pathway that ran in front of the room he rented on the outskirts of town. The officers then asked the pregnant girl if it was Yahaya who had impregnated her, which she confirmed. In his own defense, Yahaya claimed that a week before he had given the girl's mother money for the girl's medical expenses and explained that he would continue to provide financial assistance to the baby. "Work has been slow," he pleaded, "but I will provide assistance when I get paid."

The case moved seamlessly through the criminal justice system, providing good evidence for national monitoring bodies that law enforcement and the legal system in Iganga were working together and taking defilement seriously. About four months before the end of Yahaya's initial sentence, his sentence was extended by six months when the father claimed that Yahaya had defied court orders by communicating with his daughter through a letter delivered by a friend. The father, according to a court clerk, brought the letter as evidence that the defiant young man had no respect for the law or authority. Neither Yahaya nor the daughter was given an opportunity to respond to the charges. The situation between Yahaya and the girl is suggestive of various analytic interpretations. Yahaya's case exemplifies how class and age determine a man's culpability, and subsequently how the triple helix of class, age, and criminality gets reproduced and strengthened through systematic use of the defilement law. Yahaya's sentence might not have been as harsh had he not been perceived as part of the group of visibly underemployed young men who were a threat to a girl's upward mobility, and had the girl had not been seen (at least by some) as part of Uganda's future promise. The pregnancy symbolically represented the socially and morally corrupting force of Uganda's idle young men.

The image of a working-class man in dirty clothes polluting the "virginity" of a well-groomed schoolgirl is a common visual theme in anti-defilement campaigns, where it takes on the symbolic connotation of Uganda's dark underdeveloped past threatening the nation's arrival into modernity. The implication is that poorer men—who are imagined as unable to obtain sexual access to younger or older women by the historically

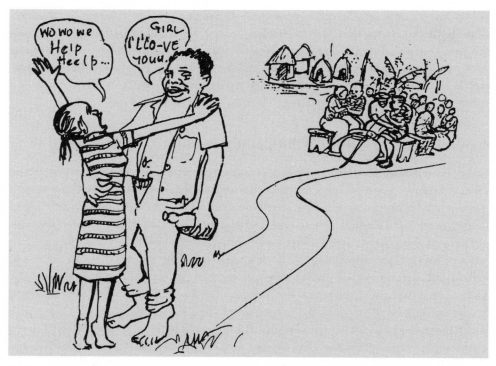

FIGURE 6.3. Defilement campaign: *Talking with our Children about Sex and Growing Up* pamphlet, Uganda AIDS Commission and UNICEF, 1990s

legitimate means of exchanging bridewealth with her appropriate clan members—will take unsuspecting adolescent girls by force or through subtle coercion (Figure 6.3). Throughout the interviews about this case, Yahaya's poor socioeconomic status and limited possibility for upward mobility were continually contrasted to Lydia's future potential and upwardly mobile status, which were demonstrated by her attending one of Iganga's more prestigious secondary schools. In order to establish the degree of violation, Lydia's father repeatedly invoked her schoolgirl status and how it had been despoiled by Yahaya's impregnation.

Shifting our analytic gaze to narratives about the transactional dynamics of the liaison offers another interpretation of why this case resulted in Yahaya's imprisonment. Both Yahaya and Lydia agree that their relationship began with a gift exchange. They met during a school holiday, when Yahaya noticed his attractive neighbor as she tended to chores in her father's house. After exchanging a few glances and smiles, Yahaya asked Lydia to visit him at his place of work, in the town's busy outdoor marketplace and transportation hub. The next day, Lydia and her friend passed by and waited for Yahaya to finish loading crates of soda onto a delivery truck. Seeing the two adolescent girls, Yahaya and a coworker waved two soda bottles, signaling for them to come closer. The girls approached and accepted the sodas. Lydia and Yahaya arranged to meet again at his home the next day.

Their stories diverge when discussing the gift exchange aspect of the relationship, which might point to their mutual acknowledgment of the problematic nature of sex-for-money relationships. According to Yahaya, "In the [initial] conversation, she asked me for some money. I told her she should come to my home for the money she wanted. She came and found me. I gave her the money and she went." Lydia's version of the money exchange was slightly different. As she explains, "Yahaya said he wanted to become friends with me and I asked him what will he do for me. He told me to come at his place on Saturday and he will show me. On Saturday when I went to his place, he told me he loved me and offered to buy me fabric from town. I said my parents would begin asking questions, so he agreed to give me money instead." A week after the gift exchange, Yahaya and Lydia began their sexual relationship. That neither Yahaya nor Lydia wants to be seen as initiating the economic aspect of their relationship points to the effects of the public critiques regarding transactional relationships—a shifting moral economy in which the gift-for-sex exchange takes on new meanings about a person's self-interested greed and desire. Hence, while the exchange of bridewealth is seen as a transaction between male and female members of two exogamous kingroups, sex-for-gifts relationships involve two parties acting as autonomous sexual agents with little regard for their *máka* (place of belonging) and or the wider moral economy that binds together a community.

While Yahaya was found guilty of defilement, young women are often seen as more blameworthy than men in transactional sex liaisons. Iganga residents' perceptions of the ways in which young women use their sexuality for material gain have left many people ambivalent about adolescent defilement cases. Many older residents feel that adolescent female sexual agency and their desire for modern goods have caused men to lose sexual control. In the words of one elder, "Our girls have gotten out of hand. They give themselves away so cheaply."

As discussed in a previous chapter, youth sexual relations defy notions of parental authority and are often classified under the general term *obwenzi*, which can be roughly translated locally as "sexual promiscuity," or in anthropological terms as "sexual impropriety." While the concept has shifted over time, during my research *obwenzi* frequently referred to the exchange of sex for modern material goods, such as makeup, clothes, and beauty products, or of cohabiting without parental consent. According to Iganga residents, *obwenzi* and the moral decline from which it stems led to and fueled the rampant spread of HIV and teenage pregnancy. However, adults also make an important distinction between *obwenzi* and defilement as defined by law: the former involves delinquent daughters who engage in *obwenzi*, and the latter refers to the sexual abuse of young girls or daughters who are seduced by men of power.

Cases of young lovers demonstrate another way in which the age of consent debate is less about age than it is about violations of obtaining parental consent. While this notion of failing to obtain parental consent is similar to sugar daddy violations, a key distinction is that young suitors are also violating age hierarchies among men, providing further evidence that youth have abandoned cultural ideas of morality that had previously kept a community socially safe. For parents such as Lydia's, the defilement law restores some control over a daughter's sexual autonomy by punishing a suitor who, from the perspective of the parents, cannot provide adequate compensation to them or care for their daughter. In the words of a local saying, "Ákúsígúla, tákúkwa" (One who entices you away will not pay bridewealth).

Contesting Notions of Consent and Blame

The notion of consent becomes further complicated when considered with a related concept, blame. The case of a fourteen-year-old girl who engaged in sexual relations with a teenage shop attendant in town illuminates how notions of consent and blame are intricately woven. As part of the girl's evening chores, her parents sent her to town regularly to purchase goods and food. A young shop attendant often offered the unescorted girl free items and eventually invited her to his room, located behind the shop. One day after returning from town, the mother noticed that the girl's way of walking had changed, and inquired about the change. The daughter evaded the topic of sexual intercourse by blaming her new stride on a boil between her legs. Concerned and suspicious, the mother took the girl to the doctor. Unable to hide her sexual activity, the girl revealed at the doctor's office that she had been having intercourse with the attendant. The girl's parents confronted the young man and his parents and explained that they were willing to forgive the boy in exchange for a fine of 300,000 shillings (about 170 USD). When the young man's mother could not produce the amount, the girl's parents became incensed: "We have been kind enough to you. What kind of person are you? You have destroyed our girl and you are not being considerate." The girl's parents then reported the case to the police, and the boy was arrested and eventually convicted of defilement. Separate interviews with the father and the grandmother of the girl reveal conflicting notions of responsibility and culpability.

According to the grandmother, both the girl and her parents were to blame for the girl's sexual activity. The grandmother noted that the girl "did not know what she was sent to town for because she was often not given enough money for the requested goods." The old woman further implicated the parents by stating, "You always hear over the radio to stop sending children out at night to buy things." The girls' parents did not heed the warning, sending their daughter to the evening market unattended and without proper instruction on "how to handle herself." To the old woman and others in Iganga, strict supervision and surveillance of adolescent daughters is the responsibility of parents. Gendered child-rearing roles dictate that the mother is blamed for raising a daughter of questionable moral character; a daughter's unchaste behavior is thought to reflect the mother's own inner moral failings. Hence, in addition to the generational tensions between parents and daughters that we have seen in the two previous defilement cases, this case illustrates a multigenerational dynamic of blame occurring in Uganda, in which adults claim youth are morally corrupt while elders argue that adults (or parents) are responsible for the moral failures of young people.

In other cases, adolescent girls' desire for modern luxuries is blamed for their succumbing to the temptations offered by men. While prepubescent girls are often assumed to be passive or naïve, pubescent girls are thought to possess the mental capacity and self-discipline to recognize temptation and resist it. In one case, a father found his fifteen-year-old daughter having intercourse with a teacher who had come to the house to tutor her. The father threatened the teacher with court action, but decided against it after finding out that prior to this incident his daughter had not been a virgin. The disappointed father explained, "I have nothing to do because the girl was not found a virgin." The daughter's virginity became the test for whether she was worthy of state protection.

In the case of the fourteen-year-old girl and the young shop attendant, the girl's disgruntled parents first tried to pressure the young man to either marry their daughter or support the child. Unfortunately for the young man, neither he nor his widowed mother had access to the amount of money demanded. The unsatisfied parents used the age of consent law as additional leverage against him. After the girl's pleading, the case was eventually dropped and an agreement was reached out of court. From the perspective of the girl's parents, it was better to get an out-of-court settlement or arrange for child support with the young man than to have him in jail, where he could earn no money.

Conclusion

Analysis of the defilement law as a planned intervention into youth sexuality highlights the competing ways that problems associated with youth sexuality, and hence ways to alter outcomes, are conceptualized. From the unfolding of national debates surrounding the proposed amendment and promotion of the law to its unintended uses within communities, the legal intervention demonstrates how stakeholders in Uganda have conflicting ideas about how the problem of youth sexuality was defined. Early anti-defilement social marketing campaigns, which drew from the rights-based idea of protecting girls from preying men, played an instrumental role in shaping public conversations and debates about youth sexuality. The sexual exploitation frame put forth by women's and children's rights advocates was an attempt to recast the prevailing narrative that located much of the blame for Uganda's social decline on the sexually free bodies of young *nakyewombekeire*. Instead of conceptualizing teen pregnancy and disproportionally high rates of STIs and HIV among girls as a result of their own individual immorality, undisciplined sexual agency, and greed, in the early and mid-1990s women's and children's rights advocates (and eventually the public health industry) partnered with international agencies to bring onto the public stage a discussion of the role of structural inequalities and patriarchal privilege in fueling gender disparities in social, economic, and health outcomes. The popular idea that adolescent girls were too sexually free was publicly challenged by the idea that structural factors shaped their risk and limited their options.

By the early 2000s, there was another visible shift in public discourse. A wave of social conservatism globally and within Uganda helped bring about the emergence of discourses of individual responsibility in solving Uganda's problems. Largely funded by President George W. Bush's PEPFAR program and broadly supported by Uganda's growing evangelical movement, this campaign conceptualized the problem less as a structural one and more as a problem with culture (i.e., African men behaving badly), and the structural change model took a backseat to an aggressive focus on encouraging individual responsibility (i.e., girls making the decision to remain abstinent). Ironically, the sexual agency of young females that had been erased in the defilement campaign's rhetoric of the innocence of girls was brought back in by social conservatives for whom the focus on individual responsibility (as well as "Christian" morals) was doctrinal.

No doubt these shifts in discourse and strategies shaped and reflected what was occurring in local communities, but in many ways they also exposed conflicts between rigid ideologies of national efforts and the complexities and histories of local communities. Whereas advocates of the defilement law proposed a structural solution (e.g., prosecute exploitative men and protect the rights of girls) and social conservatives promoted individual responsibility (e.g., abstain from sex), another solution was found in Iganga—a return to a past (and glorified) system of regulation. Specifically, for some residents the law was useful in restoring patriarchal control over the sexuality of adolescent girls as well as disciplining their young lovers, or bringing the sexuality of young people back into the patrilineal kinship system's clearly defined rules of consent, exchange, and respectability. Putting this use of the defilement law into dialogue with the previous chapter's discussion of the breakdown of the kin-based system of sexual development of girls, we can see how the law provides a legal mechanism for grounding *nakyewombekeire* and the proceeds from their sexuality (through *omutango*) back into the protective guardianship of their patrilineage. However, even though defilement cases in Iganga suggest a nostalgic return to the past, residents are well aware that this past system was never so perfect, nor is it able to respond to the realities faced by today's young people. The unresolved issue of boyfriends of daughters becomes collateral damage, so to speak, since charging young men with defilement at least temporarily stops the threat of a daughter's being impregnated or distracted by someone as poor as she is.

Importantly, then, the intersections of age, socioeconomic class, and gender have played a central role in how the law was conceptualized nationally and is used locally. Policy makers and parents are at odds regarding the socioeconomic class of men from which girls need to be protected. The law's initial advocates wanted to protect girls from older businessmen and sugar daddies, while parents often want to protect themselves from younger and poorer men who might impregnate and abandon their dependent daughters. Here we see how the universalist discourse about children's rights is in conflict with or complicated by class-based agendas, reflecting tensions occasioned by increased monetization, that have exacerbated local and national economic stratification. Unlike cases of sugar daddies, where the conflict is between two adult men, cases involving young lovers are about generational tensions. The former can be understood as a move to shift economic gain obtained from a daughter's sex liaison with a sugar daddy from her to her father, as the sugar daddy now has to negotiate with the father. Meanwhile, the latter is about the regulation of youth romance. In such cases, the law is used not only to punish young suitors who have transgressed generational lines of respect among men but also to control the sexuality and reproduction of delinquent daughters. Socioeconomic class also shapes how the female participant is perceived. The defilement law is phrased in terms of protecting "the girl child," regardless of other aspects of her identity. In actuality, class and perceived future potential are fundamental to the way that innocence, consent, and youthful sexuality are defined in any particular instance. The law was originally intended to protect young females; however, the selective enforcement has worked in some cases to undermine the autonomy and rights of adolescent girls, since it is the parents and other adults who determine which cases move through the judicial system and which ones are settled outside formal arbitration venues. As defilement is a criminal offense, it is a crime against the state and the parents technically receive no compensation for cases adjudicated in the courts (see also Hodgson 1996). Hence, the legal mechanism that some parents use to reinstate their rights over their daughters transfers authority to the state, a higher patriarchal power. Just like national reformers who are discovering how difficult it is to engineer social change in a desired direction through planned intervention, so too is the older generation in Iganga experiencing the unintended consequences of their attempts to reconstruct a Basoga notion of rights that they believe existed in the past.

PART III

Counterpublic

Youth Romance and Love Letters

CHAPTER 7

Geographies of Courtship and Gender in the Consumer Economy

> A relation of cruel optimism exists when something you desire is actually an obstacle to your flourishing. . . . These kinds of optimistic relations are not inherently cruel. They become cruel only when the object that draws your attachment actively impedes the aim that brought you to it initially. . . . Whatever the *experience* of optimism is in particular, then, the *affective structure* of an optimistic attachment involves a sustaining inclination to return to the scene of fantasy that enables you to expect that *this* time, nearness to *this* thing will help you or a world to become different in just the right way. But, again, optimism is cruel when the object/scene that ignites a sense of possibility actually makes it impossible to attain the expansive transformation for which a person or a people risks striving. (Berlant 2011:1–2)

A few months after I stumbled upon Sam's love letter, one of my research assistants ran into my office in town, urging me to come with him to one of the secondary schools outside of town. He excitedly informed me that the headmaster was about to *okuswaza* (expose, or publicly embarrass) students who had been caught exchanging love letters. My assistant had rushed to me in a bicycle taxi; we summoned a second taxi and rode to the school's morning assembly. The headmaster of the school waved the confiscated love letter in the air, subduing the morning chattering among the students. The three exposed wrongdoers—the writer, the recipient, and the facilitating emissary—were led from the administration building to the school's open courtyard and onto the weathered cement assembly block. The headmaster handed the letter to the writer and then gestured for the nervous girl to read her words aloud.[1] In a trembling voice, Annette read her letter to the eagerly listening crowd:

Hullo GE,

Happiness is beyond my control seeing that I am capable of writing these few lines exchanging greetings with you well.
    Sweet words of love with me. Really I have to say that my love with you kills me just only when I look at your structure, your behaviour and the way you shine like a star at night and the way you were brought up by your parents.
    Yours Faithfully,

Before Annette could finish reading, laugher erupted. Her head fell in embarrassment. It is difficult to know which might have been worse—being forced to read the intimate details of her desires to her peers, being caught in the commonplace act of love-letter writing, or being afraid about her uncertain fate at home and at school. The headmaster later informed me that the incident was to serve as a warning against what he thought had been an escalating sense of freedom and social mingling that was distracting students from their studies. With national standard exams approaching, he wanted to do everything he could to ensure that his school ranked high in the district performance rating. The public outing was also intended to reassert his authority and restore the proper social and moral order.

The morning assembly incident calls our attention to several aspects of the geographies of youth romance as explored throughout Part III of this ethnography. The incident highlights how youth participate in romantic practices with constant awareness of their vulnerable position to dominant adult structures and to the competing moral discourses that attempt in various ways to define, regulate, protect, and control youth sexuality. While this marginality leaves youth relationships in a precarious position, the risk involved in exchanging love letters and other youthful romantic practices elevates the significance as well as the pleasure of such acts. Pursuing romance in the face of danger not only indicates the extent to which a lover will go for a sweetheart but also demonstrates the independence from authority that the young person has achieved, hence increasing the person's desirability. Also revealed in this vignette is the contradictory position of schools and other socially sanctioned youth spaces that simultaneously represent progress but are also sites of moral corruption precisely because they offer new social configurations and ideas that challenge older lines of authority. These civic spaces are sites of dangerous intragenerational interactions that operate outside of the intergenerational, kinship-based system that has its own method of controlling sexual access and punishing those who transgress boundaries of sexual morality. Finally, Annette's being forced to read her letter aloud is a deliberate act of publicly shaming a young woman who has subverted gendered courtship conventions by displaying sexual agency (by actively articulating her desires in her letter) instead of following the accepted convention of passively speaking through a culturally designated intermediary. The punishment of the public reading can be considered a patriarchal attempt to discipline her as well as other (potential) *nakyewombekeire* before they fall to their own ruin.

Despite a variety of efforts to limit and regulate youth romance and sexual activity, as examined in Part II, romantic liaisons with peers are important features of young people's lives in Iganga, much as they are with adolescents around the world. Not only do these relationships offer youth companionship and venues for the exploration and development of their identities and sexuality, but they also provide access to new forms of respect and prestige among peers. Having a sweetheart is considered a demonstration of maturity and sophistication. More than just a private affair between two lovers, developing a relationship with a sweetheart requires active engagement with the public spheres, attention to Uganda's vibrant consumer economy of sexuality, and a fine understanding of how the world of youthful romance operates in relation to dominant structures. Hence, Nancy Fraser's term "counterpublic" appropriately characterizes the world of youthful romance and draws attention to its relationship to dominant regulatory structures as being one of complementarity and resistance. Fraser argues that marginalized groups form "subaltern counterpublics" that are "parallel discursive arenas where members of subordinated social groups invent and circulate counterdiscourses to formulate oppositional interpretations of their identities, interests, and needs" (1990:67). By conceptualizing youth romance as the creation of a counterpublic, I intend to demonstrate that youth romance is not an event or series of single events or relationships but a *process* through which young people express new forms of status among peers in an alternative romantic world that is constantly surveilled by concerned adults and thwarted by the economic and social precarities that surround them.

We now shift our analytic gaze away from Part II's examination of Uganda's sexual publics, which have been shaped by the country's active AIDS industry, vibrant mass media and consumer economy, the rise of evangelicalism, and policy reforms. These publics have influenced the ways in which the sexuality of unmarried young people is monitored and disciplined, and has made the adolescent female body the platform for public debate about morality. In Part III, I narrow my analytic focus to the inner workings of the counterpublic of youth intimacy and romance. I consider how the contours and practices of youth romance emerge in particular ways, given the historical and wider contexts described in the previous chapters, and pay particular attention to how youthful romance interacts with competing ideologies of gender and sexuality circulating around Uganda. Additional contexts that come into play include monetization of the economy, the anxiety and secrecy surrounding youth sexual culture, and persistent economic and gender inequalities. This chapter and the next provide the contextual contours of the counterpublic of youth romance, highlighting the gendered dynamics that reproduce and challenge ideologies offered to youth by dominant structures.

Analysis of the context of letter exchange shows that the counterpublic of youth romance represents more than discursive and identity politics at work; it also has an economic primacy and function. Given that youth's ideal commercialized notion of romance is out of reach for most, love letters as a form of romantic self-fashioning and foreplay are important in the creation of a youth counterpublic. Youth who participate in romantic practices gradually acquire, with varying degrees of proficiency, the ability to work around but also draw from dominant discourses, performing what I call "a localization of public interventions," and simultaneously help to fashion a counterpublic world of youth romance. In that sense, youth romance can be understood as a space for possible acts of refusing to submit to regulation and creative cultural production. Beyond a platform for creativity and resistance, the counterpublic of youth romance provides a space for young people to create collective and individual fantasies of a "good life" based on imagined attachments with an imagined romantic partner as they work through and cope with current life crises and uncertainties. We see that the commercialization of social life (through, for example, commercial establishments in town), emerging ideologies of romance (through media representations of modern love), and messages of sexual risk (through HIV and sexual health campaigns) have engendered new possibilities for youth sexuality and liaisons but have also exacerbated the gap between the ideal that shapes the pursuits of young people and what is actually achievable

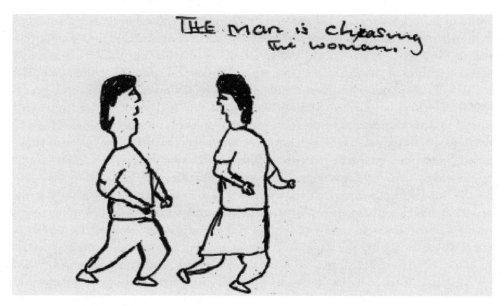

FIGURE 7.1. Youth drawing of "the chase"

in the context of uncertainty. As such, the project of youth romance becomes what Lauren Berlant calls a "cruel optimism": it is a drama of adjustment—a drama of consciousness and of mediated life—that forces into being new recognitions of what a life is and ought to be.

"The Chase": Gender and Courtship

Iganga residents conceptualize romance and courtship as highly gendered processes. The narrative trope "the chase" best captures residents' ideas of the proper gendered roles, social responses, and courtship process, as depicted in drawings by primary and secondary school students (Figure 7.1). According to this widely accepted trope, the man actively initiates and pursues, while the young woman or the guardian of her sexuality initially feigns indifference, resists, or acts coy in an effort to elevate her desirability, respectability, and ultimately the amount of bridewealth. Eventually the young woman, through her guardian or with her guardian's approval, either rejects the man's proposal or consents with stipulations. The consent process culminates in a public *kwandhula* ceremony during which the gendered chase is performed by and for the approving gaze of a wider audience that consists of kinsfolk and social affiliates on the bride's side, who (not too) patiently "wait and receive" the "visitors" on the groom's side, who have to prove that their clan is worthy of the young lady.

Elders' stories and sexual histories emphasize masculine ideal characteristics of aggression and persuasion in courtship and feminine characteristics of restraint and patience, which are to be reproduced throughout the courtship, engagement, and solemnization processes and eventually displayed within marriage. As explored in the earlier discussion of Basoga sexuality education, within the realm of sexuality women are thought to have greater sexual allure and power than men (and hence the need to culturally groom and discipline the female body); however, in courtship men are expected to actively pursue or perform direct acts of wooing. While "proper" women may and should employ subtle and deniable methods to attract suitors, both young and old maintain that a proper woman should not initiate courtship or display too much desire, as Annette did in her letter. A woman's active engagement in courtship lies at the heart of critiques about today's youthful romance, and specifically the *nakyewombekeire* (free woman) who *visibly* and *actively* participates in the chase by displaying overt (as opposed to veiled) sexual agency and therefore belying Basoga ideologies of female public modesty and the father as the authorized arbitrator for the young woman and her sexuality. The concern about the *nakyewombekeire* is not only about her transgressing gender courtship conventions by acting on her desires; she also presents a threat to the moral order of the community and to the stability of married people's unions.

From Village to Town: Romance, Consumption, and Shifting Sexual Geographies

Generational transformations around courtship and romance in Iganga are similar to those experiences in other parts of the world as written about in recent literature. Particularly useful for understanding changes in Iganga is the literature on the commercialization of romance and leisure and within shifting sexual geographies in the region. Drawing from this focus on commercialization, I offer an alternative to the common sex-for-money paradigm that dominates literature on sexuality in Africa and that effaces the significance of how the consumer market shapes *affective* (and not merely material) attachments and imaginations. In other words, unequal access to capital and the consumer marketplace might motivate transactional sexual liaisons, but this same marketplace also serves an important influence on how young people imagine romance and affective relationships. Analysis of cross-generational data shows that there has been significant transformation in the sexual geography surrounding courtship as occasioned by the commercialization of social life and sexuality since independence. The social production and imagination of romantic spaces has shifted to towns as urban spaces have opened up to Africans since colonial times and, more recently, as age-segregated commercial establishments and institutions have proliferated and replaced earlier, more familial outlets such as village functions or schools. Drawings by young people help illustrate this point. A group of secondary schoolboys drew a series of pictures that elaborates shifting notions of place and respectability in courtship (see Figure 7.2). According to the students' explanation of their drawings, in the past the man and woman met while she collected water and he herded his cattle around the village; the man was attracted to the young woman's beauty and work ethic, and she was impressed with his wealth (in the form of cattle) and "good manners," meaning he was respectful of elders and lines of authority.

Similar to elders' stories about the (idealized) past, intergenerational village ceremonies and spaces were the main venue for courtship activities such as flirting, meeting a sweetheart or new love interest, or sneaking off for a private moment, but such

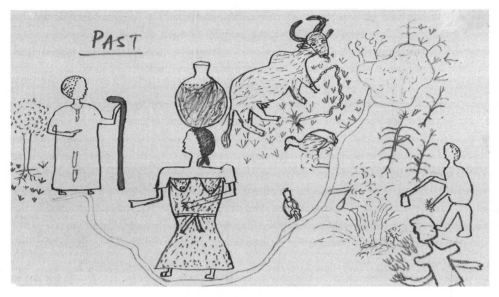

FIGURE 7.2. Youth drawing of courtship in the past, tending to tasks in the village

encounters were always under threat of being exposed. The same youth who drew and described past premarital encounters as being situated among the familiar depicted today's courtship as having shifted into public and commercial spaces in town outside of the purview of kin and neighbors and where young people can engage with a wider world of affective possibilities and attachments (Figure 7.3).

In older and younger people's discussions of romance, the "village" gets configured as an intergenerational space for romantic encounters of the (imagined) past, while "town" emerges as a dominant theme when residents talk about courtship today. The "village" and "town" in such cases are not geographically fixed locations; rather, the terms become symbolic, material, and discursive categories that residents deploy to signify the degree of attachment to the marketplace, moral propriety, and kin involvement in the courtship process. "Village" signifies that a relationship operates within the morally appropriate networks of kin groups and older people, while "town" privileges civil associations and networks (such as peers, classmates, or coworkers) as well as engagement with global flows and commercial marketplaces when forming notions of love and romance. Hence, whereas older and younger residents can invoke the term "town" to signify positive progress and future potential, when invoked in discussions about propriety, the moral signification of town becomes complicated—simultaneously indicating increased individual freedom in choosing love interests and a moral critique of the potential corrupting factors that surround sexual liaisons enacted away from watchful, intergenerational eyes in the familiar "village," as implied by the use of the term.

Shifting geographies also emerge in courtship narratives in discussions of secrecy. Since most parents in Iganga do not openly approve of youth courtship, a rendezvous has to be arranged by both the boy and the girl and often occurs away from their homes. Keeping a relationship from parents is both an act of cultural respect and an

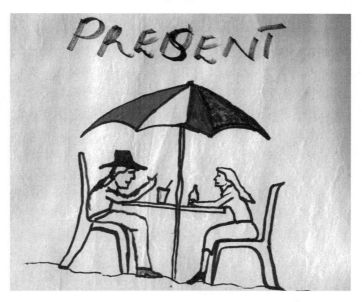

FIGURE 7.3. Youth drawing of courtship in the present, eating at a restaurant in town

act of developmental independence. Village locations such as water collection places, shops, and paths have been common meeting places for youth, and places in Iganga Town (such as alleyways, the evening *kayola* or bazaar, dances, and schoolyards) offer additional places to meet partners who reside beyond their village. However, within youth's imaginations of romance, commercial spaces in town fuel their ideas of possibilities and expectations of romance. In her essay about adolescent "love," an eighteen-year-old girl reflects on the importance of place in the romantic process:

> Now in the game of love. In the infant states everyone will have to do what he or she can do best to please the partner and to show that meeting at pubs and the private places they can think of to discuss their affairs and to make the best promises one can ever think of. It is at this stage that the two start exchanging/ offering gifts to each other, sending all kinds of cards to each other, exchanging snaps [photographs] and letters and going out for drinks in pretty cool public places say hotels and clubs.

Reflected in this essay and others is what Beth Bailey (1988) calls the "consumption-centered" romantic ideal. In her social history of changes in courtship in the United States during the twentieth century, *From Front Porch to Back Seat*, Bailey argues that the location of courtship shifted from the parents' home (or the "front porch") and into public spaces that were "removed, by distance and by anonymity, from the sheltering and controlling contexts of home and local community" (1988:3). In both Bailey's study and in Iganga, the shifting of geographies of romance to anonymous spaces allows for an exploration of intimacy between two people that extended possibilities of premarital courtship. The commercialization of leisure in Iganga and in Uganda in general has produced a variety of spaces in which people can conduct secret trysts or meetings, and youth increasingly associate contemporary romance with these commercial sites (see Mills and Ssewakiryanga 2005).

These geographic nodes also provide young people a space to conceptualize romance as an escape from everyday economic hardships and parental restrictions, such as reflected in this boy's essay on love:

> When a boy and a girl are in love they forget what they have to do especially when they are students. They just enjoy luxurious things like watching movies and going for discos. In this case a girl can convince her parents that she is going to school yet she is actually going to meet her boyfriend. And the same applies to the boy who deceives his parents to give him a lot of money and spend it with [his] girlfriends.

The coupling of romance with consumption and characterization of it as removed from mundane daily life and chores has intensified tensions between generations. As young people design strategies to keep evidence of courtship and consumption away from parents, parents are fearful that young people's consumption-centered romantic imaginations will lull them into conceptualizing a life that is out of their reach. The commercial marketplace both fuels and frustrates young people's romantic desires, and has also been a topic of great interest for scholars of romance (e.g., Wardlow and Hirsch 2006; Cole and Thomas 2009; Padilla et al. 2007). The emerging romantic ideal is not only facilitated by a consumer economy, such as the availability of goods and services, but also promoted by the consumer economy through images such as advertisements to sell goods. For instance, in *Consuming the Romantic Utopia: Love and the Cultural Contradictions of Capitalism*, Eva Illouz (1997) argues that this "commodification of romance" in the United States was promoted through narrative, musical, and visual technologies, creating an image of a "romantic utopia" that included new technologies of leisure such as movies, dance halls, and new types of restaurants. In other words, romance as an object becomes a central trope in advertising, and hence certain advertised commodities become associated with attraction and love; in turn, the commodities themselves became objects of desire and a demonstration of true affection. The attainment of romantic utopia is therefore highly classed, alienating poorer citizens from its reach, but the allure is so pervasive that it guarantees people's belief and pursuit of the new commodified romance. Hence, Illouz writes, "the ability to enact the romantic ideal in the twin domains of communication and consumption demands a *romantic competence* marked by access to linguistic, cultural, economic, and time resources" (1997:248).

Similarly, most youth in Iganga do not have access to financial resources—whether themselves or through their parents—to achieve their economic romantic ideal, leading to frustrations and sometimes, as in the case of Sam and Birungi, the ending of relationships as older male suitors are able to demonstrate that their promises have a greater likelihood of coming to fruition. Young people are aware of this economic contradiction, which noticeably intersects with age status for men. However, idealized courtship places, such as bars in Iganga Town or an imagined beach near Lake Victoria (a common spot mentioned in essays and interviews), and commercial gifts, such as shoes and photographs, remain a central part of their romantic imaginations and longings. The connection between romance and consumption is also reproduced in the popular media. For example, during a popular evening radio program, the commentator made frequent references to young couples in love visiting the botanical gardens in Entebbe, a town outside of Kampala. The show offered Valentine's Day prizes that included a trip to the gardens and admission to the executive lounge of a Kampala nightclub. Although the botanical gardens are about three to four hours from Iganga and too expensive for most youth in Iganga, they are commonly imagined and identified as an ideal place for a romantic outing.

Based on her research in Spain, Jane Collier expresses skepticism about the theory that the mass media, or specifically television in her study, has "opened up" the ways of thinking for rural residents (1997:46). She argues that the "opening up" theory is based on the assumption that the village had been previously "closed." However, as she elaborates, the shift not only is discursive but also illuminates people's perceptions of possibilities. I argue that it is not that ideas in the mass media have "opened up" local thoughts about romance, for Basoga folktales and songs indicate the wildly romantic imaginations of the past. Rather, I combine Collier's skepticism with Arjun Appadurai's consideration of how to analytically conceptualize the globalization of ideas in his book *Modernity at Large: Cultural Dimensions of Globalization*, and I posit that the various media in Uganda offer youth powerful codes and images through which they discuss and imagine romance (Appadurai 1996). In Uganda's times of economic, moral, and social uncertainty, engagement with romantic discourses allows young people to imagine for themselves affective attachments with peers despite the precarity of their immediate world.

Particularly important in fueling young people's narratives of the possibilities and configurations of affective relationships are the romance novels published by the British company Mills and Boon (Figure 7.4). Whereas scholars of the United States have argued that reading romance novels figured more prominently in the past than in contemporary women's culture, adolescents in Iganga of *both* genders read such novels for romantic possibilities and, as seen in the following chapters on love letters, for romantic scripts used in missives to love interests. Most youth I met had read several romance novels while in secondary school, and they are among the common items possessed, shared, and discussed by youth. The covers of these highly circulated novels convey ideas about love and courtship based on individualization, as well as fantasy and escape through the varied depictions of a nuclear romantic couple with man-as-hero and woman-as-recued-by-love or intoxicated-with-love. It is not that youth try to emulate the characters or plots in the novels, nor do they think they can. Rather, the novels provide youth with what Brian Larkin, in his exploration of consumption of Indian romance films and Hausa love stories (*littantafan soyayya* books) in Nigeria, calls an "imaginative space" in which the plots build on "the narrative as a mode of social enquiry," facilitating the reader's creative process of relating the romantic narratives to everyday life (1997:407). The incorporation of the plots and themes in the novels and movies into local settings creates "parallel modernities," according to Larkin, in which

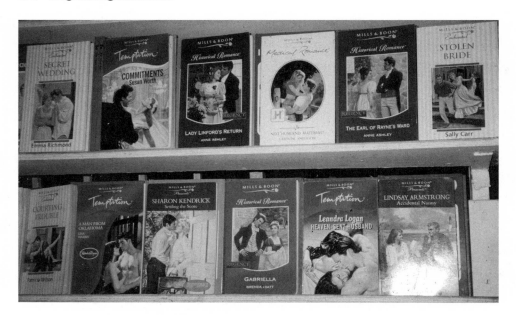

FIGURE 7.4. Mills and Boon romance novels

multiple economic, religious, and cultural flows coexist in space and time (ibid.). The idea of parallel modernities turns attention away from whether the ideals in the movies or novels are realistic in the local setting, toward an understanding of how nationally circulated cultural productions advance imagined or experienced affective attachments in ways that allow young people to cope with the uncertainties of everyday life.

In this section I have argued that young people imagine romance as shifting from clandestine encounters occurring rather opportunistically in familial-based and inter-generational village settings to relationships that are consumption-centered and located in commercial spaces that increasingly dot Uganda's age- and class-segregated sexual geographic landscape. Central to my argument is that viewing capitalism as simply facilitating transactional sex-for-money relationships ignores the important role that consumption plays in fueling young people's affective fantasies and desires. Finally, it may be tempting to conceptualize this commercialization of romance and sexuality as merely an "individualization of young love," as social histories and sociological work in the United States suggest; however, that does not adequately capture what is occurring in Iganga. Instead of an individualization of romance, there is what I would call a reconfiguring and collapsing of generational influence. Specifically, intergenerational influences (older kin over younger kin) that figured prominently in the negotiating and sanctioning of relationships in older people's stories have been overshadowed during the extended youth romance stage. Social influence has collapsed as same-age generation kin networks (siblings, cousins, stepsiblings) and civil networks (school, church, clubs) have emerged as significant in matchmaking and approval seeking. Hence, rather than a young love becoming nuclearized, the conceptual framework of the "relocation of young love" within the physical, social, and capitalist landscapes allows us to appreciate that romantic relationships in Iganga are not removed from social networks and are constantly being shaped and evaluated by their association with the consumer market, a topic I turn to next.

Social Networks, Prestige, and Reputation

To illustrate how kin and neighbors have been eclipsed by peer networks in the sexual geography of youth romance, I provide an ethnographic example. After a long week of work, ending with a particularly strenuous couple of days of research, my assistants and I decided to reward ourselves with an evening feast. Steven, eighteen years old at the time, had recently started a rabbit business at his aunt's compound, where he lived. Volunteering to manage the preparations for the meal, he rushed out of the office, proudly returning with a plump mammal.

After another assistant, Salim, slaughtered the rabbit in accordance with Muslim practice, Steven roasted our meal and the rest of us prepared the vegetables and various starches as we sang along to Top 40 songs on the radio. When the meal was ready, Janet called to Steven who told us to begin eating because he wanted to buy something from the store. "I am just coming," he assured us as he headed out the front door.

Forty minutes later, I asked Janet where Steven was. She playfully gazed in my direction as if she had been waiting to tell me a secret and giggled. Steven had gone to a dance in the village, she told me. "Without eating the rabbit that he cooked?" I inquired. "No, he packed his to go," Janet answered, mischievously stopping short of disclosing another secret. We exchanged glances, but I decided not to probe deeper. Later, while we were doing dishes, Janet could not hold the innocent secret any longer and informed me that Steven had packed some rabbit not only for himself but also for a "friend" he hoped to see at the disco. I had been there long enough to understand the coded language; knowing that she technically had not revealed his secret, I joined her laughter. Before this evening, we had repeatedly teased Steven about his new rabbit project being a ploy to impress girls, suspecting but not knowing for sure if his desire for income was partly motivated by his perceptions of how he could be an active suitor. The image of Steven smartly dressed in his disco clothes and one of his signature unique hats with roasted rabbit tucked under his arm to impress his sweetheart became the running topic of the night, and the combination of a rabbit and nice clothes as romantic accoutrements eventually became a research-long source of inside jokes.

The story about Steven represents the daily workings of youth courtship and the relatively benign aura of juvenile secrecy that surrounds it. Steven had a plan to impress a girl at a village function; Janet was a keeper of his secrets as well as one of his facilitators; I was both an unknowing enabler (because I increased his social status and access to resources) and someone from whom he wanted to keep his secret. Unfortunately, Steven did not meet his love interest that evening, and his attempts to meet with her privately over the next few weeks did not pan out. External circumstances (and perhaps a little hesitancy on her part) managed to interfere with their private meetings. On each occasion, the two young lovers could not find a way to conveniently and secretly break away from their families or the groups of peers who surrounded them. After being disappointed and frustrated with their series of failed meetings and his sweetheart's increasingly apparent lack of initiative, Steven's interest in her eventually faded and he went back to being single and "looking," as he explained to me one afternoon.

Like Janet, friends of either sex play an important facilitating role in the courtship process by serving as confidants, advisors, and alibis, helping craft and deliver love letters (as explored later), carrying messages between young sweethearts, and accompanying friends to preset meetings with romantic interests. The groups through which young people initially learn about sex are often the same networks in which they experiment with their earliest romantic encounters, whether as sweethearts or, more commonly, as facilitators and confidants. As young people relocate for school or to live with a relative, their geographic worlds transform and their circles of friends shift, overlap, and can unexpectedly converge, expanding their world of romantic geographies. Through letters, messages, or visits, many young people try to maintain relationships with former but geographically distant friends. During courtship, friends are a young lover's closest confidants and advisors; friends are aware of a relationship between two young people long before the families have formal knowledge of it.

The terms OB (old boy) and OG (old girl) are used by young people to describe a member of a civic affinity group with whom a young person shares or shared a common social space and experience. Most typically, OB or OG refers to a person with whom a youth attended school, but a relationship of affinity can also emerge from another common experience, such as a youth club or religious group. Instead of being grounded in a neighborhood or a kinship group, an OB and OG affinity network draws its association and prestige from today's civil society. It is an indicator not only of socioeconomic status but also of symbolic alignment: in contemporary Uganda, many possibilities for affiliation exist, including educational institution, linguistic group, clan affiliation, religion, parents' professional group, and the like. A person's OB or OG interethnic networks provide important links to economic and social opportunities as adults. On many occasions, when I was walking with a young adult, he or she would stop to greet someone and would introduce the person to me as an OB or OG. Although the Basoga do not have a formal process of creating age groups, as do some ethnic groups in Africa, informal age-based networks have emerged as schooling has become more widespread, and many are based on class and status as opposed to ethnicity.

As influential adolescent psychologist Erik Erikson (1968, 1970) noted several decades ago, romantic relationships play a vital role in the emotional and psychological development of young people, as these relationships become a major vehicle for working through issues of identity and individuation. While psychological perspectives provide an understanding of romance as an important stage in an individual's development of self, an anthropological perspective broadens the analytic lens, allowing us to understand the role of romantic relationships in shaping public status, reputation, and access to networks. Specifically in Iganga, participating in romantic culture allows youth to obtain status within their social networks and attain higher levels of prestige among peers, but this form of status seeking comes at the risk of being discovered by authoritative adults—a risk that can elevate status, if successfully implemented, or tarnish reputation, if a negative outcome results. Young people frequently characterize peers who are in romantic relationships as more mature and sophisticated, indexing an adolescent's degree of attaining a more senior status and being closer to adulthood. Establishing and maintaining a romantic relationship means taking on adult responsibilities and behaviors that are then revered within peer groups. Young people also talk about romantic couples as being "envied" by peers because they manage to "carry out their love," as it is commonly called, amid possibilities of being discovered by interfering adults and other structural forces working against young love.

On the other hand, whereas a steady romantic relationship can elevate the status of a youth, it can also work to a disadvantage if the relationship takes an unfortunate turn or has an unplanned outcome, such as public humiliation or a pregnancy, as explored in later chapters. Gossip about the relationships of others serves as a way for youth groups to construct and negotiate ideas about respectability and decency, which differ for adolescent boys and girls. Like gossip among adults, tales about a relationship or a person's individual behavior in a relationship serve as cautionary warnings to youth involved in the telling or discussing of the story.

For instance, the story of Ronald and Sarah was widely talked about among students in their school. The couple was considered popular as well as mature and desirable, as evidenced by their ability to maintain a stable relationship. Toward the end of their secondary education, Sarah became pregnant and the couple discussed getting married. Ronald failed to obtain employment in Iganga and went to live with his brother in Kampala in hopes of getting a job or getting enough money to pursue further education. He promised to return and take care of Sarah and their baby, but after almost a year he had not returned, and it became clear to their peers that he might not ever. Sarah remained at her parents' home with her new baby, disappointed and heartbroken. Her angry parents threatened to go to Kampala to find the boy who had impregnated and abandoned their daughter. With a baby, they worried that it would be difficult for their daughter to continue with her education or get married anytime soon, at least while still breast-feeding (see Johnson-Hanks 2002). For girls in school, Sarah's unfortunate fate served as a reminder of boys' failed promises and of the dangers of premarital sex, as well as a general warning about the deceptive and selfish ways of men. For boys, the story represented the potential complications of impregnating a girl, but even more, it shows them the possibilities of escaping responsibility and a damaged reputation. Ultimately, the story showed that it is more difficult for a girl's reputation and planned life trajectory to recover from this kind of sexual blemish than it is for a boy's, which is another reason parents are much more protective of daughters.

This certainly is not a new concept nor unique to Uganda. Literature about adolescent female sexuality suggests that there is a double standard in how boys and girls are expected to negotiate their sexual reputations (Lees 1993; S. Thompson 1995). These studies show that whereas young women are expected to maintain an aura of chasteness and innocence, young males are admired for their prowess. Categorizing women into "good" or "bad" serves as a powerful discursive technique of controlling and stigmatizing their behaviors. While the labels and gossip establish categories for females, scholars point out that in reality, the polarity is rarely so neat. The monolithic categories dissolve even further when the notion of desire is examined (Fine 1992). In

Iganga, although a girl may have earned a reputation among her peers as being "easy," she may also be simultaneously admired. Girls may see her actions as a sign of physical attractiveness, loose morals, freedom from adult authority, or as a contradictory combination of some or all of these. Boys may simultaneously be curious about, threatened by, and critical of her sexual reputation. Similarly, boys who attain ideal male prowess status gain reputations that are both envied and disdained by their peers. These gendered notions of sexual propriety and reputation motivate most parents to restrict courtship opportunities.

The story of Ronald and Sarah took a twist that was unexpected by many who knew of them. By 2006, they were living together outside of Iganga Town. Sarah was a tailoring apprentice at the shop of a well-established tailor, and Ronald was working as an entry-level office worker in town and positioning himself to take over his father's growing poultry project. Their firstborn was then around eight years old and the couple had a second child who was almost four, born while Sarah lived with her parents. Her parents were extremely disappointed, which forced the young couple's relationship to continue in a clandestine manner, hidden even from some of their closest friends. When I saw Sarah in 2006, she was expecting a third child with Ronald. They had not had a formal introduction ceremony, but now that it was clear that this was not simply an adolescent affair, their families approved of their relationship; therefore, according to widely accepted social convention, they were considered married. Sarah happily informed me that they were waiting to save more money before having a *kwandhula* ceremony—a prospect she eagerly awaited, for she believed it would finally repair the damage her reputation had sustained in secondary school.

Everyday Regulation of Romance: Denial, "Traps," and Immorality Policies

Whereas reputation management and prestige building among peers serve as important forms of internal regulation within the youth counterpublic, adults in their lives employ everyday quotidian techniques to protect young people from what they perceive as the harmful social, economic, health, and emotional consequences of the cruel optimism of youth romance. Apart from the defilement law, parents with whom I spoke pride themselves on their ability to devise creative strategies to restrict opportunities for young people's romantic liaisons.

Denying and Obstructing Youth Dating

A discursive strategy of some residents is the refusal to adopt the contemporary language of dating (including "girlfriend" and "boyfriend") that is regularly featured on the radio and in print media. This act of willfully resisting recent terminology can be read as an attempt to deny the existence of youth courtship as a legitimate experience in the first place. When I first arrived in Iganga, I would ask older people if there were a Lusoga term for "dating" or "courtship," and I was repeatedly told that the practice does not exist in Basoga culture, or occasionally I was told that it could be called *obwenzi* (which means "general promiscuity"). This act of willful refusal has a logic: If there is no term or word to name something, it can only exist outside of accepted cultural boundaries. A label's very existence indicates social recognition of a practice or belief. In contrast, refusing to name an act suggests a denial of its existence as a clear definable practice. The terms "girlfriend" and "boyfriend" have been generally appropriated by elite families, in larger urban centers, and in the media, and they are commonly used by the youth of all socioeconomic statuses in Iganga. Older people in Iganga are familiar with these terms, though they are not likely to use them with any frequency, and when they do use such words, they use them in a way that indicates their disapproval of cultural noncompliance. Some resist the terms altogether, maintaining that "boyfriends" and "girlfriends" are Western and reflect disregard for kinship roles in the premarital process. The words are a corruption, and the concepts are not indigenous or culturally sanctioned social relationships. Their evidence is that there is no Lusoga equivalent for the terms. Thus, in a society where a new linguistic competence is needed in order to discuss transformations in courtship and youth relationships, older people's refusal to appropriate the language can be understood as an act of resistance against youths' romantic relationships. Over the course of this research project, however, the English terms have been more readily adopted without the same disparaging undertones. Resisting the language of youth courtship does not prevent the practice of youth courtship; it merely shows a lack of interest in acknowledging that it has become a fairly standard social convention.

In addition to resisting the language of dating, some parental interventions to restrict courtship and romance are more direct. For example, after a long research day, I stayed at Agnes's house. As I opened the back door of the house to use to pit latrine, Agnes appeared at the entrance of her bedroom doorway with a flashlight and a broom. We looked at each other in utter shock. She explained that she had heard the noise from the dried bush above the back door and thought someone was either entering or leaving the house. She later confessed that she put the bush above the door so that she could monitor the movements of her daughters and their possible lovers. She felt defeated, however, because her two eldest daughters became pregnant by the age of sixteen. Her various methods of monitoring her daughters' activities are similar to others I heard about. Common ones included asking girls to stay on the main paths in hopes that their opportunities to secretly meet with boys would be reduced or sending adolescent daughters on errands with younger children to act as deterrents for any possible suitor. Parents also would not let girls collect firewood because it was rumored that youth would meet each other and have "affairs" while looking for wood off the main paths.

Immorality Policies in School: Pregnancy Tests, Love Letters, and Romantic Music

Schools find themselves at the center of the courtship debate. Parents can limit opportunities for courtship at home, but they have less control over what occurs while their children are at school. While expanding access to education is a policy priority and education is highly regarded as necessary for social mobility and hence an important source of social security for older people, education is also viewed as one of the greatest threats to traditions.[2] Whether evidence supports this belief or not, common wisdom in Iganga and throughout much of Uganda holds that coed schools, especially boarding schools, are breeding grounds for early sexual experimenting and decaying moral traditions. Schools offer a socially sanctioned space for young people to escape from the regulatory eyes of familiar guardians and to freely mix with youths from other areas who are unfamiliar to their parents. As a result of social fears, schools feel a great deal of pressure to closely monitor the sexual behaviors of students, which results in random acts of policing such as that experienced by Annette.

Almost all the headmasters and teachers with whom I spoke believe that schools should address sexuality and sexual relationships with students. However, most teachers did not feel that they had the cultural or social authority to discuss matters of intimacy or sexual topics with students outside of the curricula on morality, marriage, and biological development and reproduction. The few schools that did have a dedicated sex education specialist were still often wary of discussing sexuality for fear of being accused of moral corruption, and focused mainly on biological issues such as puberty, physical development (such as menstruation), reproduction, and causes, signs, and long-term effects of sexually transmitted infections and HIV. Whereas the sexuality education module has a large component on "morality," based specifically in conservative interpretations of the Bible and Koran, the discomfort with addressing the affective side of sexuality in educational settings is grounded in both the fear of being blamed for moral decline and the uncertainty of how to advise young people about the rapidly changing world of youth romance, leading to what youth experience as the bifurcation of sexual learning, as explored earlier in this ethnography.

Although administrators and teachers feel limited in their authority in this area, the pressure to police behaviors through school policies and surveillance has increased. These policies get bundled under schools' "immorality policies," which are signed by all students and frequently their parents or guardians during the enrollment process. These policies are often posted in common areas around the schoolyard and are restated by the school administration as a method of control through threats of fear. One school in Iganga has instituted an immorality policy that states: "Boys and girls should behave as brothers and sisters. The school will tolerate no other relationship between a boy and a girl. Any student found acting inappropriately may be suspended or expelled from school." When I asked the headmaster if he had ever applied the policy, he replied, "Yes, we have expelled students who do not follow this rule." The most common offense was being found in possession of romance novels or sexually explicit music or exchanging love letters. One headmaster explained that schools restrict romance novels and popular music because the sexually charged messages corrupt the minds of young people by introducing sexual fantasies and thoughts. Love letters were dangerous not only because they allowed a relationship to advance, but also because they were evidence of young people's attempting to go around adult authority.

The most serious cases for expulsion involved pregnant adolescent girls—the pregnant female body being a visible sign that the school had failed at its regulatory duties (in this case, of "saving" schoolgirls from the ruin of pregnancy) and hence the site for public discipline in order for the school to reassert the its authority. I did not encounter a school that took similar action against a male student for impregnating a female (although it was a frequent topic of conversation among feminists) because while impregnating a girl is an assault on her father's authority, it is also read as a sign of virility and masculine independence. This is another instance in which the sexuality of adolescent girls but not adolescent boys is publicly regulated, reflecting wider gender inequalities and notions of access to respectability. The youthful female body becomes the visible index of sexual immorality and a public platform upon which morality is debated and measured, while paradoxically being seen as a proving ground for male sexuality. Adolescent females and their bodies serve as the litmus test for the sexual morality of a school, as they do for society in general.

The threat of random pregnancy testing in schools serves as a way for schools to enact surveillance over girls' bodies and sexual agency and is intended to deter girls from engaging in sexual activity. Though I am not sure how regularly schools actually collect urine samples from girls or even test the urine for pregnancy hormones (for it would be a costly endeavor), the looming threat of these random tests is, as it is intended to be, a source of anxiety for sexually active girls.[3] Rumors of these tests being able to detect sexual activity in general and not simply pregnancy, hence a form of virginity testing, occasionally circulate in schools. As in much of sub-Saharan Africa, abortion is illegal in Uganda and carries a heavy religiously informed moral weight. Therefore, girls who suspect that they are pregnant are often hesitant to seek advice beyond their social network and their male sexual partners about how to access one of the few safe underground abortion doctors in town. In desperation, they resort to risky abortive measures on their own, such as taking certain pills, inducing a miscarriage by physical injury, or attempting to puncture the fetus with a stick or other instrument through the vagina. The illegal and unsanitary "bush" abortions that are available put a girl's health at great risk, but this *possible* health risk is weighed against the *real* personal and social risks of being a pregnant teen (Coeytaux 1988; Silberschmidt and Rasch 2000). I knew of several girls who were expelled from school because of pregnancy. Most, such as Sarah, were unable to continue with their education during the years after delivering; a few were sent away from their parents' homes because of the shame or because the additional financial burden was too much for the parents to afford. Many others simply "sat at home and waited to marry," as was frequently said of unwed adolescent girls. Stories circulating locally and in the newspapers and on the radio vilify girls who "dodge" school pregnancy tests and then "ruthlessly" abandon newborns in pit latrines or near rubbish lots. Other horror stories involve girls who have died, either while attempting abortion (commonly through taking fatal doses of chloroquine, a cheap and readily available antimalarial medicine) or from postabortion complications such as excessive bleeding or infections. These stories often portray the girls as merciless and nasty creatures. Girls are punished for subverting gender norms and flouting kinship rules by getting pregnant before marriage or for using pregnancy as a strategy to maintain a relationship. Whereas youth sexual activity can be treated as a public secret, pregnancy makes visible what many parents and authorities would like to ignore: that youth are sexually active, even though adults have made access to sexual health services, information, and contraception very difficult.

Folktales: Reproducing Ideologies of Female Obedience and Masculine Determination

The gendered ideology underlying the chase and the consequences of breaking with cultural conventions becomes part of a young person's worldview and subjectivity long before the influence of peer groups and globally inflected ideas of a consumption-centered romance. Young people learn about Basoga gendered courtship ideologies through proverbs that regularly make their way into conversations of older people and through local folklore recited in various functions and settings. Cultural performers hired to perform at ceremonies enact Basoga folktales through songs or animated interpretations, but indirect acquisition through informal storytelling and commonly recited tales and proverbs remains an important way for parents, other relatives, and neighbors to convey messages about gendered ways of being a respectable Basoga person. These informal settings serve as veiled conduits for transmitting cultural ideologies about a young person's responsibility and the consequences of not following prescribed gender etiquette. During my research project, for instance, older people might use informal discussions with me as a convenient and seemingly neutral vehicle for transmitting cultural knowledge and their own agendas to their younger kinfolk who were curiously lingering and listening to our conversations or watching as older people participated in one of the participatory research activities. These research instances both legitimized the contemporary value of old folks' knowledge for the groups of youthful onlookers and created unplanned opportunities for transmitting that knowledge to otherwise indifferent youngsters. Hence, adults were often not only giving me information in response to my research questions, but also cleverly using the opportunity to gain cultural authority and to strategically insert commentary and advice for youth to overhear.

Although many of the over forty folktales we collected could be used to illustrate the common themes of female obedience and masculine determination, I have decided to present one of the most widely known folktales—the Basoga origin story involving Kintu and Nambi. In examining this story, I am interested in how cultural ideas about courtship, gender, and intergenerational relations are constructed in folktales in ways that promote particularly gendered notions of premarital sexual propriety. I adopt the framework Thomas Beidelman used in his ethnography of initiation practices and moral education among Kaguru speakers in east-central Tanzania. Beidelman distinguishes between a folktale's "explicit moral conclusion" and "deeper meaning." Explicit moral conclusions are the immediate take-home messages of the story, while the deeper meanings may be unspoken and slowly manifest during the initiation ceremonies and beyond the ceremony as a person matures (1997:112–13). The deeper meanings represent a slow embodiment of cultural conventions but also can refer to the process through which ideas become taken-for-granted, or hegemonic, social beliefs.

There were variations on the story of Kintu and Nambi, but the general storyline and character construction remain fairly consistent. The version I use here is taken from a folklore pamphlet published by the (Busoga) Cultural Research Centre (1998), a center in Jinja started in the mid-1990s and dedicated to the "cultural revitalization" of Basoga traditions—or, more accurately, to cultural reinvention, as Terence Ranger (1983) reminds us, particularly since precolonial Busogaland existed as fragmented chiefdoms with conventions and practices that varied significantly by region and by clan. According to the director of the center, a major aim of this institution is "to promote a Basoga way of thinking" in a contemporary context in which foreign solutions and ways are unable to meet the realities of most Basoga. At its heart, the center is a research, educational, and archival institution that codifies, validates, and advances *a* particular set of Basoga cultural traditions and epistemology. The Adam-and-Eve-like origin story of Kintu and Nambi is one folk narrative through which the center carries out its aim.

The Story of Kintu and Nambi

Kintu comes to Buganda and finds there is no food. But he comes with his cow. The dung of his cow becomes his food and its urine becomes his water. Kintu sees people coming from above. It is Nambi, the daughter of Igulu [the ruler of another place], and her brothers.

Nambi falls in love with Kintu and wants to marry him. The brothers tell their father that Nambi wants to marry the man who eats cow dung and drinks cow urine. The father instructs them to take Kintu's cow away from him to see if he dies or if he might be worthy of marrying his daughter. Nambi finds out their plan and brings Kintu to Igulu's place to get his cow.

When Kintu arrives at Igulu's place, Igulu builds him a house and puts him through a series of tests or tricks. The first test is to consume an enormous amount of food and beer. The second is to split rock with a steel axe. The third is to catch a pot full of dew. An invisible force helps Kintu fulfill the tests. Igulu allows Kintu to marry his daughter, but before they leave, Kintu has to pass one last test: to select his cattle from a herd of thousands. A beetle assists him and he identifies his cows from amongst thousands.

Igulu is impressed and says, "You are a rare species; you even see what is hidden! Kintu, here is your wife who brought you this way. I have given her to you so that she becomes your wife." Igulu's only warning is for them to leave early in the morning so that Nambi's brother Walumbe (the brother of death) does not follow them.

Early the next morning they begin their journey to earth. Nambi tells Kintu that she has forgotten her millet for the chickens. Kintu orders her not to go, but she insists. Her brother sees her and demands that she take him to earth with her, to Busoga.

After some time on earth, Walumbe begins to kill the children of Kintu and Nambi. Kintu asks his father-in-law for advice. Igulu tries to assist but is unable. They remain on earth and Walumbe continues to be Kintu's enemy and kill his children. Walumbe's presence on earth caused suffering and conflicts. That, according to the legend, is how sickness and death started.

In the pamphlet, the origin story is followed by a commentary written by the center's staff. The commentary informs the reader of the culturally appropriate manner in which a young woman should express her desire.[4] According to the commentary in the pamphlet, Nambi is "an enterprising woman who falls in love with Kintu, but in accordance with tradition, *she does not express her love directly to Kintu, but tells her brothers and father*" (30; emphasis added). Similar to the youth who witnessed the fate of Annette, (female) listeners of this story are reminded that the proper way for females to express desire is through restraint and a supervising male. Nambi's assertion in selecting her own mate is palpable only because she, perhaps not completely willingly, follows prescribed gender expectations—not approaching or interacting with her love interest directly but instead deferring to the authority of her male kin in approving of the suitor. Before Kintu can marry Nambi, he first has to demonstrate his masculinity by gorging on consumables and by displaying strength, cleverness, and his prowess as a provider—all indicators of his worthiness. This demonstration of masculinity could be read symbolically as equivalent to the practice of a prospective bride's family setting the terms of the engagement or bridewealth with the young man. Similar to Adam in the Bible, Kintu has yet to master his skills of controlling the willfully enterprising woman, and she disobeys orders, acting of her own will and selfish desire. Nambi's disobedience leads to the continued suffering of Kintu, Nambi, their children, and the world in general. This theme of female disobedience and its consequences on the wider social order is commonly reproduced in Basoga folktales, when either a wife disobeys her husband or a daughter rebels against parents' advice in the selection of a mate. In the narrative act of telling and audience listening, the social consequence of female disobedience gets transformed into a warning about the need to control female agency and sexuality, and this narrative twist from freedom to bad fate stands as a firm warning not only to a girl but to those who have authority over her. Given the highly gendered messages in these talks, it is therefore not surprising that the consequence of being disobedient to parents is much more common in the folktales I collected from adolescent girls than it is in those collected from boys. In fact, virtually all the stories I collected from girls had the theme of obedience to kinfolk and then to husbands as a major moral lesson.

Even though elders bemoan their decreased significance in the process of selecting mates for younger people, both young and old people still believe that elders have special insight and wisdom into the character of people. The story of Kintu and Nambi also underscores the importance of the official *kwandhula* ceremony in the vetting of potential marital partners by wider kin and social groups and ensuring that there is no violation of endogamy. Interestingly, in most folktales I heard, there is little if any mention of the male suitor's clan or family in the agreement process, which is similar to Fallers's (1969) findings in the 1950s, in which he observed that the arrangement to marry took place primarily between the father of the young woman and the suitor, with the suitor's kin assisting in the acquisition of bridewealth and acting as formal representatives through which the young man articulated his intent. Also consistent with Fallers's observations is the idea that daughters should be kept under the watch of parents and have limited opportunities to meet male suitors, which can be witnessed in everyday acts of regulating daughters' movement as discussed above. While the surveillance of daughters' actions is certainly more intense than that of sons' and was most likely more intense in the past, several elder women told me of secret visits from and encounters with young suitors, such as in the stories below.

Premarital and Romantic Histories of Elders

I end this chapter with a brief historical flashback to premarital romantic stories of elders in Iganga to remind readers of the complicated ways that the pursuit (or at least their performed retelling) of romantic attachments both did and did not conform to Basoga courtship ideologies of gendering the chase—ideologies that include female obedience and masculine independence. They also demonstrate how ideologies and individual strategies of courtship in Iganga have long invoked a relation of "cruel optimism" for elders, who like young people today once held onto a belief that a "good life" could be achieved by pursuing a particular romantic project that seemed to promise a certain return (Berlant 2011). The two stories I present are not particularly fascinating. Rather, I select them precisely because they are not extraordinary. Instead they represent the ordinarily mundane ways elders construct and remain nostalgically committed to particular versions of their premarital romantic selves while at the same time being fearfully critical of current young people's affective desires and independence. Their critique of young people's romantic fantasies can be read as older people's realization of the cruel optimism of a romantic utopia.

Babirye was in her late sixties when I conducted my initial interviewed with her; she eventually became one of my key informants and friends (in a grandmotherly way) in Bulubandi. She began her romantic history with fond memories of a young suitor in her village. Their flirtatious glances and subtle communication were carried out during her trips to the fields to pick cotton with her mother and younger siblings. She enjoyed the attention from the attractive young man and had imagined him to be the type of man for a future husband. Soon after her eighteenth birthday, she was surprised to learn that her father had arranged for her to be engaged to a young man from her father's home village some thirty miles away. She staged a mild but unmistakable protest, but her father convinced her that the young man was from a good family and that it was time for her to marry. According to Babirye, "I was given to that man by my father because he was very friendly to my father. I was just told that you will marry that man. He told me that the man was well behaved and rich. I could not refuse what my father told me, though I had thought I had started to love the other boy in the village." When I asked if she ever told her father of her interest in the young man from her village, she smiled and suggested that in those days such a direct statement would lead to a confrontation between the father and the young suitor. She hoped that statements she made to her cousin about the boy in the village would be delivered to her father, who would in turn pursue her marriage with that man. That did not happen. She staged an illness to delay the engagement that her father arranged. When that strategy had run its course, she eventually "obeyed" her father and became the fifth wife of the wealthier man in her father's home village. I later found out that her father's family had a long-standing patron-client relationship with the wealthy man's family—a hierarchical relationship that had been established before Babirye was even born—and the betrothal to Babirye was one way to pay off the debt. For Babirye, like other older women, her semi-arranged marriage came at a time in her life when she still thought it would be possible to have a role in selecting her spouse. Other contemporaries of Babirye imply that by the time their fathers introduced them to their future husbands, they were ready to leave their fathers' houses and their strict supervision and begin lives as independent women. Although the marriages of their mothers, aunts, and neighbors hardly represented independence, as younger women they had held onto the belief that their marriages would unfold differently. Many elder women had stories in which their first and often lingeringly true love, who was not the person they married, became an idealized symbol of an affective bond. The earlier years of her marriage were made bearable by an imagined promise, which allowed her to hope that she would marry her village sweetheart, but as the years went by, Babirye's dream faded into a "cruel optimism" that structures romance in a place in which the utopic consumption-based idea remains unobtainable.

Analysis of other women's chronologies shows that it was not infrequent for women to begin their reproductive history before their marital history, indicating older people's amnesia about premarital sex. A common community explanation is that premarital pregnancy was (and still is) a way of proving a woman's fertility and therefore worthiness before solemnization (note the gendered assumption about infertility). Less often talked about at the community level but emerging from elder women's individual stories is that premarital pregnancy was a strategy for a young woman to push her father's hand. Sometimes a woman carefully and secretly planned her premarital reproduction with the aim of compelling her father into considering or even insisting that the young man marry his daughter rather than obeying her father's marital plans. Such women hoped, as Babirye did, that they would eventually reunite with their love interest. Regardless of evidence of histories of premarital reproductive strategies and realities, there is a general collective amnesia about women's sexual encounters and agency. This collective amnesia of Babirye's generation is necessary for the durability of the contemporary critique of today's sexually free *nakyewombekeire*.

Constructions of "self" in older men's premarital narratives are packaged quite differently than women's reconstructions. Unlike narratives of elder women, in which agency is fleetingly but fondly remembered and always tempered with tales of obedience and patience, individual will and determination are main themes running through sexual histories of elder men. Detailing their active role in selecting and winning the attention of a mate features as a predominant performative technique in men's histories. This emphasis on individual efforts and abilities overshadows the role of a young woman's father in brokering the deal and the importance of the man's own kin in raising the wealth necessary for the *kwandhula* ceremony and required bridewealth. The case of Kagoda, the father of Nakagolo from Chapter 3, illustrates this point. While working as a janitor in Iganga's British-run district hospital, he met his first wife and married her in 1961 at the age of forty-one, which was considered a late age for someone to marry at the time. He proudly says this of his long bachelorhood:

Life was not very difficult for me during my single time. It was easy for a person of my class at that time to get a friend to get along with. When I got married, my parents' response was good. They felt good that I was becoming responsible and able to get a wife without their financial assistance. My father and mother started to respect me very much after that. I also started to help them financially as I got promoted at work. In fact, after I got a wife, my father confessed that he had been worried because I took long to get married.

Like other men during the colonial era, Kagoda had a paid position at the district hospital that put him in a higher socioeconomic category than his parents, who participated in a combination of subsistence and cash farming. The prestige of a position in the colonial structure afforded Kagoda greater access to women before marriage, perhaps with his lovers or their fathers intrigued at the possibility of the young woman marrying someone with a wage job and a government pension. The status difference from his parents also motivated his desire to "get a wife without their financial assistance," further sign of his having achieved a higher status. It was also not unusual for men who were entering into Uganda's emerging middle class to delay marriage until they amassed enough wealth to stage their own wedding and maintain their family at a middle-class standard. The characteristic of economic and social independence became an important marker for the emerging African Christian middle class. (According to my interviews, Muslims still involved the extended family).

Kagoda's story also highlights the gendered value placed on family involvement in courtship. Whereas elder women often portray themselves deferring to their parents' thoughts on a suitable partner, the readiness of men to emphasize their ability to make their own wise decisions stands in stark contrast (see also Hunter 2010). According to Kagoda:

> I met my first wife in the hospital where I was working. One day she brought a sick woman in the hospital. She was admitted and when I was moving around the ward, I spotted this young black beauty who was taking care of a sick woman. I approached her and after some time I convinced her to be with me. . . . What attracted me to her was just her dark skin, her red lips and her teeth were as white as milk. She was still young and well built. I was very much attracted to her beauty. By the time her grandmother was discharged after three weeks, she was already mine.

For Kagoda, the idea of identifying his desired qualities in a partner and using his own resources and determination to win her was at the core of his courtship narratives. He had a total of nine "wives," although he officially married only four (the other five being informal or "trial") and never had more than one at a time, for his strict Christian upbringing frowned upon polygyny. He was a consummate serial monogamist, so much of his adulthood was spent courting and testing out women. Kagoda either divorced or "sent away" the women with whom he had conflicts until he settled upon one that got along well with him and his way of doing things. Throughout his story, Kagoda emphasized that he negotiated all nine of his marriages and subsequent divorces himself. Kagoda considered the number of wives he had an indication of his masculine courting abilities of aggression and determination, which were facilitated by his engagement with Uganda's emerging capitalist labor force and market. While his solidly middle-class status at the dawn of the colonial era gave him greater access to women and promises of new forms of masculinity, his fate would reverse as Uganda's postcolonial economy ushered in a larger crop of professional and educated younger people. His status in the workforce quickly declined as younger generations received more education and starting jobs that outranked his. He saw himself go from a middle-class janitor during British colonial times to a rural farmer with a relatively meager paycheck after independence, eventually being too old for the manual labor of his hospital job. He separated from his last wife around 1984 and did not remarry. Although he reflected with great pride on his romantic abilities and full love life, he ended up dying "alone" (a phrase residents use to imply dying without demonstrations of affection from a wife, offspring, or grandchildren), at the age of ninety-three years old. While he was particularly successful in terms of his romantic and marital pursuits during his younger years, his story conveys the consequences of a lifetime of masculinity based on capitalist consumption, or what I call "the lonely old man" syndrome, where wives, children, and extended family have little loyalty to a man who pursued his own interests. Specifically, Kagoda's desire to achieve the masculine acquisition of women came with the cost of his being unable to secure and maintain the loyalties and affections of a network of caregivers (wives and kids) to tend to him in his old age—a tradeoff repeated in many other narratives I collected. There are two versions of masculinity that clash here, partly but not completely differing by age: for younger men, success is measured in the number of lovers and romantic successes as well as economic success, while for older men it is being able to call on a large network of kin and other people. Both of these versions of masculinity are dependent on a man's wealth.

Conclusion: Geographies of Youth Romance

I use the concept "geographies of youth romance" to draw attention to the ways in which globalization during the postcolonial era and Uganda's recent 1990s postconflict liberalization policies have shifted the contours of youth courtship not only spatially (from village to town) as mobility and commercial leisure establishments have increased, but also socially (from multigenerational kin groups to age-segregated social networks) as civic society has become an important place where people establish their identity and status. The commercialization of romance, as influenced by the marketplace as well as the media and advertising, has also led to an imagined individualization of romance and courtship, engendering two cultural displacements. Specifically, the shifts of the orientation of social life and civic engagement from intergenerational, residential settings to more age-segregated and anonymous locations in town have changed the contours of social geographies of courtship in such a way that youthful courtship practices have greater opportunities than in the past of taking place away from chaperoning kin. This social production of space has interacted with emerging civil associations in ways that have displaced or delayed the role of kin in the courtship process. Compared to elders' memories, today young people's peer networks, and particularly the OB and OG school and civic networks, have partly displaced the role of extended family in facilitating the union of young people. Family and friends may be involved (either facilitating or constraining), but youth ultimately imagine the courtship desire and experience as concerning the two main lovers, diametrically opposing more "traditional" routes to romance, love, and marriage. Despite elders' own stories of premarital romance and particularly men's tales of their own courtship abilities, older people maintain that romance is much different today, and in so doing they express their moral disapproval of contemporary youth sexuality and their concern about the social impact of this shift. At the heart of generational tensions about youth romance is the declining significance of family involvement in the courtship process and the increasing agency of young women. The focus on dangers of female sexual agency is motivated by long-standing gender inequalities while also serving as a reason for continuing (male) control and rights over the female body. Stories that elders tell of their own version and pursuit of the romantic ideal of their time, however, indicate a longer historical reality of the cruel optimism of a consumption-based romance that promises, but cannot deliver within Uganda's postcolonial context of economic precarity and social change, a particular construction of a good life in which the individual and his or her intimate relationship is privileged over other relationships that continue to structure everyday life in Iganga. Despite their awareness that many of their romantic relationships will not materialize into a permanent union, young people continue to invest much imagination and energy into developing affective ties, for through them youth reflect on their current situation and future possibilities.

CHAPTER 8

"Burn the letter after reading"

Secrecy and Go-Betweens

When I give a lecture on the love letters, the first question is inevitably, "How did you get the love letters?" I often tell the book's opening story about fortuitously stumbling across Sam's letter at the point in my research when I was struggling with how to methodologically access youth romantic practices and desires. Coming upon Sam's letter was that "aha!" ethnographic moment in which an "opportunistic event," as Sally Falk Moore (1994) terms it, offers an analytic revelation and methodological breakthrough. Then the "dangerous exposure" at the morning assembly occurred, making it abundantly clear that these romantic missives were important to my topic and could provide a window into the contemporary functioning of the counterpublic world of youth sexuality that I sought next to understand. I had been conducting research and facilitating sessions on HIV and sexual health at one of the local schools, and I took the idea of collecting love letters from the students at the school to the headmaster. Knowing that love letters were prohibited at his and other schools, as seen in the "immorality policies" mentioned in the previous chapter, I was not sure how he would respond to my request in his role as a headmaster. I was surprised when the headmaster not only agreed but responded to my request with mischievous laughter as he reached behind his desk to pull a yellow binder from the shelf. Opening the binder, he began pointing to the letters that were inside. I could start my collecting of letters with the batch of letters he had confiscated from students, he told me, as he proceeded to offer me his commentary on different letters. A couple of male teachers from the next room overheard and joined our conversation. What ensued was a discussion about the significance of and nostalgia for their first adolescent sweethearts and relationships, which highlighted their knowledge of the hypocrisy in their own strict prohibitions against love letters and youth romance.

In four schools where my research assistants and I had been working, we got permission from the headmaster to ask students who were interested in participating to bring in their own letters or to ask friends, siblings, or other relatives if they were willing to share their letters for this research activity. I also collected some letters outside of the school setting. Many of the students had participated in other research activities or in one of the health sessions we conducted at the schools, so they were familiar with my research assistants and me. We gave them one day to submit letters, which my research assistants suggested as a way to reduce the chance of participants writing letters specifically for the activity, and received their permission and the schools' to use the letters. After we collected the letters, my assistants decided to go through the letters and identify those that appeared to be written specifically for this activity, or to weed out what my assistants called "fake letters." They felt such letters were fairly easy to discern since "authentic letters" presented signs of wear and tear, dirt, and wrinkles from being secretly concealed and stored. I offered letter collectors forty cents for a letter I could keep and thirty cents for a letter that the youth preferred that I photocopy and return, an idea I borrowed from linguist Niko Besnier (1995), who collected letters from migrant men in the Polynesian atoll of Nukulaelae. Because of the personal value of the family letters he collected, Besnier felt it important to remunerate residents for sharing them with him. The amount we set to remunerate young people for a letter would be respectful but not coercive, and it certainly did not seem high enough to warrant the level of excitement and involvement the letter-collecting project received. When I asked why the project was met with such enthusiasm, my assistants as well as students speculated that participants were delighted that an adult was actually interested in the letters they had labored over, and that the adult thought that their youthful liaisons were meaningful and worthy of positive attention. I remain unsure how we were able to collect over three hundred letters in such a short amount of time and to speak with many of the recipients about their letters, but I would like to think that in addition to reflecting young people's interest in the topic, their willingness to participate has something to do with the familiarity and trust they had developed with our research team over the previous months.

As Lila Abu-Lughod discusses in her ethnography on Bedouin women's lyrical poetry, the meanings of cultural productions cannot be separate from the context in which they emerge (Abu-Lughod 1986; see also Ahearn 2001). Therefore, when possible, I discussed the letter and the relationship with the person who gave me the letter, which in most cases was the recipient of the letter or someone who knew the recipient (but not necessarily the letter writer). During these discussions, I gathered information about the sex and age of writers and recipients, circumstances surrounding the exchange of the letters, the relationship itself (such as the nature and duration of the relationship and results of the letter exchange), and the young person's interpretation of the sample letters (with the names and identifying characteristics deleted) to discuss common terms, strategies, and discourses in focus groups of young people. Not only were the focus group sessions invaluable in deciphering the coded language of romance that I could not always comprehend initially, but the gendered debates that emerged over the intent, meaning, and sincerity of a letter indicated that youth romantic discourse and practices are indeed contested even among the young participants themselves. It was clear that both boys and girls saw themselves as victims in relationships—boys having little to offer in the consumption-based romantic ideal, and girls having something every male wanted for the cheapest price (access to another man's property).

The cultural expressions and sentiments contained in the letters are not, as Johannes Fabian (1978, 1998) reminds us, evidence of how a culture *works* but of how social problems are *worked out*. This unfolding of culture is particularly true for love letters, for in these letters young people not only discuss their feelings and desires for their sweethearts, but also spend a significant amount of time reflecting on and seeking advice on the precarity of life and everyday hardships. Here lies the real methodological

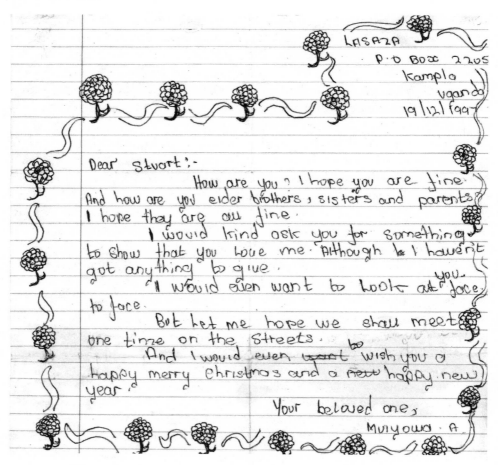

The letter reads:

LASAZA
P.O BOX 2205
Kampla
Uganda
19/12/199?

Dear Stuart:-
    How are you? I hope you are fine. And how are you elder brothers, sisters and parents? I hope they are all fine.
    I would kind ask you for something to show that you love me. Although I haven't got anything to give.
    I would even want to look at you face to face.
    But let me hope we shall meet one time on the streets.
    And I would even want to wish you a happy merry Christmas and a new happy new year.

                        Your beloved one,
                            Muiyowa · A

FIGURE 8.1. Decorated letter

contribution of the letters—they provide a window into youth intimacy and into how young people experience, understand, and cope with the everyday uncertainties and difficulties that shape their lives.

Courting through Love Letters

Young people's imaginations of romance are deeply consumption based, and love letters emerge precisely because they cannot afford commercial tokens of love. Or, since purchased gifts, money, and commercial outings that structure young people's ideas of a consumption-centered romantic ideal are financially out of reach for most Iganga youth, their carefully crafted and secretly exchanged love letters become important symbols of love and affection, and they provide a vehicle for the fashioning of romantic selves. Youth often put great effort into the creation of love letters, as discussed in the next chapter, for they become a reflection of the person's romantic self and intent. As such, they can be read as not only a written text but also a performance.

Like any form of communication, the meaning and significance of love letter exchanges is culturally and socially specific. Writing about changes in the courtship process in Nepal, anthropologist Laura Ahearn (2001) found that love letters have become a new way for young lovers to initiate and build a relationship with a future spouse without the traditional assistance from or arrangement by family. In some cases the love letter exchanges formed the basis for the couple's future elopement and entry into a modern marriage based on individual agency rather than family involvement. While Ahearn observed that clandestine romantic courtships carried out through letter exchanges frequently turn into marriages through elopement, Amy Shuman found that love letters played a very different role for working-class youth in a city in the eastern United States. Of the various written texts created by the youth Shuman studied, love letters "were the most playful of messages. . . . Furthermore, some letters were intended as serious but were received as a joke" (1986:88–89). Based on Shuman's research, love letters among youth are used to initiate and "feel out" or test romantic possibilities; maybe a few short notes are exchanged, but then letter writing gives way to young people continuing their relationship through meeting up and "hanging out," as youth call it. Love letter writing in Uganda falls somewhere in between the Nepalese beginning of conjugality and the eastern US playful exploration. Whereas love letters in Iganga do not necessarily lead to marriage or elopement, as in the case of Nepal, they are taken seriously as a venue for initiating and conducting courtship.

Once received, love letters are often kept, cherished, and read again and again. From their appearance it was evident that some letters had been unfolded and refolded many times, and the burns on letters indicate that some were read by candlelight or a lantern at night. Like other sentimental items such as photographs, greeting cards, and small nonutilitarian gifts (such as a needlepointed cloth), love letters are typically kept in the bottom of a person's metal trunk. Many adolescents receive a locally made metal trunk to store and transport personal belongings throughout their young adult years as they shift from one residence to another. For women, these locally made metal trunks are ideally replaced with purchased suitcases as part of the bridewealth exchange during the *kwandhula* ceremony. To demonstrate their commitment to their new husbands and their transition from youthful romance to the seriousness of marriage, my married female friends told me they are supposed to dispose of love letters from past boyfriends. Some, however, did not and risked the ire of jealous husbands. For men, their more frequent shifting around during young adulthood (commonly in search of work or to pursue advanced training or education) makes it much harder to retain the trunk and its contents.

Secrecy and Discretion

Courting through love letters occurs in a context in which private and one-to-one interaction among opposite sex adolescents is constrained. A couple may arrange surreptitious meetings behind the schoolyard, at a watering hole, the evening market, or a village function with prospective romantic partners, but they find it difficult for such encounters to go beyond nonverbal flirtations and exchanges, since the scene often includes other people, such as friends, younger siblings, or random bystanders. Arranging these brief meetings has become slightly easier with the use of texting, which has increased as young people gain greater access to mobile phones, borrowed from an older friend in some cases and owned in others. During these brief semipublic encounters, young lovers are often too inhibited to speak to their sweethearts, as cultural conventions of public restraint make it inappropriate for sweethearts to engage in conversation beyond prosaic and casual topics. In this context of supervised interactions, letters become their romantic voices, allowing young people to fashion a romantic self, develop a relationship further, and work out issues in the relationship. Letters also allow young people the graceful expression of words they might otherwise be unable to articulate, whether because of nervousness or for fear of being found out by curious bystanders. Cathy, an eighteen-year-old girl residing with her aunt in a village beyond Iganga Town, had a chance encounter with a love interest in a public transportation park, during which they felt too self-conscious and hesitant to speak with one another. Later, she wrote a letter to the young man, recounting the fortuitous encounter and her disappointment that they were unable to speak:

> By the way, do you still remember a day when you were in a taxi/bus (Jinja Bus Park) and all of a sudden you glanced at me? I never thought of meeting you anywhere (esp. Jinja) but only it was just a surprise to see you trying to communicate to me. It made me sad for not saying hullo to each other since the bus was leaving and I was left in suspense. I really miss you, my dear. (letter G:46)

Cathy's words reveal the power and ambiguity of subtle flirtatious glances, and the role that private letters play in conveying deeper meanings and anxieties that young people have toward romantic partners. Attending different schools separated Cathy from her potential sweetheart, and their unexpected encounter reminded Cathy of their short romance and her initial pain after their separation. She asks her sweetheart: "Remember those days we used to stay together and never thought of finishing a whole week without seeing each other? Can you imagine? On my side it took me time to live lonely without you. What about you?" Communicating sentiments of longing and desire for more physical interaction is a common purpose of love letters. In written declarations, romantic feelings and personal thoughts are delivered without interruptions or the threat of having a relationship discovered by others, unless the letter is confiscated.

As the morning assembly event illustrates, while letters are supposed to be private missives between two people, communicating intimate feelings through the written word always runs the risk that contents will become public. The writer of a letter willingly defers discretion and the rights of circulation to the addressee or another person who might find the letter. Letters often have instructions not to share the letter with anyone or to destroy the letter. In the top left corner on the back page of a letter, one boy writes: "Remember to burn the letter after reading; let it be privy." Letters are too precious to dispose of, and the girl obviously did not follow his instructions to burn the letter. Girls and boys hold different reasons for wanting letters to remain private: girls risk the embarrassment and scrutiny of their messages (such as in the case of Annette) and boys risk the consequences of being caught by the girl's parents, particularly if their letter contains references to sex. For instance, a boy writes: "Remember to demolish this sheet after reading by any means, as it might cause problems. . . . My view of writing this letter is to request you to 'come friends with me.' I hope you know the use of friends because it is difficult for me to express how I feel for you babe" (letter B:29). He is likely asking for the letter to be demolished because of "problems" associated with his not-so-encoded request for sex, "come friends with me." If this evidence of a request for sex falls into the hands of a girl's guardians, it can be used against the writer in the future—a consequence that young men are continually reminded of through local gossip and stories about defilement cases. One such story circulated around Iganga regarding a Probate Office case in which the guardians of a girl used a love letter from a boy as evidence of his paternity. Since the girl was under eighteen years of age, the boy, who was also under eighteen, was to be charged with violating the age of consent law. Fortunately for the adolescent boy the case was dropped, most likely, we were told, because of either the girl's pleadings or a satisfactory financial settlement between the girl's guardians and the young man who was charged with impregnating her.

A different adolescent male took care to directly highlight the risk associated with carrying on an affair through letters, and he advised about the caution with which he and his lover should proceed. His cautionary note was based on an actual event that happened to him. He writes:

> As I am concerned, I am saying that I shall be talking with you through letters but the bad thing is that when I came there, they told me that my letter which I send to you was opened by the teachers in the office and it was read. So it seems that I may stop writing to you b'se everything will be known to them. So give me advice to such. Because I can write my words and they know also what I have written. As you know love is love. (letter B:41)

Although the boy had already been caught once, he was not deterred from jotting new missives to his love. Instead, the two devised other, more clandestine methods of communicating, which pushed their courtship into deeper secrecy.

In another case, seventeen-year-old Sophia attracted the attention of many young male suitors and received numerous love letters from boys. Her parents were aware of their daughter's popularity and were known for keeping a close watch over her. In a note to Sophia, a potential suitor, also seventeen, seeks Sophia's advice on how he can court her without her parents discovering: "I didn't mean you to decide either to give up or to go on but asked you to suggest which method can we play when carrying our love affairs in order to avoid being netted by your parents who are bitterly in need of netting me" (letter B:11).

While young writers gamble against the possibility that adults will get hold of incriminating letters, most youth were concerned that their private words would become the topic of schoolyard gossip or that their failed attempts at romance would be exposed in front of their peers. Such a fear is the main theme woven throughout a letter in which a boy of nineteen pleads with his sweetheart not to share their relationship or the letter with anyone because he does not want people to "spread rumors." He writes:

> Another thing, don't tell anyone about our relationship because if you tell anyone, she will start spreading rumors which some of them will not be true and for my case I don't want people to be concerned with our relationship. That's why I'm avoiding them. On addition to that, if there is any misunderstanding just come to me so that we can solve those problems don't tell even your heart (Katima) if there is any problem. And don't tell the whole dorm as you did within those days and that thing hurt me up to now. (letter B:8)

The boy cleverly entitled the letter "Forgiveness," positioning his stern plea for secrecy after his kind gesture of forgiveness. Like much rhetoric of forgiveness, the boy appropriates a Christian framework in order to establish a hierarchical relationship between the sinner (his love interest) and the saint-like forgiver (himself). He writes, "I have forgiven you in God's name, because Jesus said that forgive those one's who do bad to you." To wrong him once, he advises, is forgivable but to wrong him twice, he threatens, is not. He warns: "I request you kindly that not to make me annoyed any other time becoz you will be making me to remember what you did to me." Youth must navigate the concerns they have for being embarrassed among their peers (which has immediate reputational and status consequences) with the potentially more serious consequences of being caught defying their parents or other adults.

Letter Writing as the Elaboration of Sentiment

Not only does the written word provide evidence of defiant or embarrassing acts of romance but letters can also serve to bolster romantic sincerity and thought. Unlike face-to-face speech acts, the process of letter writing and reading serves to elaborate sentiment by allowing both the writer and recipient an extended and solitary time for reflecting on thoughts, feelings, and intensions, and for contemplating the ways in which to best express oneself (Ahearn 2001; Giddens 1992; Goody 1998). Whereas face-to-face communication compels immediate interpretation and reaction, communicating through letters inevitably slows down dialogue, enabling the writer and reader to reflect on sentiments and strategically compose the written missive. Through the extended elaboration of sentiment a sweetheart can become idealized as an object of perfection, affection, and attention, a location for the writer to posit optimism or despair about the future and intimacy. Particularly useful in understanding the role of love letters in youth romance is Niko Besnier's exploration of why certain emotions are found more frequently in letters that migrant men write to family members than in regular face-to-face conversations among residents of a Polynesian island. Borrowing Robert Levy's (1984) distinction between "hypercognized" and "hypocognized," Besnier explains that letter writing and reading "hypercognize affect" in such a way that some "emotions are referred to more overtly and frequently than in other communicative events" (1995:110–11). Through letters, he argues, people can express emotions that in other social contexts they may be reluctant to share because of cultural norms or personal inhibitions. Likewise, in her study of nineteenth-century love letters in Britain, Karen Lystra (1989) found that love letters reveal more about a romantic relationship than other archival sources precisely because they were presumably private communications between sweethearts, written in isolation from others, including the intended recipient. Similarly, youth in Iganga often use letters to convey feelings of attraction or desire that they hesitate to express in face-to-face encounters. An eighteen-year-old boy appends this postscript after declaring his love:

> I had a thought of
> talking to you physically
> but I thought something
> will go wrong (letter B:2)

As the passage above demonstrates, written requests spare the embarrassment of rejection or having to face an uncomfortable power imbalance. Beyond the elaboration of sentiment and the pragmatics of escaping embarrassment, within the Basoga culture of respect, in which indirect or circuitous requests represent deference, letter writing as the chosen form of personal communication signifies the humility and sincerity of the letter writer. In such contexts, the written word as an indirect form of communication indicates both respect and sincerity. For instance, in a patron-client relationship, if a client makes a request directly to a patron, the client is crossing lines of respect by positing the two on the same level. Sending a message through another person or in writing allows the client to humble himself or herself by signaling that the requestor is not worthy of directly communicating with the patron. In romance, conveying sentiments in writing also intensifies feelings, making sentiments more heartfelt and genuine, and the writer more humble. Phrases written in love letters such as "I just feel like looking at you all the time" or Sam's "Lover why do you make me cry" are easily articulated and invoke strong romantic feelings in the recipient in a way that the spoken statement might not. Furthermore, submitting requests in writing, rather than verbally, shows respect for the person and establishes, even if temporarily, a hierarchy in the relationship. Hence, male suitors can demonstrate respect for their sweetheart while simultaneously requesting sex. I too have been the recipient of letters in which the writer wanted to emphasize a sentiment such as appreciation, or make a humble request for a favor or money.

Merely receiving a love letter, regardless of its content, is itself a valued expression of admiration among Igangan youth. When I asked one adolescent girl about the meaning of a letter written by her admirer, she explained that the letter said he liked her and wanted to establish a relationship. In the letter, in fact, the boy wrote less about his admiration for her and more about recent prosaic news (e.g., his mother's sickness and his lack of money for school fees). But to the girl, the main message behind this letter was less the actual content and more that he was sharing this news with her as a way of showing his interest through this act of intimacy that requires a deliberate investment. It was the act of taking time to write a love letter that said he had a romantic interest in her.

Love letters are a particularly useful window into youth relationships because—unlike purchased gifts that are frequently unidirectional from male to female (but even this is changing)—both parties must participate in the exchange of letters in order for a relationship to continue. This leads to two important distinctions between the exchange of monetary gifts and the symbolic token of love letters. First, the gender hierarchy produced by commercial gifts gives the purchaser (most often the male participant) greater power over the recipient (most often the female), particularly in instances in which the recipient cannot provide a gift of equal monetary value. In such a case, the social contract might dictate that the value of the material item given be returned in the form of indebtedness or a favor—for instance, sex—and hence the gift signifies the giver's power over the receiver. However, in the exchange of love letters the value is not material but symbolic, and power is shifted to the recipient, who is in a position to respond, reject, or delay reaction to the letter. While love letters are not devoid of gender hierarchies, as explored later, feminist scholars have noted that letter writing and journaling offer women greater expression and ability to state their desires than in courtships, in which they are merely recipients of male advances and gifts. This leads to the second distinction of letter exchange. Love letter relationships require the full participation of young females for the liaison to progress and last, meaning that young women are required to exert agency and clearly state their intentions and desires. From an analytical standpoint, the reciprocity involved in love letter exchange allows for the exploration of both men's *and* women's sexual agency and active participation in the romantic project. Women are not just passive recipients of proposals of love, but they must actively interpret suitors' requests, construct their own ideas of romance, and communicate their feelings, which is ultimately what makes letters so threatening to elders' notions of premarital liaisons.

While adolescent boys most often initiate an exchange of love letters, girls draw from gendered cultural mannerisms to subtly attract male suitors. Some of these culturally appropriate acts of demurely making oneself desirable and open to a suitor—which often allow a girl to deny that she is doing so—include passing by a place that he frequents (such as a storefront or the market), giggling, making eye contact, or walking in a slow and sexy manner. A letter written by a boy of sixteen reflects cultural notions of female attractiveness: "I fraternal [admire] you the way you talk, stand, smile and bend. . . . I want to tell you that I love you with all my heart and soul and . . . you are going to be taken as queen with reconciliation" (letter B:43). As explained to me during a group discussion, when an adolescent boy is interested in a girl, he might choose to "become friendly" with one of her female confidants in hopes that she will pass on good messages about him, in a sense temporarily emasculating himself with the aim of gaining a girl's interest. Girls are less likely to employ this strategy for fear that the boy's friend will misread her motives. Ultimately, though, whether near or far, and within the context of secrecy, young people manage to communicate heartfelt emotions and sentiments of desires with their sweethearts through letters. Tucked away from the chaperoning eyes of adults, the letters are part of an elaborate underground world of youth courtship wherein the letters and romantic sentiments become semi-public property.

The Contemporary Intermediary: Go-Betweens

The use of go-betweens to deliver letters and verbal messages between two lovers is crucial to a relationship, particularly during the early stages, when each party is uncertain of the other's interest. Although letters are private and often extended communications between lovers, intermediaries help move the relationship along and help in negotiating and relaying the intentions of young lovers. As explored in the previous chapter, the use of a third party in romantic liaisons builds on traditional conventions in which two lovers declared their intentions to each other through a spokesperson. This is most clearly seen in the engagement process, during which a spokesperson for the prospective groom, not the groom himself, expresses the desire or intent of the young man to marry the bride-to-be.

Edward T. Hall's (1976) discussion of high-context versus low-context communication styles is useful in understanding the use of go-betweens in Iganga. Like many other groups in Uganda, the Basoga practice an ideology of respect that neatly follows a "high-context" communication style, which Hall describes as being more indirect and formal and requiring the receiver and listener to decipher nonverbal clues and coded messages. The use of go-betweens to deliver letters and messages follows the high-context cultural model. Not only is indirect communication, such as speaking through another person, thought to be more respectful, but it also allows for flexibility in meaning, enabling either party to easily escape or deny an unwanted or offensive situation. Like all surrogates in indirect communication, go-betweens are carefully selected; the spokesperson is considered a reflection of the writer's social network and capital and also needs to be a trusted confidant.

Regardless of the careful selection of a go-between, courtship complications often occur. Requesting the assistance of one who has not yet perfected the art of being a sneaky and reliable messenger can have unforeseen consequences, such as incorrectly relayed messages, letters left with the wrong person, or go-betweens caught in a feud between lovers. One girl had a letter from her lover accidentally delivered to her step-mother. A common mishap in schools is for letters to be intercepted by teachers, as seen in Annette's case. In another case, the female recipient of a letter hoped that her lover's female go-between would reveal more information than divulged in the letter as an act of gender solidarity. The unsuspecting courier encountered a barrage of questions from the letter recipient, becoming the target of the adolescent girl's anger when she refused to disclose or did not know the requested information. The frustrated teenager wrote back to her lover: "Thank you for your message. Anyway I received it but I was furious with it becoz I was deceived by the person who delivered it to me. I don't know whether she just feared to tell the facts because of my reactions or she was ordered by the writer" (letter G:17). The frustrated girl advised her lover to not use another female student as the go-between and to select his messenger more carefully next time: "Reply if you're willing but never give it to my fellow girls to bring to me."

Some youth use the go-between system to deliver written or verbal missives to their lovers across long distances, since few have easy access to post office boxes. The regular mobility of many young people from the residence of one relative to another for school or financial reasons means that a network of go-betweens is required not only to deliver messages and letters but also to provide updates on a sweetheart's fidelity. Newer electronically mediated communication relies less on go-betweens but facilitates other dynamics of romance.

High-Speed Romance in the Age of Electronic Communication

Readers familiar with contemporary Africa might wonder about how cell phones (and specifically texting), e-mail, and social media sites (such as Facebook) fit into this hand-written romantic counterpublic. No doubt the increased availability and access to electronic technologies over the course of my research has expanded and transformed the discursive space and possibilities of youth romance. Dating even further back, pay phone booths have been sites for arranging romantic meetings and have been mentioned in the local press and academic writing for their role in extramarital liaisons among adults. Since the turn of the twenty-first century, mobile phones as vehicles for advancing romantic liaisons and intentions have presented a different set of issues. As opposed to phone booths, in which sexual discussions leaked out to the overhearing ears of entrepreneurial operators, mobile phones allow for greater discretion, at least in theory. During the beginning of my research, hardly any school-age youth in Iganga owned or had regular access to a cell phone. By the early 2000s, there was a notable increase in the emergence of pay-by-minute cell phone stalls in both rural and town locations around Iganga. Some of the young adults I knew opened up stalls as one of their income streams. In this entrepreneurial venture, a person with a cell phone would set up a table and would charge customers by the minute to use the phone. Throughout much of Africa, the first decade of the twenty-first century saw a great proliferation in cell phones as competition among providers drove down prices for phones and services and increased the service area, number of retail outlets, and trained technicians and salesforce. Having access to a mobile phone became a social expectation among young adults and a symbol of status. Today, many young people who do not own a phone can easily find an older friend or cousin who will allow them to send a text message. A similar proliferation of Internet cafes, tablets, computers at local shops, and the like has also increased access to web-based communication.

Although I did not systematically collect courtship text messages to conduct a meaningful content analysis, the few exchanges I did collect and discuss with youth allow me to offer a few insights into how electronic technologies serve a different purpose and enable new types of practices and possibilities. Compared to love letters, main differences in courting through texts include greatly abbreviated messages, the elimination of the go-between, the immediate transmission of a message and a response, the possibility of an archive of bidirectional exchanges (as opposed to a person's retaining only one side of the letter communication), and an extended communication range that is no longer limited by the geographic proximity of two people. The elaboration of sentiment found in most love letters is absent in texts, as desire is reduced into sound bites and SMS textese (including acronyms, abbreviations, pictograms, and emoticons). Messages of love become prepackaged and standardized. Mobile phones also make it easy for a person to send the same message to multiple recipients, increasing the pool of potential partners and the chances of getting a positive response. I spoke with several boys who regularly sent the same "I am interested in you"–style message to various adolescent girls in hopes that at least one message would prove productive. Adolescent and young men explained that this practice of casting a wide net when seeking romance was used so frequently that they too felt compelled to do so in order to compete with other boys. If a relationship does take root, texting makes arranging a meeting much easier and allows lovers a new level of secrecy and discretion, which has led to the emergence of a more ephemeral type of relationship (similar, in some ways, to US "hook-up" culture). In addition, whereas letters allow lovers to build a relationship through the process of reflection and the letter writers' ability to address a variety of topics in one letter (e.g., from updates about health, school or family to detailed descriptions of emotions, as explored in the next chapters), extended self-representation and communication in a single text is greatly limited.

Another difference we observed between texting and writing a love letter is that the sincerity and intent of "I love you" text messages are more likely to be questioned than the sincerity of the message in a letter (in which the writer has to expend the energy of constructing a letter and recruiting a third-party go-between) or an e-mail (which still retains some element of the personal). However, in Iganga access to the Internet is more limited than access to mobile phones, with cost, computer knowledge, and location of Internet cafes being key factors in accessibility. While texts are used for short messages, such as declaring interest and soliciting a response or arranging a meeting time and place, e-mails tend to be used to elaborate on the happenings in a person's life, much in the way that letters allow. E-mail has also opened up the communication range nationally and globally, which is something I repeatedly heard from youth when I asked about their e-mail use. Not only does e-mail provide a way for former classmates or lovers to stay in contact after one has relocated, hence extending the possibility of a future relationship, but it also has become a new technology through which the older practice of international pen-pal relationships operates.

Social media sites offer yet another venue for romantic connections and explorations. Facebook, for instance, allows youth to keep up with both romantic partners and platonic friends who post pictures, "share" links, and post comments without the observing person reciprocating information or declaring his or her presence on the person's site. This act of intimate voyeurism provides youth with important information about potential or past lovers that they can use when deciding whether and how to proceed with a relationship, and they can keep the possibility of a relationship open by periodically posting on a person's wall. A person can appear and disappear from another person's electronic life by deciding when to make a post, send a message, or recognize a birthday. Much like e-mail, the end result is the possibility of an increased network—both geographically and quantitatively—of extended intimate relationships, some of which might be the source of jealousy, suspicion, and insecurity in marital years. Whereas electronic communication technologies offer young people new spaces for romantic practices and self-fashioning, they also highlight, more so than love letters, economic inequalities and hierarchies among youth themselves.

Hence, an analysis of electronic technologies might demonstrate ways in which romantic practices and discourses are becoming increasingly segregated by socioeconomic class and geographic location, but because of their condensed messaging and ability to mass-produce messages, these technologies might be limited in what they can tell us about young people's developing of romantic selves and relationships. Methodological challenges are also present, which might lead to new ethnographic innovations and creativity, as well as a new set of ethical considerations. Precisely because of the wider accessibility of letter writing, the greater investment and effort required to participate, and the space for reflection and careful selection of words, love letters lend themselves to understanding how the romantic imaginations about the future interact with and are shaped by the dominant public and the precarious realities of everyday life.

CHAPTER 9

"B4 I symbolise my symbolised symbology"

Packaging and Reading Love Letters

> B4 I symbolise my symbolised symbology symbologically I would like
> to write multiplying love b'tn me and u. My love is as lasting as a gravity
> stone—I love u b'se u are beautiful, charming and my best friend. I will
> always love you until the sea dries. Your shining face attracts and affects
> my feelings and make me even mix up my chemical wrongly. (18-year-
> old male)

In this chapter, I examine the format and the key features of love letters, and argue that these elements are just as critical as the main body of the letter in the creation of romance and expression of sentiment. As reflected in this chapter's epigraph, young people strategically use certain literary techniques (from the grand effect in boys' letters to the deployment of invented words and local metaphors) to perform romantic modernity and acquire romantic capital. I also explore the role of the "peripheral aspects" that youth use to package letters—the return address, margin art, and quotes, the song dedications at the end, and other elements—to illustrate how youth interact with and draw from a variety of regulatory publics and discourses in imagining romance and crafting affective subjectivities and selves. In examining the peripheral aspects of love letters, this chapter continues to introduce readers to excerpts of letters in order to draw attention to the writers' romantic hopes, imagination, and hesitation.

During my initial research stint, "Un-Break My Heart," a 1996 Toni Braxton hit, became the romantic theme song among youth in Iganga; it was constantly played on the radio, in discos, and in karaoke competitions. The frequently repeated words in youth letters and casual conversation—"Un-break my heart / Say you'll love me again"—are not simply begging a former lover to undo the pain he or she caused. Rather, they represent a broader belief in romance as a cure to everyday struggles, that an escape to a better life is indeed possible. The title of the song symbolizes the tremendous hope and belief young people have in the transcendent power of romantic imagination—a hope-filled belief that romance will lift them out (whether temporarily or forever) of their current context of persistent community poverty and illness. Hence, what I am arguing is that romantic sentiments are about not only a relationship with a person, but also the process of imagining a future life in general.

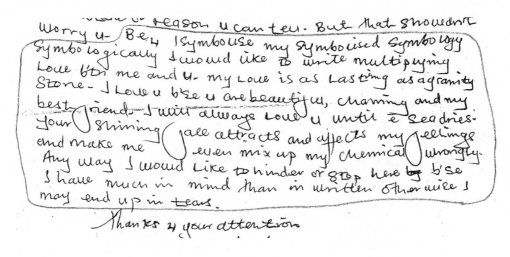

FIGURE 9.1. Love letter and creative English

Writing Romance: English, the Grand Effect, and Invention

English is the standard language of love letters. Even with deliberate effort I was unable to collect any love letters written in Lusoga, though this does not mean such letters do not exist. There is a practical explanation for this. Most young people do not formally learn to write in Lusoga. It is not taught in schools, and there was no standard Lusoga orthography developed when colonial missionaries were translating the Bible into the languages of neighboring ethnic groups.[1] The lack of standard and written Lusoga and the subsequent gradual adoption of Luganda (the language of the neighboring ethnic group) have left some Basoga leaders feeling as though their group has been subject to cultural imperialism. In response, the (Busoga) Cultural Research Centre was in the process of developing an official Lusoga orthography during my initial research, and the director informed me that many instances arose when the committee had to decide which of several options to adapt. Hence, young people's ability to write in Lusoga is often very limited and correct Lusoga spelling of words constantly under debate, as I experienced when my research assistants and I translated our interview guides and consent forms into Lusoga.

In addition to practical reasons, the use of English carries affective and symbolic valence. As English is the language for instruction in formal education and mastery of it is required for succeeding on national standardized tests, linguistic competency in it indexes a young person's potential social mobility and future status. English also affords youth greater cultural license and freedom to express sentiments of desire than their mother tongue. This is not because love and desire are foreign, but rather because English allows young people to break free of local sexual mores and conventions that govern what it means to express desire and to imagine romantic possibilities beyond cultural boundaries. For instance, while direct declaration of intimate sentiments or sexual interest might be read as crude and culturally inappropriate in Lusoga, or

unride wooded plain thus, always have the guts to look ahead of the present.

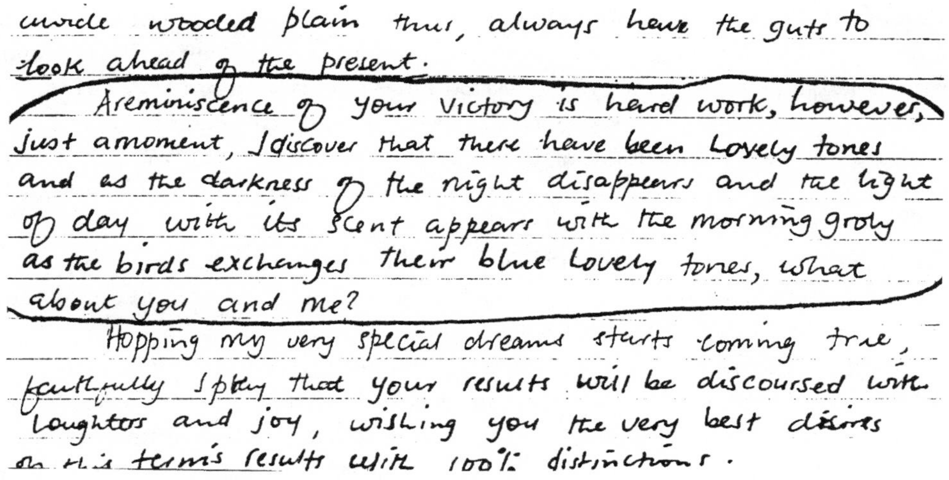

A reminiscence of your victory is hard work, however, just a moment, I discover that there have been lovely tones and as the darkness of the night disappears and the light of day with its scent appears with the morning glory as the birds exchanges their blue lovely tones, what about you and me?

Hopping my very special dreams starts coming true, faithfully I pray that your results will be discoursed with laughters and joy, wishing you the very best desires on this term's results with 100% distinctions.

FIGURE 9.2. Grand effect

a breach of conventional routes of obtaining permission, by using English a young person can temporarily suspend cultural prescriptions. By using a foreign language and borrowing English idioms, phrases, and references acquired from Western movies, books, and songs, youth can create a romantic space that transcends (even if discursively and temporarily) the constraints of local precarity and regulation. On the other hand, English as the standard language of love letters also excludes or limits some young people from fully participating in the counterpublic of love letters. As a result, most letters I collected were written by adolescents who either currently were attending or had attended at least some primary school. That said, even young people with minimal written ability in English (such as primary school students) manage to use letters as a form of communication. In such cases, the young person might use an amanuensis (a friend or the like) or simply supplement the limited written text with greater attention to decorating the paper, adding scent, using colored paper, or attaching dried flowers.

The most skilled love letter writers artfully employ what I call a "grand effect," meaning sentiments expressed through strings of alliteration, hyperbole, melodious phrases, assonance, and metaphors.[2] There is a high premium on eloquence, sophisticated vocabulary, and melodramatic effect, which can be seen in an artful passage admired by a group of students in Iganga (see Figure 9.2). While the passage evokes beautiful images of nature and change, it is also valued for its harmonious and sophisticated sound. The phrase "reminiscence of your victory," rather than referring to a specific victory, is understood to indicate a general positive state of being or encouragement. By employing a grand effect, the writer aims to elicit romantic thoughts and emotions from the recipient through skillful use of linguistic registers. The grand effect is also commonly found in other speech events, such as impromptu narrations of dramatic stories, local gossip shared with a group of people, or public speeches. In the last, for instance, through often verbose rhetoric, the speaker carefully performs dramatic eloquence in hopes of impressing the audience with the display of grand effect or winning election votes by demonstrating great showmanship. Grand effect is a cultural act of persuasion. Such is the case with love letters, particularly by boys at the beginning of a relationship, when they are trying to woo a love interest with romantic charm.

The English of love letters is dynamic, reflecting wider cultural shifts and inventions. Adding to the romantic tone is the strategic use of invented words, in which writers invest great effort when they are unable to adequately call upon standard words to convey their emotion or sentiment. This lyrical proficiency is an art and increases with experience or with greater competency in English. Since creating this effect is a time-consuming task for most young people, some authors choose not to invoke it at all or use it only in part of a letter.

The repeated variations of "symbolise"—"symbolised," "symbology," "symbologically"—in the epigraph of this chapter, and the turn of phrase "reminiscence of your victory" in the passage the students admired, are intended to convey strong romantic feelings for which the author might lack the words to express. The writer may have learned the word "symbolise" in school or through the mass media, thought it sounded eloquent and sophisticated, and, with much effort, decided to creatively construct a sentence around it, thus producing a grand effect. By leaning on the assumed shared understanding of the word in question, the poetic writer lets the word do the work for him by simply using various inflections and conjugations of the word and creating an expansive romantic affect. The word "symbolise" is found in another letter written in the same month by a boy from the same school, suggesting how words acquired in school or through the media become a part of a collective love letter lexicon at a particular moment. The highest compliment to any letter writer is to have his or her words reproduced in the love letters of others, becoming part of the written counterpublic. Young men and women commonly attempt to re-create a particular grand effect or word that they have read or heard; for example, a derivation of this chapter's epigraph was found in a love letter written by a girl. It is difficult to tell who the original author of the passage was, since one of the letters does not have a date, but the original author or source is often of secondary importance to youth who reuse the words or phrases.

Metaphors and similes are a regular and important part of the language of love letters. They help establish a romantic ethos by removing the writer and reader from the everyday and relocating both in an imagined space or by emphasizing declarations through drawing on familiar or recently learned references, such as "my love is as lasting as a gravity stone." Romantic space can be created through references to nature, such as "I will always love you until the sea dries," or by the use of elaborate passages, phrases, and words, such as "B4 I symbolise my symbolised symbology symbologically I would like to write multiplying love b'tn me and u." The distinct high-tone literary style in these letters is reworked from various sources. When I asked about the origin of hyperbolic phrases in letters, I was told by a group of adults that these were the same ones that they used to use. One laughingly said, "It seems they just stole our words." Some phrases are gleaned from subjects learned in school, such as this familiar opening adapted from earth science class: "How is the atmospheric pressure over there?" Other language is borrowed from popular songs and romance novels, and some is newly invented.[3] A letter writer who can skillfully blend familiar phrases and words of love while creating new ones is regarded as a master in the written language of romance.

There are some marked differences between the language of girls and boys, the motivation of which will be explored in subsequent chapters when discussing the themes of love letters. Grand effect, invented words, and metaphors are more frequent in letters written by boys. One possible explanation is that boys have a greater motivation to demonstrate literary dexterity, as their letters are often intended to woo a girl and convince her of his romantic worthiness. Whereas boys are more likely to use grand effect in order to impress, girls' letters tend to sound more hesitant in their declarations, often seeming less committed and more skeptical, maintaining local gender conventions and strategic gendered positions surrounding romance. When girls do employ the grand effect strategy, their intent seems to be similar to that of boys, to woo or impress their love interest, as in the case of Annette, whose letter was read at the morning assembly. The language of both girls and boys becomes more direct and less grand when they are explaining their own problems or when confronting their love interests with suspicions or accusations. Gender differences in the use of language also point to how gender inequality manifests itself in creative freedom or, conversely, linguistic constraints. Specifically, it is likely that boys' sense of gendered entitlement translates into greater poetic license to invent words and employ grand effect as compared to their female counterparts, who may fear being mocked for using embellishments or nonsensical words. Hence, generally speaking, while boys' gender privilege allows them greater poetic license in this particular genre and the assumption that girls might not question an invented word, girls' awareness of their place in the gender hierarchy makes them more cautious and fearful that their linguistic inventions will be further evidence of their inferior status. Girls such as Annette, who challenge these gender constraints, are both admired and put under an increased critical gaze.

Packaging Love in Letters

The physical presentation or aesthetic packaging of the letter provides insight into how youth draw from the public spheres in creating romance. Although the format is highly standardized and structured and is based on the formal letter writing they learned in school, youth individualize letters with creative elements. The packaging and creative elements of a letter, or what Besnier calls the "peripheral aspects," serve to set the tone for the letter as a whole and are often as important as the main body of text, with some writers taking great care to decorate their letters with margin art or sayings. Peripheral aspects, Besnier argues, "are often neglected in descriptions of letter writing because of their non-textual nature." He argues that "non-textual aspects of letters deserve close scrutiny, since they provide a 'frame' to the text, i.e., 'guidelines' for its interpretation" (1995:84–85). When analyzed according to the gender of the writer, the packaging of love letters reveals only slight differences in the frequency of each element.

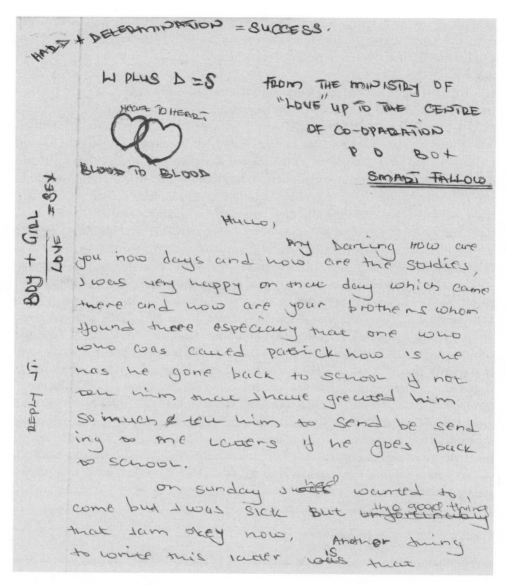

FIGURE 9.3. Peripheral elements

Return Addresses and Senses of Belonging

Following conventions of business letter writing their writers learned in school, love letters typically begin with a return address and a date at the top right corner of the letter. Some letter writers use the post office boxes of their parents or other relatives. However, since most youth either worry about privacy or do not have access to family mailboxes, more typical is the use of an institution or civic association that reflects their status and upward mobility, most commonly a secondary school, vocational school, college, or university. Or they might use the address to construct a style or aspiration, such as the boy employed by a taxi park using "Love Is Toyota" as his address, or another who uses

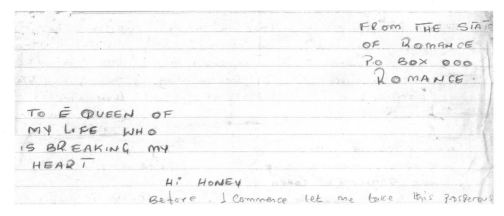

FIGURE 9.4. Romantic return address

"NGO States, #7091." The return address can also be used to invoke the sentiment or purpose of the letter, such as a writer who sends his letter from a space named "Forgiveness." The return address provides such writers with opportunities to create imaginary locations of their love and set the tone of their letters, such as in the one pictured above: "From The Ministry Of 'Love' Up To The Centre Of Co-Oparation, PO Box *Smart Fallow*" (Figure 9.3). Another technique is invoking a romantic device not only in composing the sender's address, but also when establishing a relational place for the companionate partner, such as when an adolescent boy indicates that his letter is originating "From the State of Romance, P.O. Box 000, Romance," and being delivered "To Queen of, My Life Who, Is Breaking My Heart" (Figure 9.4).

Salutations and Closings

The salutation is an important and standard aspect in love letters. According to Basoga convention, it is considered abrupt and rude to begin a conversation without a proper (and often extended) greeting. Love letters frequently take on this characteristic, particularly if the intent is to persuade or impress, and less often if the letter is intended to convey anger. Writers use the salutation to set the tone for the rest of the letter, such as the formal and sophisticated tone here:

Dearest Batty

Hullo

The jumblication is towards beyond human degree rather for to write to you this simple cominiant piece of letter. (letter B:46)

Slang words for "hello" are quite common in everyday-speak as well as in love letters. Derivatives or variations such as *hi, hullo, hallo, hai, hark*, or *hey* indicate a young person's engagement with the youthful culture of invention and are followed by the recipient's name, pet name, or another term of endearment.

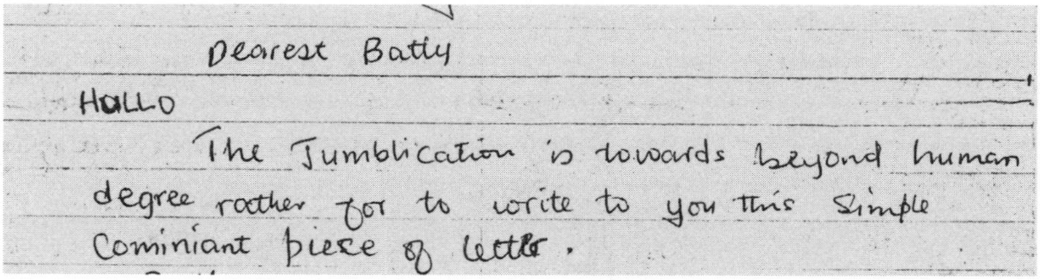

FIGURE 9.5. Romantic salutation

> Hallo Daddy;
>
> Before I pen the point allow me to send warm greetings to you with great pleasure over to you . . . that how are you over there?

The salutation can also be incorporated into part of the opening paragraph or sentence as one complete phrase. For example:

> Hey Irene, allow me to say this word of hullo and love to you in addition to how are you these days?

As seen in the passages above, opening phrases are typically very formal and polite, even when the tone of the rest of the letter is anger or disappointment. Many young people refer to the process of writing in their letters, such as "before I pen the point." Another common tendency is for the writer to refer to himself in third person—that is, "back to the jotter's main aim," as is often found in verbal speech acts. According to Basoga custom, putting too much direct emphasis on oneself appears conceited and suggests self-importance, belying the cultural expectation of humility.

   The introductory greeting in both written and verbal speech has the aim of showing respect and is often directly followed by a series of uninterrupted questions about the addressee's health, family, studies, and life in general. In Lusoga greetings, questions about the person's well-being are a gesture of politeness and an important cultural display of concern for others. Unique to the written word, as we see in the greetings above, are rhetorics of love and tenderness (e.g., "warm greetings to you," "love to you," and "hallo daddy"). While this romantic rhetoric is not typical of face-to-face greetings, a young person might use it when greeting a peer with whom he or she is very familiar. Another purpose of openings is to convey how overjoyed the writer is to have the opportunity to communicate with the addressee—another demonstration of romantic sincerity. Openings are also used to illustrate a writer's proficiency in the language of love (a form of boastful posturing) in hopes of gaining valuable romantic currency. David, a nineteen-year-old, writes an elaborate introduction to his sweetheart in a neighboring town. His pet name for her in the letter, Complex, both reflects his perception of their relationship and foreshadows the elaborate rhetoric he is about to employ:

Dear Complex,

Indeed I am with preferential interest and vividatude happiness to get this ingince of jokes trying to jot to you these few lines, words at this melodious threne of the year. However, how are your preponde rating the life under classification of the environmental aspects of the family at large? (letter B:2).

In this salutation we see use of a pet name, grand effect of language, and invented language. Young men use these elaborate introductions significantly more often than their female lovers. This difference not only is due to the intent of boys' letters, but also reflects a pervasive gender difference in confidence with English proficiency. It is a common belief among youth that boys have greater scholastic ability, and as a result, many girls are hesitant to use elaborate language or to experiment, both in academic settings and in the language of their love letters. Below are two examples of adolescent girls' opening lines. As in boys' openings, in girls' letters we also find an expression of being grateful for the opportunity to communicate with their sweethearts and elaborate language:

Hullo GE,

Happiness is beyond my control seeing that I am capable of writing these few lines exchanging greetings with you well? Sweet words of love with me. (letter G:12)

Another girl opens her letter with

Waawo

It is actually my concern & with golden chance among my views to kill the prance and pick up my pen to jot to u. But be4 I split the macabre, let mi say Hai to u. How is life treating you around? On mi side life is just mediocre. (letter G:17)

There are striking gender differences in opening passages that provide insight into how young people conceptualize their embeddedness in wider social obligations. Adolescent girls are more likely to relay information about recent events in their own lives or ask for specifics about the recipient. For instance, girls might inquire about burials, sickness, information about mutually known people, or events in school. Girls also tend to be more direct about the purpose of their letters when dealing with conflict or misunderstanding, while adolescent boys are more direct when their intent is romance and courting. I return to these gendered patterns in subsequent chapters, but in general the gendered patterns of inquiring about the lives of others point to how females are socialized to view their identity as connected to systems of reciprocity and care.

In closing phrases, we see definite youth romantic subjectivity in which, depending on the purpose of the letter, many humbly identify themselves as romantically

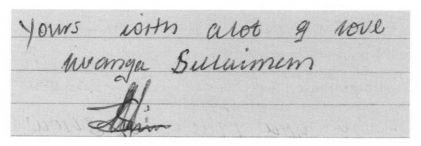

FIGURE 9.6. Romantic closing statement

belonging to the addressee. Others may simply refer to themselves as being in a particular emotional or romantic state. For example:

> I will always remain yours forever,
> Isabella

> I remain your's in love and blood
> Doubtless that sends me sleep
> with honey in my heart,
> David

Request for Reply

Requests for reciprocity are another key feature of love letters. Even though the assumption is that a reply is wanted, many youth end their letters with reply statements such as "Please, a reply is needed kindly." Another commonly used request-for-reply technique is the use of alliteration by which the writer can create a fancy design such as: "Remember, Record it, Read and Reply" (Figure 9.7) or "A Reply is Needed. Long, Lasting, Love" "Read, Rest, Remember to Reply." The request for a reply indicates the writer's desire to have the letter reciprocated sooner rather than later and also assesses the recipient's level of interest. If a relationship is further along, writers may request the recipient's help in formulating a next step in moving the relationship forward, such as arranging a time and place to meet or directly asking how the other person feels about the relationship. Given that face-to-face interaction is often limited or takes place around others, a request for a reply also serves as a way for the writer to either probe the interest of the receiver or affirm his or her own continued interest.

No reply is translated as an insult and an indication of lack of interest, both potentially angering the writer. For some, not receiving a reply letter is a great frustration. Kagoya, a seventeen-year-old girl, had been courted by a fellow student for a short time, and they had exchanged a series of letters discussing their feelings. When Kagoya was dissatisfied with the delay of the student's reply, she wrote about her disappointment and exasperation in this introductory passage: "It seems that you're just playing on my head because how can I write a letter to you and you don't reply" (letter G:1). Kagoya ended her letter by giving the young man an explicit deadline for replying: "I need a

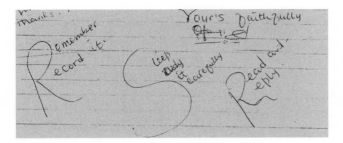

FIGURE 9.7. Creative request for a reply

reply before Friday." This strategy allowed Kagoya to assert her desire while maintaining the expectation of putting suitors to a test to prove their interest.

Boys tend to ask for replies more frequently than girls, given that their letters are often the initiating letters and involve asking the girl if she is interested. Along with requests for replies, writers often ask for photographs. If a person responds with a photograph of himself or herself, the writer knows that there is definite interest.

Margin Art: Song Dedications and Quotes

Two final packaging aspects—song dedications and quotes—are common features in the margins or at the end of letters, serving the dual purpose of being aesthetically decorative and demonstrating a young person's familiarity and connection to interaction with popular culture and discourses in the public sphere. Song dedications reflect the strong association that youth have between romance and music. Most songs are popularized by their continual play on one of the Kampala-based radio stations or on large sound systems that surround the taxi park and market areas. Most of the songs listed in letters are pop music from playlists by popular Ugandan disc jockeys or global lists such as Casey Kasem's or Rick Dees's weekly Top 40 countdowns. The playlists comprise a mix of dancehall reggae circulated throughout the black diaspora (from the Caribbean to Africa), US hip-hop and R & B, country and folk music, and local folk music played on a guitar called *kadongo kamu* (one little guitar).

But there is also a common set of popular songs that have come to represent love and desire at any particular time; hence, more so than other elements of a letter, the songs listed change from one year to the next. One boy lists fourteen songs for his love interest, the list becoming a sort of written mix tape:

DEDs '4 'U'
In ma'life (D.J. Bob)
I Make Love to You (Boyz II Men)
As, I lay me down
Maama (Boyz II Men)
Maama (Brenda faso)
Woman I love (Chaka Demus & Pliers)
Love me with reason (M.J.)

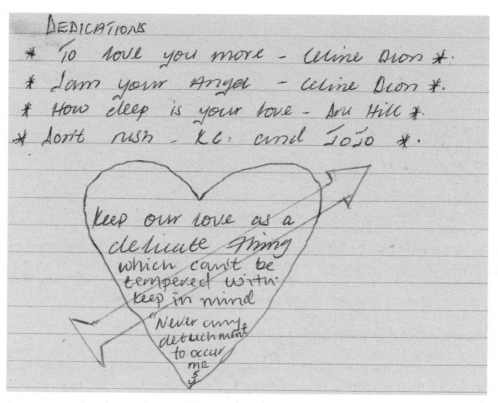

FIGURE 9.8. Song dedications and margin quote

I believe I can fly (Lucky Dube)
Where do 'u go' (No mercy)
I want somebody (Dr. Victor)
Dombolo (Wenga Musica)
Ekumuli kya Roza (F.M)
When I think of "U"
Red on Red

The above dedications are less a reflection of the boy's feeling toward the girl than a symbolic gesture emphasizing that he is an authority on music—a sure sign that he is an experienced and true romantic lover. Having knowledge of contemporary popular music and being able to select a song to reflect a particular sentiment also implies that a writer is engaged with the public sphere and has both access to a radio and leisure time to enjoy it—additional indicators of status and modernity. In the initial batch of letters I collected between 1998 and 1999, common songs included Braxton's "Un-Break My Heart" (discussed earlier), Usher's "Nice & Slow," and Brandy and Monica's "The Boy Is Mine," indicating the speed at which songs travel globally and signaling the way ever-evolving globalized popular culture gets appropriated and retooled in specific local settings alongside more local items. By the 2000s, common love songs were Jennifer

Lopez's "My Love Don't Cost a Thing" and Faith Hill's "The Way You Love Me," as well as songs by Celine Dion, Destiny's Child, and eventually Beyoncé, Pharrell Williams, Jennifer Hudson, and Rihanna. Boys dedicate songs more frequently than girls, not only because boys have more extensive exposure to areas where popular music is played, such as discos, public transportation areas, storefronts, and bars, but also because familiarity with recent regionally or globally produced pop and hip hop music is sign of masculine competence. Dedications in love letters have been further popularized by various radio shows that play song dedications over the air, cuing each dedicated song with a note from the caller. According to the station manager of one of the earlier radio stations to take on this practice, the idea for the show came from the existing practice of dedicating songs in love letters, suggesting a relationship in which the counterpublic affects and becomes practice in the public, and vice versa.

Another peripheral element that appears with great frequency is the margin quote, saying, or equation. Like other peripheral aspects, quotes are used to convey the emotions of the writer or to evoke emotions in the reader. Quotes are not necessarily famous sayings by others, but are typically invented or overheard by the writer of the letter. Some youth create fancy enclosures for their quotes, especially if there is blank space on the page. Many of the quotes have become part of love letter dialect. For example, one of the most commonly used sayings is "Love without sex is like tea without sugar." One of the teachers involved in my initial discussion of love letters with the headmaster and his staff told me that when he was young they used to write, "Love without a kiss is like tea without sugar." When I told him the current version, he laughed and said, "Boy, they have really gotten advanced." In their eagerness to impress, some inventive youth make interesting transpositions of foreign sayings. One girl wrote to her distant lover, "Out of mind doesn't mean out of sight." Another boy cautioned his love interest to "never cross a bridge before you come across it."

Finally, in addition to margin quotes functioning as a place to establish romantic expectations, they also provide the opportunity to indirectly warn a lover, serving as a device for regulating the behaviors of current or potential sweethearts. In particular, youth draw from HIV messages to warn their interests about the disease, often invoking the virus to deter sweethearts from engaging in sexual activity with *others*.

AIDS is AIDS please watch out

AIDS HAS NO CURE

You be there knowing that AIDS is killing in Iganga too much. Be careful about my body. B'se it is not yours.

While all three quotes invoke fear as a plea for their partner to remain faithful, the adolescent female author of the last quote employs another public discourse. Specifically, she combines health warnings about HIV with feminist discourses of sexual rights, autonomy, and integrity of the female body. In short, she is asserting her independence and declaring ownership of her own body. We clearly see in this case how youth call upon discourses in the public sphere to create a youthful counterpublic and develop authority for their own romantic ideals and desires.

Conclusion

When they participate in love letter exchanges (whether as writers, receivers, or go-betweens), young people in Iganga contribute to the creation and transformation of a youthful counterpublic while interacting with public discourses and moralities. Their letters provide insight into how a variety of interventions around youth sexuality—including HIV and public health messages, popular and local cultural productions, and other regulatory regimes—are absorbed into local imaginations about romance and structures of affect. The larger purpose of this chapter has been to bring attention to the striking ways that these youth create romance in their love letters, not only in the main body of text but also in the construction or packaging. Youth put deliberate effort into the selection of language and the peripheral aspects of the letter. Rather than being just a preoccupation to fill time or to pursue hopeful sexual encounters, writing love letters is an investment in a process that reveals young people as optimistic, active agents in forging their futures despite their awareness of their marginalized position in the world. Such an insight into the desires and imagined possibilities of youth is crucial for appreciating why people hold onto hopes of love despite conditions of precarity and evidence that their desired "good life" is likely unachievable (Berlant 2011).

CHAPTER 10

"I miss you like a desert missing rain"

Desire and Longing

This chapter and the next examine the main body of the letters in order to tease out commonly occurring themes that shape the intimate experiences, lives, hopes, and anxieties of Uganda's young people. This chapter focuses on sentiments of desire, longing, and hope that motivate the initiation and subsequent exchange of love letters between two young people, and the following chapter examines sentiments of disappointment that youth confront and express. In my examination of sentiments of desire that youth grapple with and work out in letters, I am interested in what these sentiments tell us about the gendered nature of youthful subjectivities and constructions of future possibilities. As stated earlier, I take seriously the position that despite our academic writings, development reports, and donor agencies, which tend to use discourses of vulnerability to characterize youth in marginalized communities, these youth are also intentional social actors. As I demonstrate, they work within their constraints to actively appropriate, rework, and make sense of conflicting local and global ideas about the pleasures and dangers that come with the so-called modern sexuality and sexual freedom of young adulthood.

I argue that an analysis of discourses of desire shows that young people's pursuit of affective attachments is not an indication of their lack of knowledge about their precarious position in today's society but rather is an enactment of their remaining hopeful about a future in which they imagine becoming full citizens, having rights and control over their destinations. Nor do I see romance in Iganga as a halfway house on the young people's road to autonomy and separation from their natal families, as Sharon Thompson (1995) suggested about relationships among teens in the United States. Rather, despite their witnessing of breakups around them, romance, particularly as an imagined hopeful state, offers Iganga youth a temporary escape from everyday realities and hardships. A closer look, however, provides us insight into how gender and status shape possible future trajectories. More than just affectionate missives to sweethearts, love letters can be read as living diaries in which youth reflect on the mundane details of their daily lives and demonstrate their deep belief in the possibility of a different outcome. In love letters, youth provide glimpses into how they understand and negotiate their marginal and uncertain position within contemporary Uganda, a state of precarity exacerbated by wider processes of increased socioeconomic stratification and by interventions aimed at protecting youth from the harms of their own sexuality.

"The Books": Individual Responsibility, Determination, and Uncertain Futures

Obtaining a formal education is a primary and constant preoccupation among youth in Iganga and throughout Uganda. Youth often use the term "the books" as an idiom for "education," with the main focus on being literate. This likely reflects the localization of global development measurements. More than simply referring to education or literacy, "the books" symbolizes the promise of educational attainment—a bright future, social mobility, an escape from poverty and dependency, and entry into the global economy of goods and ideas. Encouragement to work hard in school and reminders of the sacrifices necessary to achieve future success are scattered throughout the letters of young people. Ronald, returning from Iganga to Makerere University to take the final exams for his first semester, provides an example of this:

MAKERERE UNIVERSITY
NSIBIRWA HALL
KAMPALA

Hai Sarah,

Welcome back. Hope you had a nice time and enjoyed. How are you doing? Hope you're fine and doing well. Thanks for that time.

Sarah, I have arrived safely yesterday and have embarked on serious studies here at campus. Hope you too arrived safely and have also resumed serious reading, this being your third term. Remember it's hard work and sacrifice that enables one to reach the desired goal. I will be very glad being with you at campus preferably sharing the same room (if possible any way).

At this time, I would like to inform you that I am very eager to receive my message I was promised yesterday through Peter. I have been unfortunate for not seeing Peter before writing.

So I exactly didn't know what he had for me from you. If you didn't write then I don't know.

Otherwise I met Alice yesterday. I told her to pass on my greetings to you. Tell her that I wish her success in her Exams.

Nothing much to say only to caution you revise carefully, read hard and discus where necessary. Have ample sleep to refresh your minds. This is how we used to go about with books and I think you saw the end justifying the means. Please campus is for none other than you. I hope to provide you with some Econ, Div, and History notes after getting them from the people I had given. Otherwise I am expecting a message from you not later than this Saturday.

Wish you the best.
Bye
Yours,
Ronald
MAKERERE

For many youth such as Ronald, hopes about their romantic relationships and futures with peers offer them motivation to continue through difficult times as well as a discursive space for working through their anxieties. In working through the uncertainty of their lives, the themes of individual responsibility and consistent hard work underlie young people's messages about the connection between educational success and social mobility, and thus failure or success are indications of an individual's level of determination. The enactment of hope and determination through letters is a gendered practice. In this particular letter, for instance, while Ronald's message to Sarah contains sentiments of affection, it also demonstrates how a male suitor uses a romantic relationship as a site for the performance of confidence, a key aspect of masculinity. Specifically, Ronald's letter to Sarah provides him the opportunity to assert his masculinity amid the emasculating anxieties produced by upcoming final exams. He performs gender by reminding Sarah (as well as himself) of his great achievement relative to hers and assures her that she too can achieve his level of success if she takes his advice: "Remember it's hard work and sacrifice that enables one to reach the desired goal." Hence, whereas encouragement during difficulties is an important aspect of youth relationships, the gendered way this is carried out demonstrates how youth romance often draws upon and replicates (and at times challenges) gender hierarchies operating in the public sphere.

The Uncertainty of the Future

While for most adolescents in Iganga education is highly desired precisely because it is seen as a necessary route out of poverty, the costs and the performance expectations associated with that education also make it a source of great uncertainty and anxiety. The costs of education are both economic and social. On the economic side, there are school fees, charges for uniforms and educational supplies, and other expenses. On the social side, families lose contributions of labor: students are less available to help with the running of the household, working on the family farm, or caring for the sick, elderly, or young. These economic and social costs are constant obstacles to young people attempting to advance through the education system.

Another challenge is passing the standardized tests required to advance through the system. Administered by the Uganda National Education Board (UNEB), these national exams are written in English and are taken as students advance from primary school (Primary 1 to Primary 7) to secondary school, which comprises Ordinary level (O level, or Senior 1 to Senior 4) and Advanced level (A level, or Senior 5 and Senior 6). A large number of students fall out after O level, like Sam. After each exam, students are ranked against all students in the country and based on their results can gain or be denied admission into one of the higher-performing schools in their region or in the country. Similar to the British system, the level attained the exam results determine what type of higher learning institution a student qualifies for, the most prestigious option being admission with funding into the state institution, Makerere University.

The exams are notoriously difficult, and hence youth in rural or poorer schools are at a great disadvantage: they are likely to have missed topics on the exams because their schools might lack books and supplies. Additionally, these schools often have abbreviated terms because they lack money for teachers and lack school fees from students. The results of the A-level exams are public, and the country's top-performing students (likely not from a school in Iganga) are listed in various media outlets, increasing Iganga residents' awareness of their marginality and lower socioeconomic status within Uganda. The feelings of stress and anxiety caused by the exams appear in letters frequently. A girl writes to her love interest about her exams, requesting his sympathy and support: "By the way about UNEB results for my side, I don't see that I did well because I wanted to be in first grade. So I am really reading very hard in order to a first grade in my UNEB. I will be very grateful when I receive a success card from you" (letter G:31).

Given the importance of schooling in opening up future possibilities and prosperity, school success, working hard, and determination are key aspects of youth's emerging work ethic and means of rising out of poverty. These are ideals drilled into students through government, development, religious, and school discourses that position hard work and economic achievement in opposition to laziness and poverty. However, even if a student qualifies for a top school, the higher costs associated with the top schools are impossible for youth from poorer families. The emphasis on education and the public ranking of schools have further exacerbated stratification among young people. Students who fall out of the education system for economic or social reasons or because of test results might hope to end up in a vocational training program, but many search for income in other ways.

The stress generated from the uncertainty of educational paths can be exacerbated by periods of interrupted schooling, such as that experienced by Sam. These interruptions are the result of either poor performance on an advancement exam or a family's lack of funds. In both cases, a student may sit out of school for a while. Regardless of obvious economic constraints, neoliberal ideas about individual effort leading to personal progress remain a fairly hegemonic attitude underlying residents' ideas about why their area remains poor. While school success and hard work are typically not the main purpose of letters, these themes are prominent secondary topics and are invoked to convey a particular association with a modern (capitalist) work ethic. In their letters, most youth simply ask, "How are the books?" not only out of a genuine concern but also to fashion themselves as modern subjects. These letters show us how youth struggle to balance their romantic relationships with their desire to do well in school, both of which consume much of their thought and time.[1]

Youth's notion of an ideal relationship is similar to what scholars have called a "companionate" relationship, characterized by self-selection of a mate with whom one can communicate and share leisure time. This observation is supported by a survey we conducted with two hundred school-age kids and by semi-structured follow-up interviews in which girls consistently rated as a high priority communication with their partner, specifically being able to share their problems with their sweethearts; for boys, problem sharing and solving was mentioned less often, but there was still emphasis on general communication and leisure. In one instance, Lucy is feeling increasing pressure at home and in school, and is unable to discuss her problems with her father. She uses a letter to express her frustrations with her situation at home with a potential romantic partner:

But still I can't concentrate with all those problems at home. One of these days I have to write a letter to my father and tell him a piece of my mind. It seems he doesn't know much about what is happening [with my stepmother and stepsiblings]. . . . In case I take long to reply, don't get worried because it's hard for me to fix time for writing letters. I've written this during a physics lesson. I wish the teacher knew my struggles. Anyway, hope to hear from you. (letter G:27)

For Lucy, writing a letter to her lover becomes her venue for self-reflection—for expressing feelings about her school and her father that she has been otherwise unable to articulate. Letters are often an ideal setting for reflecting on and sharing disturbing events with lovers, transforming letters into personal diaries. Commenting on the role of journaling in the subjective reflections of young people in the United States, Shuman writes: "Diary writing was one of the only ways in which the adolescent could set up a distance between themselves as authors and the ongoing situation. Diaries provide seemingly unlimited entitlement to express a point of view" (1986:174). The concept of entitlement is useful for thinking about how youth use letter writing to convey thoughts in a manner that cannot, at least immediately, be disputed or challenged; the writer is the authority over the contents and the construction of the "facts."

Unlike other topics in love letters, there is no expectation that a reader will respond to the writer's introspections on school or other problems. Such reflections serve as a pieces of personal history and context for the letter and are usually only passing thoughts. In another example, Nangobi, the firstborn child of a well-off businessman in Iganga, had recently switched to a school in another town. Her father had hoped that she would get a better education, but her transition there has been difficult. In a letter to her companionate partner, Nangobi writes, "Life here is half crazy due to the hell at which books are really proving to be challenging but always with hope to overcome them instead. Otherwise expecting everything to be quite fine as we push on with the term" (letter G:15). In the remainder of the letter, as well as in other letters, Nangobi reflects on the difficulties of trying to meet her father's high expectations. The tone of subsequent letters indicates an increasing frustration with the pressures felt at home. In attempt to deal with her father's expectations of perfection, she falls deeper into romantic imaginations with her love interest, in one letter writing, "If only we could take a week-long vacation to Mt. Kilimanjaro after our exams." Like many youth in Iganga, letter writing provides Nangobi a venue not only for reflecting on her anxieties about education and success, but also for making such states bearable by imagining a life beyond the immediacy of family pressures.

Performing Gendered Success and Giving Advice

Determination is a striking tone in many letters about school, even when students are faced with daunting challenges. Determination is found equally in both boys' and girls' letters, but compared to girls, boys do not easily admit to struggling in school except when the difficulty is financial. Admitting to scholastic difficulties runs counter to constructions of masculinity based on success, confidence, and superior intelligence over girls, and therefore admitting being scholastically defeated can tarnish a boy's image. Admitting scholastic defeat to a girl is further inhibited by the idea that boys are innately more intelligent than girls, a belief that many youth have accepted as a biological truth. For adolescent males, maintaining the image of scholastic acumen is largely posturing or performative, but vital for their construction and maintenance of masculine desirability. Boys' letters often read as an elaborate performance, not only through the invocation of grand effect and elaborate language, but also through acts of boasting in an attempt to position themselves above their hapless lovers. While I collected no letter in which a boy discussed his own scholastic problems with his lover, I have many letters in which boys follow the convention of establishing a gender hierarchy in the relationship by serving as advice givers to women. When boys position themselves as naturally wiser than girls, the social organization of gendered inequalities in relationships takes shape: "I cannot tell you enough how difficult the exams are, even for me. I advise you to get extra help in the subjects that you are weak in. I can even give help in your times of difficulty with your books" (B:95). Others remind their lovers to stay focused. A seventeen-year-old boy writes: "I warn you, dear, to take your studies as seriously as I do. I see you getting distracted but you have to keep on your books. Remember, success is through hard work" (letter B:79). This hierarchical relationship of male advice giver and female advice recipient is further fueled by the age difference that structures many youth (as well as adult) relationships, such that a boy derives higher status not only from being male but also from being older than his female love interest. However, while the gendered structure of advice giving reflects gender and age hierarchies, it is also about a young man proving that he is a useful and worthy partner of his love interest: for, as one girl commented, "what woman would want a man who can offer nothing?" The act of giving advice becomes a key strategy in demonstrating masculinity and dedicating time to the needs of one's female interest.

Intellectual Reputation

The idea of reputation building is useful in understanding boys' attempts to fashion a certain image. In her analysis of ideals of masculinity and femininity in northeast Brazil, L. A. Rebhun suggests that the theoretical concept of masculine reputation refers to "a set of social ideas about the relationships among masculinity, power, and respect. They are subject to contingent interpretations, creating a structure of possibilities within which people negotiate status" (1999:112). She argues that reputation is less a standard intended for actual practice than "symbolic vocabularies through which to judge status" (ibid.). Offering a slightly different perspective, Sue Lees's (1989, 1993) work on British girls' sexuality reports the great extent to which feminine identity and social relations rest on a girl's sexual reputation. The sexually derogatory word "slag" (similar to the word "slut") was used both for social control and as a normative basis on which girls would reflect on sexual decisions. In examining the role of reputation for youth in Iganga, I couple Rebhun's idea of "symbolic vocabularies" with Lee's notion of reputation as a social control that guides behavioral choices. In Iganga, authors of love letters can craft an image of themselves, filtering out certain pieces of information and highlighting others.

As discussed earlier, according to elders, past characteristics of an ideal mate were based on family background and an individual's reputation, which had different signifiers for men and women. A man's reputation was based on his wealth, intellectual ability, and "popularity." For a woman, it included modesty, sexual propriety, reproductive ability, perseverance, and work ethic. In the context of capitalist attainment, in which a dual income is often required to meet needs of households, young women have the burden of being judged on both historically feminine characteristics and "male" characteristics such as intelligence, worldly achievement, and popularity. For example: "Let me assure you that I have never been stupid. If you thought that I am stupid girl, I am not of the type please. And I am the best English speaking girl in our class and the good thing I am not stubborn like you. Anyway, being stubborn is not bad. But why are you so stubborn like that?" (G:44). The writer sets out to accomplish two purposes in connecting female desirability with intelligence. First, she reminds the boy that she is not to be deceived (because she is not a stupid girl); and second, she seeks to remind the boy of her desirability, as she is the top- performing girl in English. Yet while male qualities are valued in both men and women, there is a lingering social desire and expectation for men to appear intellectually superior to their mates. In their letters, girls struggle to balance flattering a boy for his intelligence with reminding the boy that they too are intelligent partners who are desirable (because of their intelligence) and who cannot be easily deceived by boys' ways.

Declaring Love in the Written Chase

A main purpose for sending love letters is to declare love or respond to a declaration of love. Expressing love in face-to-face interactions is difficult, as discussed earlier, because of fear of rejection or punishment, nervousness, or lack of privacy. Youth are aware of the role that letters play when verbal declarations are difficult, as seen in this letter written by an adolescent girl: "It is really impressing and joy to inform you of my love in you. It is really hard to tell someone how much you love him or her. I really can't express or rather I don't know how I can express my love to you. I tried the other day after school, but failed to speak the words. This is why I chose to write a letter" (letter G:21). As the gendered narrative of the courtship chase suggests, there are considerable differences in the use of letters by boys or girls to declare love or initiate a relationship. In the letters that I collected, 45 percent of the boys' letters were used to initiate a relationship with or declare interest in a girl, compared to only 6 percent of girls' letters that did so. Conversely, girls affirm or reciprocate love in letters more than boys, though with a less dramatic difference—34 percent versus 25 percent of letters respectively.

After being introduced to a girl from another school and interacting with her a few times, one writer uses a letter to reveal his feelings in hopes of starting a relationship. It is an example of a common declaration of love: "I would like to inform you that my heart had never settled since I felt thoughts of love with you, ever my heart can think in heaven of love, Mary, your sight makes me think of nothing but your talking treats me like injection" (letter B:2). The term "injection," found in other love letters, is adopted from common medical language in Uganda. It is commonly believed that the potency of medicine increases when administered through injection, for it gets directly into the blood system, a vital source of life and regeneration. Hence, by equating his reaction to his prospective love to the potency of an injection, the young man hopes to demonstrate how the thought of her takes over his entire body.

When I presented groups of young people with sample letters and asked them to select the most beautiful passages, almost all chose a letter in which the writer was making a declaration of love. Most writers put much effort into writing embellishments of love, attempting to impress potential lovers and convey their intense feelings. This boy makes such a declaration to his interest: "Penny, why I have taken time to hold a pen and paper writing to you is to show how much I care and love you. I want to show you and get you contented that you are the only vessel of my life. Whenever, I recall your smiles and romantic behaviours, I feel as if I am one of the angels in heaven. I wish you knew how much I love you Penny" (letter B:18). The romantic technique of declaring that someone is "the one," or "the only vessel of my life," is common. Another boy tries to convince a girl that he has chosen her as his "first choice": "Since a period of time I have been looking for a partner to whom I could share with but I have discovered that you are of my choice" (letter B:28). Beautiful discursive phrases for referring to a love interest and for indicating that she is whom the writer has willfully selected as his object of affection and attention are romantic strategies commonly invoked by boys. The emphasis on *one* love interest borrows both from recent public discourses on monogamy as circulated by HIV campaigns and from Christian messages but also does not preclude the boy from pursuing other relationships that are less loving but perhaps sexual, as we will see in the next chapter. In other words, declaring that someone is your one *love* does not necessarily mean that other forms of relationships with females have ended or will not be pursued.

Adolescence provides an ideal period for young boys to practice and perfect their use of romantic discourses and devices in order to achieve their desired outcome. One boy directly asks of his interest, "What can I do to prove I need your love? What will it take to believe I won't give up? Open your heart and let your feelings show. And I think of ways that I can win your heart. But I am so confused I don't know where to start. It's more than love had some bad luck" (letter B:19). Other boys use love letters as what one boy calls an application for love. The general idea behind these love letters is: "I like you. How do you feel about me?" In applications for love, a boy and girl may flirt a bit in a public place, such as school or in youth gatherings, and become interested in taking the relationship to a higher level. In one example, a young couple met during an event in town. The boy writes to the girl about his new feelings of love for her, asking for advice: "I have been forced to fall into love with you. But . . . for I it is doddle to become your lover as u also become mine. But I don't think you will bare with my ways because I am a character which is simple but complicated. You will excuse me to say so but facts are bitter and truth is better than deceit. Basing on that information above what is your suggestion?" (letter B:33). While the description of "simple but complicated" may seem contradictory, the boy is playing on the admired qualities of being humble ("simple") and the assumed association of intelligence and masculinity with "complicated," casting himself as a type of mystery man. He is, as discussed earlier, attempting to construct himself as both compelling and alluring. His letter clearly reflects the idea that falling in love is perceived as a predestined state that takes over one's mind and body—the lover has no control over such feelings and therefore cannot take responsibility. The writer is pained by his love, and it is the responsibility of his love interest to relieve the pain caused by the inevitable condition.

Applications for love made by older boys (or more experienced boys) tend to follow a basic format, indicating a shared notion of romance. The suitor convinces the girl that he is truly interested in her, giving her reasons for his love. He describes the extent of that love through grand effect and literary tropes, humbly asks for her love, and finally asks for her response to his application. A boy of twenty has perfected the format, writing:

> I am fine and my temperature is rising day and night whenever I think of you. With a lot of pleasure which I am full with I just want to tell you that the aim of writing to you this letter is to come in friendship with you, boylover.
>
> So I want to tell you tell you I love very much. So much that my heart keeps on pumping a thousand times a day whenever I think of you. However I imagine your picture my heart just keeps on pumping and I want to tell you that I love you very much and you are the most peerless girl according to my choice. Really I would like to tell you that my love towards you will never end until the end of our life! It can be separated when one of us have gone to hell or one has gone to heaven.
>
> I would like to tell you clearly that my love towards you is not for concupiscience but it's for marriage after when we have all finished our studies. I want to tell you that I don't love you for sexual desire but I love in heart and I want to be with you as my wife for forever and ever. In fact I want to tell you clearly that my love towards you can't be expressed in anyway. I fraternal you the way you talk, stand, smile and bend. . . . So you see how I have love you and I'd like to tell you that if you have put my message which I have delivered you as a momentour issue as I did to you I will be very happy and I'd like to tell you there's no regret after only being in a luxurious place until death with reconciliation only.
>
> I want to tell you that I love you with all my heart and soul. I'd like to tell you that, you are going to be taken as queen with reconciliation.
>
> . . . . So I want to assure that if you have put my application about boylover in consideration I guarantee to marry you; to be with you in reconciliation throughout the years; I don't mind no matter tribe you are. Love isn't for tribe. With those love words I beg you to pen here.
>
> I wish you a victorious studies and happy staying. Your reply is highly homologated with pleasure of love and kisses forever and ever. (letter B:43)

The promise made by this boy, to love not for sex but for marriage, dovetails with various campaigns and messages about respecting girls that circulate through a variety of development, gender equality, and sexual health interventions. The subject of

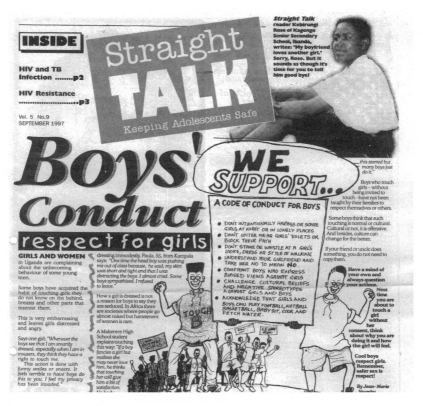

FIGURE 10.1. *Straight Talk* article on respect for girls, 1997

boys' behaviors and attitudes toward girls has been a recurring topic in *Straight Talk*, a monthly sex education insert geared to adolescents that started in 1993 in *New Vision* newspaper. On the cover of one issue is an article entitled "Boys' Conduct: Respect for Girls" (Figure 10.1). The marketing strategy of the article includes a drawing displaying two boys dressed in urban-inspired clothes and labeled as "cool," leading a parade of boys as they hold aloft a placard with the words "A code of conduct for boys." The drawing portrays a bandwagon effect, subtly acknowledging that sexual attitudes and behaviors are learned, shared, and reproduced within wider social networks. The article, code of conduct, and drawing infuse an image of urban modernity with the new concept of a right of sexual consent for girls, challenging the notion that men (or boys) have unrestrained sexual access to girls. In attempting to disrupt the common masking of certain behaviors toward women as cultural, the article tells boys "culture can change for the better." Furthermore, the article encourages boys to follow their own standards, which the editors hope will be informed by the ideas in the article, instructing boys that "if your friend or uncle does something, you do not need to copy them." The message promoted by *Straight Talk* competes with other sexual agendas circulated in peer groups, religious institutions, families, and popular culture, and is undergirded, like many other agendas, by the notion that boys initiate the chase. Hence, while it pushes for changes in gender roles and conduct, it simultaneously relies on these familiar ideas in its attempt to appeal to youth, thereby reinscribing the gender norm it seeks to challenge.

When I compared letters collected in 1999 with those collected in 2002 and 2004, I found an increase in the number of girls who initiate a relationship through letters. While reputational risks of transgressing gender norms still keep many girls from overtly initiating a relationship in a letter that can easily become the topic of gossip among peers, some girls feel empowered to initiate a relationship through a letter as opposed to the accepted female ways of subtle flirting, giggling, and making oneself visible to the boy of interest. Older girls are more likely than younger ones to make the first move directly, particularly if they feel the social stigma of *nakyewombekeire* is bearable or, better yet, avoidable altogether. For example, one girl was inspired to initiate a relationship after reading the controversial leisure magazine *Spice*. She informs her selected love interest of her intentions: "I decided not to stay without a pen pal, as it's difficult to stay without a boy lover or a girl lover that's why I have written to yo' this letter as I read from Spice this evening, in order to get some entertainment from yo' young guy" (letter G:23). It is precisely this conscious decision not to conform to Basoga gender ideologies that leads to intergenerational tensions. The adolescent girl below initiates and declares her love for her sweetheart, which she asserts by suggesting her willingness to engage in physical intimacy:

HELLO D.J.

Let mi take gracious moments to dot to you this massive note which I hope won't sabotage your mind at any rust. Anyway how is life plus the situation there? However I am not pushing on well b'se. I miss you. I can only say that I have got great affinity for your love. In fact, if I had proximity to you at this moment I would kiss you b'se you are a special person to me if you know that I was deeply lost in yo' love you would do something but I am not meaning.

   Hence let our love begin now and ever more because I am ever dreaming about you and ever thinking about you honey not only that but also you're so cute and pretty. (G:74)

Declarations of love in letters reveal the desire young people have in entering into romantic liaisons and their ideas of love. Despite the many forces that seek to thwart young love—from parents to teachers and religious messages to sexual health campaigns—the youth counterpublic is characterized by explorations of intimacy and sexual companionship. In their imaginations of a better life, the tenderness that romance offers gives young people comfort that they will share their dreams with another.

Prove Your Love for Me: Managing Reputation and Desire

Responses to declarations of love also follow gendered patterns. While boys feel little risk in responding positively, girls' responses are more measured. Receiving an elaborate declaration is definitely flattering for girls, who are simultaneously curious and

insecure about their sexuality and fearful of the consequences of being in a relationship, including both reputational risks (such as being labeled a *nakyewombekeire*) and
health risks (such as pregnancy). There are also positive reputational rewards in being
in a relationship that is working well, such as being seen as a mature female who can
attract a man *and* keep him in love. Hence, given the range of consequences, it is not
surprising that responses from girls to boys' declarations of love are extremely varied.
Some girls may choose not to respond to the declaration, which itself is an implicit
reply. Other girls are doubtful of boys' claims of love, with their skepticism likely
based on the behaviors of males in relationships around them; some are hopeful but
want more proof. This girl replies to a request with a series of questions challenging
the boy to prove his love:

> By the way what do you mean by love?
> Give me five reasons why you want to fall in love me.
> Supposing I fall in love with you what will you do to the rest of yours?
> Do not deceive me that you don't have any.
> Reply if you're willing. (letter G:17)

Here we see a reworking of the historical courtship expectation in which a male
suitor has to overcome a series of challenges before proving his masculine worth and
winning his female love. However, instead of these challenges being established by
the girl's father within the counterpublic, this burden has shifted to young women
themselves. For many girls, taking on the responsibility of screening potential suitors, which in the past their parents would have done, leaves them in a double bind:
on the one hand, being in the precarious position of the socially derided category of
nakyewombekeire, and on the other hand, interested in experiencing and participating in youth dating.

Girls' constant awareness of the need to balance the management of their public
reputation with their personal desire translates into girls frequently responding with
skepticism or hesitancy to written declarations of love. The tension between reputation
and desire also keeps many girls from overtly initiating relationships, although as we
saw in the case of Annette, the ideal courtship convention of boys chasing girls is slowly
unraveling.

The majority of letters I collected from girls can be categorized as affirmations of
their love for a boy, in which they either accept his offer to pursue a relationship or
remind him of their love. As we will see in the next chapter, the latter frequently occurs
after a boy's attention or wooing has waned. After expressing her deep longing, the
following writer encourages her romantic interest to keep up his love for her:

> However, my dear, the main objective of writing to you this letter is that I really
> miss you a big deal and I think you know that with the beloved one even a
> minute seems a year without seeing you anymore. And my heart is paining for
> the search of your love.

Otherwise I didn't have much say but I just had a word of love for you because I landed on you and I love you. And please, my dear, always remember to keep a loving corner in your heart for me and me only.

LOTS
OF
LOVE,
(letter G:7)

Analyzing girls' intended messages is often complicated, because their desire to explore their sexuality and sexual relationships with boys is constantly balanced with their desire to protect their reputations. This discursive tension between romantic pleasure and reputational danger is found throughout girls' letters. Boys' love letters, on the other hand, tend to follow more neatly a single equation: love equals sex. Although I have separated the two themes of love and sex for purposes of examining the themes in love letters, in reality the two are very much intertwined in letters. However, despite these gender differences, it is clear that both boys and girls employ several techniques and rhetorics in order to elicit responses from prospective lovers, to proclaim their love, and to persuade love interests to reciprocate such feelings.

Sentiments of Longing, Strategies for Meeting

Given that parents in Iganga face daily problems in supporting their families, the romantic concerns of their adolescent dependents are a low priority. Furthermore, youth perceive themselves as living in a world very different from that of their parents, for the youthful world is influenced by global, social, and economic changes and can exist as an imagined space with multiple possibilities. Young people seek comfort and understanding from their peers; their lovers become confidants and help ease feelings of isolation and insignificance. Even if two young lovers live near each other, feelings of emotional longing because of social distance created by supervision are common. Youth desire someone with whom they can privately share their problems and find consolation, such as demonstrated by the boy whose love interest lives in a nearby village. He borrows a line from a popular song to express feelings of loneliness: "Days and nights are becoming centuries due to your absence. In fact, its u're absence that I miss you like a desert missing rain" (letter B:31). Similarly, a girl writes to her distant love interest: "Thinking of u is so easy but missing u is the most heartache, dear" (letter G:3). Another girl writes a letter to her new boyfriend, expressing her burning desire to be physically close with him: "However dear this precious note is to let you know I have accompanied ma' cousin to Kaliro road. I will back in a meantime coz whenever u're out I feel to kiss you in that distance but what is impossible. I miss you every hour you're out but with time it will be solved" (letter G:5).

The longing and desire for physical closeness often ends with a suggestion of how to arrange a meeting. Boys, more so than girls, tend to initiate these meetings. One boy arranges a secret meeting with his girlfriend after school: "I do not want to tell your sister or anyone that you love me. On Saturday after lunch I will meet you behind the lab and discuss more about it" (letter B:37). Young people's desire for physical closeness and face-to-face time with their love interest is complicated by older people's fear of physicality inevitably leading to sexual activity, and hence adults' various attempts to regulate youth romance and encounters. The obstacles surrounding youth romance often have the unintended consequences of heightening young people's desire for exploration and inspiring the creation of the secret counterpublic.

As discussed earlier, elders perceive school and town as responsible for the loosening of sexual mores. From their perspective, these locations offer youth unlimited opportunities to meet, mingle, and carry on sexual affairs—a perspective, though simplified and one-sided, that is supported by contemporary adolescent courting habits. A boy writes: "I have much to tell you but let us meet today and I have a small discussion with you in any executive bar you will want, which is the best in town. So reply and tell me where we can meet and what time to meet. But I suggest to meet at around 4.30 p.m. after your exams. And reply my letter first to show me that you really love me by telling me where and what time to meet?" (letter B:25). The short after-school detour is easily explained to parents as after-school activities or late classes. Boys are encouraged by their friends or older siblings to make arrangements to meet girls, but during the actual meeting, boys might become shy or uncertain what to do next. Like many boys, this suitor wants to confirm the girl's interest before the meeting in an effort to reduce the chances of an unrequited interest. Sometimes letters discuss what might take place at the meeting—whether the sender can expect a private moment away from others or an intimate touch.

Scheduling a secret rendezvous presents complications for youth who reside in distant towns. Leaving parents' homes for extended periods to visit lovers requires not only ingenuity but also nerve, especially for first-time planners. A girl of seventeen was asked by a suitor to visit him at school. In her reply, she expresses her apprehension about visiting him, a virtual stranger: "About coming to check on you I really don't know b'se to me that is a very impossible thing. First of all there is no way I can leave school or home for Mbale. It's a place where I have never been and know no one at all. And I also think its too early to be thinking about such a step. We hardly know each other but here we are planning a visit" (letter G:20). According to widespread beliefs about sexual availability, an unmarried young woman who visits a man's house unaccompanied is sending a signal that she is open to having sexual relations with him. This logic informs the decisions a young female makes when visiting a suitor at his home, oftentimes leading her to bring a friend along to act as a buffer or chaperone. A more common arrangement is for boys to visit girls at their schools, as boarding schools are thought to be generally safe and girl students are more likely to accept such offers to visit.

For adolescents who frequently shift between houses of relatives (whether to attend a certain school or because their parents are temporarily unable to economically support the number of dependents in the household), there is a constant threat of departing from newfound love interests, causing some romances to advance quickly. Nampina, an eighteen-year-old girl, became acquainted with a boy who was temporarily residing with his uncle in her home village. When it came time for the boy to leave, Nampina wrote him this letter expressing her sadness about his nearing departure. She hints at secretly "escaping" or eloping with him:

> My friend u may think that I don't love u but I do. My friend in our culture they keep us seriously but when you love somebody you escape. When I love someone he takes all my mind. Without admiring at him I feel sad. My friend this is not your home village and then if you go back to your home my minds will goes on becoming mad. How can I love u when it is time for u to go away from Busembatia? (letter G:19)

While in the past long-distance relationships eventually faded and were replaced by newly formed and more convenient ones, the electronic technologies discussed in the previous chapter (such as text messages, e-mail, and Facebook) allow youth to more easily maintain a larger network of peers and potential lovers.

School holidays are ideal occasions for young people to visit past or current lovers. Many parents work away from home during the day—farming, marketing crops, or working in town—creating brief windows of opportunity to meet with lovers. This boy expresses his feelings about a holiday romance: "Please Leatisha, I miss you plus your company you offered to me during holidays because at this time we enjoyed a lot and I will come back. Not only that but also you showed me a good heart during the visit and may God reward you accordingly" (letter B:15). This boy's letter was intended to maintain a relationship with Leatisha in hopes of rekindling it when they meet again. During an interview about this letter, Leatisha explained that he referred to a private, shared experience when he wrote, "You showed me a good heart." Using a cryptic reference allows the writer to deny accusations of wrongdoing advanced by an unforeseen or unintended reader.

God as Moral Authority

Religion plays a major role in lives of people in Iganga. Reflecting this shared deference to a higher power, young people in their love letters strategically invoke God to gain moral authority with the aim of shaping their partners' behaviors. In the following letter, the female writer calls upon God to help her and her lover not stray and look for other partners. Through an invocation of God, she attempts to regulate the behaviors and temptations of the recipient while positioning herself on a higher moral ground where she has achieved a state of restraint. She writes:

> Setan is also there. He can show you a good girl/boy who is beautiful in color, lovely in figure, short in size, between black and brown. Who is more beautiful? But my friend she/he is not a life in body and Christ Jesus. So you have to pray and say God I don't want to see a beautiful girl/ boy, and "AIDS" also is with beautiful girls / boys. My dear, pray. Do not sleep such that our promise can remain the same.

> I don't want to leave you, and I don't want God to show me a good boy who is not you. I am praying that you're mine and be mine forever and ever. I pray to God amen!!
>
> NB: try to look in these books Mark 1:35 (the weaknesses of youth). Eph 6:1–3, Rom 12:1–2, 1 peter 5:2–3, Job 9,10:21–22: 23–24 you can go on reading state of 9 and 10. (letter G:34)

The writer puts the relationship in the hands of God, asking that he not lead either of them astray. By suggesting that she is also asking God for assistance in helping her avoid temptation, she reminds her sweetheart that her commitment should not be taken for granted. God is also a romantic device whereby young people call upon a higher being as a metaphor for their love or destiny to be together. Another girl writes: "Your love to me has been welcomed in my heart as Jesus was welcomed in Jerusalem. I have already suggested that you are the one whom God has given me, the first one, and the final one and I think our love is one hundred percent pure love" (letter G:91). Letters collected in later years made more references to God, and the increase was most significant in girls' letters. This increase might be stimulated by the growing public presence of the evangelical movement in Uganda and the turn toward discourses of religious-based morality in HIV prevention campaigns, particularly as international faith-based initiatives were privileged during the George W. Bush administration's PEPFAR policies; the initiatives have continued through the morality crusade that peaked during the wave of marriage equality bills under Barack Obama, which to fundamental Christians were evidence that evil was winning out. For women and adolescent girls, these newer, socially conservative religions provide a recognized, higher authority to call upon when negotiating relationships and sex with men, as explored in the following chapters. While God was often invoked for the purpose of regulating a lover's behaviors, in a large number of letters the writer portrayed God as a supportive and nurturing figure as well. This supportive figure helped guide the writer through tough times and gave hope. Again, this language is more common in girls' letters and follows Basoga gender ideologies in which a woman is subordinate to a man (either a father or husband) who offers advice and guidance.

Conclusion

This chapter has explored sentiments of desire, hope, and affirmation in youth love letters and has examined what those themes reveal about how young people make sense of the world around them. Youth turn to their romantic partners for self-realization, support, sex, and companionship as they begin to experience feelings of neglect from parents, who are burdened with other household problems. Love letters become a space through which youth can imagine and express their desire not only for their sweethearts but also for their futures. We see much anxiety in their writings about their uncertain educational futures and economic situations. These concerns are expressed throughout their relationships, but as we see in the next chapter, the expectation that their lovers will assist them takes on new dimensions.

Many of the letters examined in this chapter were written at the beginning stages of a relationship, and in them we see the enactment of the gendering of "the chase" that both older and younger people describe. Many adolescent and young males do not have the financial means to achieve the consumer-based romantic ideal, and therefore they attempt to woo a love interest with eloquent declarations of love and careful crafting of romantic selves. This romantic foreplay competes with the economic foreplay offered by a young woman's older suitors, motivating adolescent males to go to great lengths in their letters to construct themselves and their future potential as something worth waiting for. Adolescent females, on the other hand, tend to express hesitancy during earlier stages out of fear of risking their reputations, a tendency that can be understood as defaulting to Basoga cultural norms of female restraint and respectability. Girls often respond to boys' initial declarations of love with skepticism and request more proof of a suitor's love. In their letters, we also see how adolescent girls eventually, after additional effort from boys, gain confidence and comfort with expressing their own romantic desires, thereby allowing the relationship to progress and further eschewing Basoga norms. Letters also contain evidence of how young women are increasingly transgressing gender ideologies of women as demur and passive romantic subjects, and deciding instead to initiate a relationship. Yet since love letters are material evidence of individual acts of female sexual agency, many adolescent girls choose not to display such bold initiation in letters, saving it instead for flirtatious encounters or verbal messages delivered by a go-between. In short, girls use letters to navigate the continuum between Basoga conventions and newer romantic norms and, in some cases, manage to satisfy both, as seen in the appropriation of Christian ideologies. Young male suitors, on the other hand, demonstrate an awareness of the precarious position of today's adolescent girls and, in their letters, appeal to these conflicting norms. As scholars of romance have suggested, during early stages in a relationship there is an inversion of gender inequality, in which the young woman has the upper hand while a male suitor tries to convince her that his love is sincere and that he is the best choice of all her suitors. As we see in the next chapter, however, this gender inversion is temporary, and girls struggle to hold on to their once-dominant position.

CHAPTER 11

"You're just playing with my head"

Disappointment and Uncertainty

In *The Origin of the Family, Private Property and the State* (1884), Friedrich Engels chronicles how state interventions into the family have been fundamental to the advancement of capitalism. Engels demonstrates that the labor and consumer needs of capitalism thrive best when society is organized into nuclear and monogamous family units with a (male) household head through which wealth can be accumulated and passed down and with (female and child) dependents who provide productive and reproductive labor. Engels's argument about the relationships between the privatization of property and accumulation of wealth and the subsequent bolstering of men's domination over women was particularly compelling to feminist scholars in the 1970s who were interested in the origin and universality of women's oppression (see Sacks 1974). More recently, Engels's analytic perspective has informed investigations on romance, provoking scholars to question the extent to which romantic love and nuclear-family relationships under capitalist conditions are liberating for women, and whether such relationships reproduce and mask gender inequalities. While initially relationships based on individual choices may appear to provide women with freedom and rights, scholars have questioned this assumption and have demonstrated that nuclearization of relationships may increase women's vulnerability precisely because nuclearization tends to confine women to the domestic sphere and alienate them from economic resources and previous sources of social and kin support (Beauvoir 1953; Cancian 1986; Collier 1997; Constable 2003; Parikh 2007; Rebhum 1999; Freeman 2007). Not only are women bound to the domestic sphere and denied access to control over property and wealth, but their reproductive and productive labor becomes the property of their husbands. Scholars examining the premarital stage of nuclear marriage suggest that the process of premarital romance serves to seduce women into the belief that love equals gender equality (see, for example, D. C. Holland and Eisenhart 1992). Other research examining the intersection of gender inequality and love shows how the notion of a companionate relationship encourages women's silences or willful ignorance of their lovers' less desirable behaviors (such as extramarital affairs or abuse) as women strive to preserve both the public appearance of a modern relationship and their own trust in a mate (Rebhun 1999; Sobo 1995; J. S. Hirsch, Wardlow, Smith, et al. 2010; Parikh 2007; D. J. Smith 2007; Phinney 2008; Wardlow 2007; Bailey 1988; Padilla et al. 2007).

This chapter takes up the issue of freedom of choice in mate selection within the context of gender inequality and a market-based economy in which men have easier access to social and economic resources, or in the case of youth, in which adolescent males have future gender privilege. In this chapter, I examine themes in love letters that frequently emerge after a relationship has been established or in later stages of a relationship, with the aim of understanding how shifts in the dynamics of a relationship are shaped by gendered reputation, expectations, and inequalities. While some of the themes examined in the previous chapter could also fall into this category—for instance, God, sex and AIDS, and affirmations of love are all found in established relationships—the themes in this chapter revolve around the general idea of disappointment. These themes reveal how affection might circuitously, negatively unfold and often eventually fade among young companionate partners who were once romantically hopeful that their relationship would allow them to transcend everyday precarity and warnings of young love.

Sex, Pregnancy, and AIDS

Letters written after a relationship has been established frequently contain direct or indirect references to sex, and are typically gendered. These letters are fairly formulaic: an adolescent boy attempts to convince a girl who in a previous letter or gesture has shown interest in him that sex is the ultimate proof of their love and commitment, or that sex is a demonstration of their (but mostly, her) maturity. The tension between girls' unresolved conflict about their desire to explore their sexuality and romantic relationships and their anxiety about protecting their reputations becomes increasingly salient as pressure to engage in sex intensifies. As explored in Part II of this ethnography, the tensions between the ideas of sexual desire and risk of disease and pregnancy in Uganda have been occasioned by the multiple messages about sex circulated in the public sphere—in AIDS education, the media, religion, and the like. Love letters reveal how youth draw on sex and AIDS messages, reworking them either to protect themselves from the risks of sex or to deter lovers from wandering to other romantic relationships.

Boys and Sex

Sexual intercourse is a source of anxiety for both boys and girls. For boys, the anxiety concerns when they will *start* having sex, which is a particular concern given that boys often are not able to engage in the economic foreplay associated with men's sexual success. For girls, the anxiety is what will happen *after* they have sex, in their relationship with both their sexual partner and their circle of friends and family. Viewed by boys as their entry into a mystical and pleasurable world of manhood, sexual activity is seen by girls as necessary (for they expect to reproduce one day) and potentially liberating and pleasurable, but also as the dreaded exit from innocent childhood into the social burdens of womanhood that they see their mothers and aunts carrying. In discussions and interviews, older and younger men represent sexual desires as uncontrollable urges that need to be satisfied or else an "unfortunate condition" will arise. The "unfortunate condition" is seen as the result of not releasing sperm, which, many believe, causes penile shrinkage, lower back problems, dwarfism, and laziness. During a discussion I had with students and teachers, male teachers talked about the belief of backed-up sperm and asked me what I thought. I turned to the medical doctor who had accompanied me on this particular visit. He stated that there was no scientific evidence to support the idea that backed-up sperm could cause problems and that it is absorbed into the body without side effects or difficulty, but the teachers appeared unconvinced, maintaining the belief that not engaging in sexual activity or specifically releasing sperm has negative physical and mental health consequences. When the doctor mentioned masturbation as an option, the room grew silent with a cloud of suspicious embarrassment quickly followed by a collective laughter of denial. Reasons for not masturbating ranged from it being a same-sex act to it being un-Christian to waste sperm to it not being a practice within Basoga culture. (Although the idea of ejaculation through self-stimulation is publicly frowned upon, I have no reason to believe that the act of masturbation does not exist. The Lusoga word for and concept of "wet dreams"—i.e., the nocturnal emission of semen—is commonly known, which indicates that emission occurring without stimulation from a partner is socially accepted.) Whereas negative consequences for not having (or delaying) sex similarly exist for girls, more common are beliefs about the biological importance of women giving birth and the possible health complications that could result if they choose not to have sex, or if they delay it for too long. Both sets of gendered ideas are commonly circulated, providing, particularly for boys, powerful peer-pressure techniques and reasonable justifications to engage in sexual activity. The necessity for boys to have sexual intercourse is further fueled by the pervasive adage among boys, "practice makes perfect." In addition, the belief that love—particularly love not acted upon—can lead to physical and mental conditions is commonly reflected in boys' letters and in their discussions about love and desire: "Even I feel like running mad. . . . My love for you in future might drive me crazy" (letter B:29). As boys attempt to reconcile their sexual desires with their emotional ones, many are left with unsettled and unidentified feelings toward their interests. Boys eventually learn that they cannot directly ask a girl to have sex (for proper girls are expected to resist direct requests as indicated in the chase narrative); rather, boys share and practice veiled requests for sex that draw on cultural logics detailed above (such as the biological or emotional need for sex), flattery, or manipulation. Revisiting a passage presented in a previous chapter, we see that this letter writer combines two of these strategies, initially flattering his love interest and then explaining the uncontrollable sexual desire he experiences when he sees or thinks about her: "My love is as lasting as a gravity stone—I love u b'se u are beautiful, charming and my best friend. I will always love you until the sea dries. Your shining face attracts and affects my feelings and make me even mix up my chemical wrongly" (letter B:12). What stands out in many boys' letters is an emerging sense of male sexual confidence or privilege—the assumption that girls will respond positively to their requests for sex or that girls will not be offended or report them. This boy expresses a deep, uncontrollable yearning he has for his love interest: "You break my heart sincerely when I look at you. It is so obligatory for me to have something with you. Let me fast jot the main issue/ideal. It is about love and sex actually. Ashex, when I look at you, I feel like doing an action with you" (letter B:32). To many boys, this desire can be resolved only by "doing an action." Most boys assume that courting a girl will lead to sex; their supplications for sex become more persistent over time.

In addition to cultural logics about sexual activity and flattery, boys also use social manipulation as a strategy for requesting sex. The idea that being sexually active is a sign of maturity and, conversely, that being a virgin represents a state of immaturity or childhood becomes a tool for pressuring love interests into having sex. For example, one boy ends his request for sex with the postscript, "I hope you are mature and do what is expected of you." The term "mature" is commonly used by adults as a justification for youth's inability to partake in certain "adult" activities, whether relationships, tasks, or decisions. When used between people of the same age group, invoking maturity is a power play of peer pressure. According to Cindy Patton, "the pressure is applied on the fault line between the quest for autonomy through shared disidentification with parents and the group performance of the very behaviors that mark their parents as adults" (1996:46). The strategy is often effective between age-mates because it touches on the very divide that separates youth from adults (sexual activity) while creating equality between two adolescents (the decision to engage in sex).

Virtually all the youth with whom I spoke discussed the pressure from and possible disappointment of lovers as primary reasons for engaging in sex. Alex, a nineteen-year-old high school student, has been courting his love interest for some time. After many failed attempts to convince her to have sex, he takes a different approach: "I long to have some romance with you because several times I ask you for romance you always tell me the other day. But on the point of sex as you had told me that you're not prepared for it. I agreed that I'll wait until the time comes when you're prepared for it" (letter B:5). Through a subtle sleight of hand, Alex's letter conflates the words romance and sex. For what girl would refuse romance? His assumption is that his love interest will eventually comply with his request for sex when she is "prepared for it." Not all boys pressure girls into having sex, but from my discussions with boys, it is believed that sex is a natural outcome of love. Love is the feeling; sex is the proof.

Girls and Sex

The double standard for girls and boys leads to different sexual strategies in love letters: while boys pursue sex with respectable girls to gain status, girls attempt to postpone sex to avoid pregnancy and a bad reputation. One girl tried to explain to her boyfriend why she is cautious about sex: "Another thing to write this letter is that I love you and you love me. But the bad thing is that if to be with you which I am meaning is to have sex with you. For me I fear to conceive, but if you try another way I will be with you but if not that we shall forget about that" (letter G:13). Her suggestion to "try another way" is likely connected to contraception, probably in the form of condoms, since they are easier than hormonal contraception for youth to acquire. Although youth know the risks of sex and the protection that condoms can provide, according to public health research they are not very likely to use them. Whereas for long-term or permanent relationships the suggestion of condoms is often associated with distrust of the other or an admission of one's own infidelity, in newly established youth relationships the expectation to use a condom is present. However, the simple gesture of a lover agreeing to use a condom is often enough proof of intent; the use of one does not need to follow. Observing a similar tendency among lower-income African American women in the United States, Elisa J. Sobo (1995) argues that women in her study were aware of sexual risks that lead to HIV infection and of ways to reduce their risks; however, when it came to evaluating their own risk and using risk reduction practices, her informants relied upon two narratives to rationalize and deny their risk of contracting HIV from partners. The first is the "monogamy narrative," in which women convince themselves that they are in a monogamous relationship with their partner, even if evidence suggests otherwise. The second is the "wisdom narrative," in which they believe they have the knowledge and wisdom to select safe partners and practice safe sex when necessary. When women deny any risk in their primary relationship, Sobo argues, they elevate or maintain their social status and associated self-esteem. Sobo's analysis is useful for understanding the relationship among condom use, trust, and the status of a relationship for young people. Similarly, girls in Iganga might choose to deny the risk that a lover might pose in order to preserve the status derived from a relationship, putting them at greater risk.

Another girl, Amina, offers these lovely passages to her lover in explaining why she cannot engage in sex. Amina struggles to refute his earlier pleas for sex:

And I think as we are little flowers, I mean as we are still young I suggest that we should abstain sex before we are old-ups that's before marriage because you never know such slight mistake may occur and then it causes other probs all together (how do you see it?)

And my dear George it's not true when you say that you won't believe whether we are lovers before having sex. Let me assure you having sex with someone does not mean that you love that someone but it's just by heart that you vocal out that expression of love to someone.

And now time and again you've been telling me that it seems I have another boy I love which boy I don't know. But to be sincere I have no any other boy lover apart from you and except friends as usual. (letter G:22)

Amina's ability to support her decision not to have sex is evident and is consistent with messages youth hear from sexual health campaigns, parents, and teachers. Notable in her letter, however, is the delicate manner with which she deploys the common public health and cultural arguments for delaying sex. While boys feel empowered to ask for sex directly, girls feel less empowered to stand their ground, because they fear that denying sex might end a relationship and also because they have accepted the notion that they are obligated to fulfill men's sexual needs.

From the above letter, it appears that Amina's boyfriend, George, has been accusing her of having sex with another boy. Implying that Amina has thwarted his requests for sex because she is having her sexual needs met by another male (perhaps an older man) is a strategy for pressuring her to have sex. In order to prove her commitment to him, she should also have sex with George. On a more general level, the idea that a girl who has already had sexual intercourse (and therefore is already "spoiled") should demonstrate her love for a new boyfriend as she did for those in the past both leads many girls to want to conceal their sexual pasts and becomes a key bargaining strategy in boys' requests for sex.

Gender and HIV

The risk of contracting HIV is a well-known outcome of sex. However, youth view it as less likely to occur if their significant other is of their own age group. One explanation may be that transmission among youth is overshadowed by the more prevalent public association of HIV transmission through intergenerational relationships between older men (sugar daddies) and younger women. Although boys know that intergenerational sex increases the risk of HIV among their female peers, I saw little if any evidence in love letters that this deters them from requesting sex. One explanation could be that boys are less likely to actively pursue romantic liaisons with girls who are thought to be at risk for HIV because of their relationships with older men. In other words, a girl with an already sullied reputation may not be worthy of the investment required in love letter romances. Whereas, as mentioned above, boys made minimal, if any, references in their letters to the fear of contracting HIV from the recipient of the letter, boys did invoke the possibility of contracting HIV as a way of convincing their lovers to remain faithful and patient. For instance, in a letter written to his love interest who is attending school in a different area, a boy writes: "But don't waste a lot of time thinking about me b'se a disease may develop into your body which is incurable. I advise you to read books because boys are the causer of failures in girls and also girls are the causer of failure in boys. So both of us we must have enough concentration on book. . . . I emphasize many good boys are around and many girls are around the world but let us keep ourselves from HIV" (letter B:24). Given that adolescent boys cannot compete with older men's ability to offer girls money and gifts, the younger men utilize romantic strategies to make themselves more competitive suitors. They also creatively invoke the idea that intergenerational sex puts girls at risk for HIV. The following boy argues that although his "pocket is light," he is a better choice than a rich man who may be HIV-positive:

> I have concluded in all ways that there is nobody better than you except God in heaven. But although my pocket is light I am better than those rich men around b'se they are diseased (HIV). . . . By the way anytime you will get money in your life. . . . In addition you should be wise because all eyes of men are on you. But to conclude remember me. Whenever you budget put me number one I also put you number one on my budget. But since God is in heaven, long live serving me. (letter B:24)

After attempting to frighten the reader with his talk of sugar daddies and HIV, the letter writer's invocation of God can be interpreted as serving two purposes. First, calling upon God allows him to make a moral critique of older men who have more economic power, thereby establishing his own moral authority. His invocation also allows him to deter her from accepting the advances of other men by leaning upon Christianity's conservative sexual mores. This clever one-two punch is a demonstration of how young people appropriate and deploy public discourses in advancing their romantic projects. In sum, boys often use the AIDS messages to scare their love interests from other men, yet ignore the messages themselves when it comes to having sex. Girls, on the other hand, borrow the three-part AIDS message of abstinence, monogamy, and condom use to negotiate terms of a relationship or to resolve conflicts.

Gender Inequality and Infidelity

The ending of a relationship is difficult for youth, particularly for girls. Girls might be skeptical or hesitant when a boy first declares his love, but once involved, many are reluctant to let an unhealthy alliance go. When a relationship does dissolve, other youth (both male and female) often assume the girl is the one who ruined the relationship. This parallels the tendency of elders to say of failed adult marriages, "The woman did not persevere." In conflicts, girls are more likely to initiate discussion and to assume and accept blame. However, crafted away from lovers, letters allow girls to assert a greater voice in articulating their concerns. The following example demonstrates how letter writing as an act of communicating intimacy removes the immediacy of gender hierarchies and provides a space for girls to challenge this idea of ultimate female blame. The writer quite assertively assigns equal blame to her young lover:

> But in the actual sense darling I tell you I think I don't have any greater problem which can not be solved . . . but I am mentally disturbed by those few statements we use to frighten each other. . . . So please my dear one, in order to avoid that I think the solutions we can use may be identified in this way. Let us avoid talking about what happened in the past you know that will cause chaos. I swear Sam not to ever frustrate you at any single moment and I want to promise me that you will never do that again to me. In deed Sam for today's case, I was really disturbed by your words which you may call minor. I went back home, I don't get super but I just got a pen to jot to you but I need to talk to you personally not by letter before going to the afternoon exams. . . . Let me think you will respond positively to my letter. . . . I will always remain yours in deep luv. (letter G:33)

Girls struggle to understand why their love interests had changes of heart, what they did wrong, and how much pain they should endure. After a relationship has turned sour, this girl writes a letter to her love interest asking why he is avoiding her. Her love for him, she explains, is still strong: "We are all born weak and helpless, then why do you bring bitter charges against me even on simple issues. I love you but maybe you are excited with glare of anger. Why do you want to avoid me dear? There is hope for us, let's enjoy our bitter life together b'se like rivers that stop running and lakes that dry, people die, never to raise to life. But ma' love for you is unavoidable" (letter G:5). Judging from the letters I collected, girls more than boys tend to write about deteriorating relationships and a lover's change of heart, often pleading with the loved one to provide a reason for his shift in affection so that she can adjust to better meet his needs. Girls often respond to their lovers' anger by accepting blame, even if they are unsure of what they did:

> If I annoyed you somewhere it would be better to tell me than making me empty promises. However Sam I can never find another lover like you, sweeter than you, more precious than you. Husband to be you are closer to me just like my mother, I pray for someone like you and I thank God that I finally find you; and I hope that you feel the same way too, I promise to never fall in love with a stranger. You are all I am thinking of. (letter G:39)

Compare the deferential tone of this letter to the next letter, written by a boy. A common strategy is for boys to draw from the gendered nature of blame and guilt by transferring the cause of a relationship's deteriorating into their lover's actions—the girl was not meeting his needs, he thought she was cheating, or some combination of the two. In the letter below, the boy has grown tired of being questioned about his suspect behavior, and strategically turns the situation around by arguing that her continual questioning of him is the source of problems in their relationship. He writes: "Please Aisha, I have all that time singing the same mistakes but you have failed to change. Instead you continue with the same. On this note therefore, I'm sorry but it's unavoidable, are you continuing with me? If you are continuing with me is this how you are supposed to behave? Please madam, it is a high time for you to change" (letter B:1). Aisha's "mistakes," as he details later in this letter and in subsequent ones, center around how she is dealing with rumors that he has another girlfriend. The male writer skillfully deflects the accusation of infidelity, turning attention instead to her continuing socializing with people he had requested she not—presumably the same people spreading rumors about his other girlfriend.

Suspicions of infidelity are the source of many problems in relationships among youth, and are dealt with in gendered ways. As in the letter above, boys are not necessarily compelled to disprove their girlfriends' suspicious and might turn the criticism back on the girl (e.g., she's overly jealous or her behaviors are driving him away), whereas girls accused of having extra lovers are often expected to address the accusation directly, particularly if they want the relationship with the accuser to continue. While this general pattern exists in the letters I collected, messages about monogamy and infidelity circulated in the public sphere offer girls a language and a rationale for them to confront a straying boyfriend. Girls witness their mothers struggling with cheating husbands and with rivalry between co-wives, and they do not want to fall victim to the same fate. Juliet firmly expresses her disappointment to her suitor:

Dear William,

Sorry for having let you down because you were showing me disloyalness. Remember I told you that if I find you with another girl, that will be the end of our love. Remember that the bible says in (Hebrews 13:4) "Let marriage be honorable among all, and the marriage bed be without defilement, for God will judge fornicators and adulterers. And in (Peter 3:7) try to read. (letter G:11)

Use of the Bible to justify monogamy and faithfulness is common in Uganda. As discussed earlier in this book, there is a visible increase in religious (mainly Christian) fellowship groups for single and professional young people. These fellowships have great appeal in the time of AIDS, especially with young working women who fear the possibility of contracting HIV from cheating men and who want a man who will be faithful.

Like Juliet, this next girl is not ready to tolerate the unfaithfulness of her man. She has other options in suitors, she states, so she demands reassurance of his loyalty. She writes:

> With no wastage of time as the proverb says that "facts are bitter" . . . Your love between girls is very rampant and I can't tolerate. Another thing is sharing. I understand you are booked by many. Moreover some of them are my friends. Now how will I, the whole me, start sharing with them. . . . There I will look like an idiot; uneducated person and a person with no thinking capacity. Maybe there jokes, or you wanted to experience my reactions.
>
> As I know village girls yet I am also a villager but not as such. You only wanted me to be beaten by your girls. I understand they fight for guys. Will I manage that situation? (letter G:17)

"I will look like an idiot," she declares, if others know that her man is cheating. "Sharing a man," according to this letter, is done by women of lower status ("village girls") who perhaps are unable to control their mates or do not know better.

Many young girls desire a monogamous and faithful man. According to my survey data from youth, almost all girls consider a "good" marriage to be a monogamous one. Some girls, however, do not feel completely empowered to present a monogamy ultimatum. This next girl, a primary school student, confronts her love interest about his cheating but maintains that she wants to remain in the relationship. She explains her suspicions:

> I am not fine why? Because you have me to be annoyed because you have a girlfriend in primary five but let me tell you Alex I love you so much but you don't no why I love you because of your beautiful body and face that is why I love you so much and that matter of having very many girls in the same school for me I don't want that and you will make me to leave you . . . again please as I don't have much to say I only end my letter by saying that Alex I love you so much but I want you to show that you love me.
>
> From your girl friend. (letter G:25)

The feisty tone of this girl is an example of young girls' developing sexual agency—their uninhibited ability to state their needs and desires. Her reasons for "loving" him (his "beautiful body and face") are also notable, as they are more in line with boys' stated reasons than with those of older girls. As she ages, her interest in boys is likely to shift to more emotional and economic needs.

As we saw earlier, promises or hopes of marriage keep some girls in relationships. Historical continuity is found in the idea among girls that the safest route out of their parents' home is through marriage. This route becomes more pressing as girls age, or as their opportunities for schooling decrease. The girl below writes about her confusion over her lover's change of behavior in a poem. In a desperate attempt to move past their conflicts and his change of heart, she suggests marriage, a promise he had made to her in the past. She writes:

> Hallo Daddy;
> *RE: MESSAGE OF FOR CIVILNES*
> Before I pen the point allow me to send
> warm greetings to you with a great pleasure
> over to you, that How are you over there?
> I believe you are not fine due to what you—
> did to me everyday.
> ***
>
> I am sorry you told me that you never
> did it again but you're still going on.
> What is the problem now?
> ***
>
> I want to know the truth you said your
> coming everyday time to time what is
> the matter. Tell me the truth.
> ***
>
> If you're busy come and you tell me—
> face to face.
> If it's impossible receive a letter.
> but I am sorry you're absent minded.
> If there's another problem tell me.
> ***
>
> You said if I want marriage you're ready
> to capture on it.
> On which day of the month?
> Really are you sure?
> For I am ready on it.
> ***
>
> Lastly, really I am sorry to say that my love with
> you impresses me so much it wants—
> marriage. Help me on it.
> Let me pen off you reply today or tomorrow.
> Yours,
> (letter G:6)

For this girl, like others, she does not want to lose her boyfriend. She is ready to commit to a relationship, even though she senses that his feelings for her have changed. Her plea "Help me on it" reflects a prevalent idea that marriage is often a favor that men bestow on women to legitimize their love or relationship.

Importantly, the longer a relationship lasts, the more a girl is willing to tolerate, be it cheating, unmet promises, or physical abuse. After a relationship goes public and is known to family and friends, this tolerance seems to increase. The girl's sexual identity becomes increasingly associated with her lover, and ending the relationship can threaten her reputation and, from her perspective, diminish the chances of a new relationship.

Aisha and Peter: Infidelity and Gender Violence

I use the relationship of Aisha and Peter to examine how gender dynamics change over the course of a relationship as structures of inequality create a greater gap between young men's and women's ability to manage their public reputation as well as their access to and control over economic and social resources. When I met them, Aisha and Peter were both in their early twenties and had been dating for several years. Their relationship began during secondary school while Peter was dating someone else. A year into their relationship, Aisha went to university in the capital, and Peter attended a teacher's college, but he had to withdraw after one semester because of lack of money for tuition. Aisha had suspected that Peter was sleeping with young women in her absence. In particular, she suspected that his neighbor, Merisha, was one of those women. Peter denied the accusations and even had Merisha corroborate his story. One day during a surprise visit, Aisha found a note from Merisha in Peter's room. A disappointed Aisha wrote the following note on the bottom of Merisha's note:

> Peter is that what you are trying to show me, someone you really promised that I'm your future wife and we made vows but I don't know because I've found very many changes even some clothes maybe for your woman.
>
> Why are you doing all that to me? We would have quarreled and another thing but not cheating on me. The other box of condoms you said that I must complete already is half yet I have not even used a single condom.
>
> Peter remember I'm your wife. I was just sitting there and your girlfriend came asking for you and holding the other yellow jean jacket for Gerald. But I'm ready to abide by the conditions of you came of dreaming.
>
> Peter darling, stop cheating me. You are even advising me that this is a deadly world but to my surprise I don't know.
>
> I still remain your wife,
> Aisha

NB: How come I found this note inside the room? It implies that she also has a key. (letter G:40)

I am not sure how Peter handled this particular incident, yet I do know that despite this and other evidence of Peter's infidelity and Aisha's insistence that he stop his philandering, Aisha continued her relationship with Peter. As the relationship progressed, so did the power struggles. The impact of wider structures of gender inequality on their relationship and their individual strategies became apparent. Aisha attempted several times to regain the power she had at the beginning of the relationship, and at specific moments she found herself in a good bargaining position (such as when she was accepted and later entered into the prestigious state university). But for most of their relationship, Aisha found herself negotiating status differences *between* herself and Peter's other women, on some occasions directly confronting his suspected extra-relationship trysts. Similar to the way younger men vie with a sweetheart's older suitors for status, romance functions as an articulation of both gender and class politics for women as well.

Gender violence also played a part in the couple's relationship, as Peter resorted to physical force when frustrated with Aisha's accusations and his own jealousy of her accomplishments. In a letter written after Peter hit her, Aisha takes responsibility for provoking Peter's temper and abuse. She writes:

> Anyway darling I have admitted that I was the trouble causer but then to some extent you need to sympathise me just b'se I wasn't in mai senses. As you know that I had already sipped some ESB [beer] I hereby apologise to forgive me all what I did as I forgave you.
>
> I was hurt in the ears where you slapped me but then I had to forgive and forget all those issues and I had only to remember your sweet love and good life as many people admire our couple why to ashame ourselves. Anyway I have much to say but I can't express it all on this paper so good bye. (letter G:35)

Violence against women is a commonly recognized problem in Uganda but, as in much of the world, it is represented in the media and in everyday talk either as a result of a woman's actions (such as the way she dresses, behaves, or moves) provoking the violence or as isolated instances of a man's misbehaving instead of the result of structural gender inequalities. Gender violence is in fact the extension of patriarchal domination over women's bodies. Within intimate relationships, domestic abuse is considered a private affair between the two people, and it is thought to be most effectively handled by older family members. Adolescent girls face an additional complication in cases of abuse. Specifically, because they often do not want their families, teachers, or other familiar adults to know that they are in a romantic relationship (for it will bring about unwanted critique), girls often feel that they have no adult that they can turn to for advice or assistance, making them more vulnerable to relationship violence. Like Aisha, many young women accept responsibility for the abuse by their lovers; some claim it is a sign of love, as older generations were taught to believe. The situation becomes increasingly difficult for women who are financially dependent on their lovers but is also complicated by social norms and gendered expectations.

The Economy of Love

The strong association between a woman's romantic interest and a man's economic ability often gets woven into popular discourse as a story of ruthlessly greedy and money-hungry women preying upon innocent male victims. Stories of barmaids or "detoothers" who take advantage of drunken men for their money, mistresses who are kept by powerful politicians, and university girls who sell their bodies for sex are common portrayals of "bad" girls. Local talk suggests that every woman has a money-hungry person lurking inside her. If sex is the proof of love, money is the supposed motivator of love. Life histories of elders underscore this connection between a man's money and a woman's love for him. For example, Yiige, age fifty-five, narrated his life history as a string of four wives who left him for men with more money. Underlying his narrative is an association between his financial hardships and his wives' departures. His neighbor added a missing element to Yiige's failed marriages—domestic abuse and excessive drinking—but also maintained that inadequate finances were the primary reason for the wives' running away.

For boys in Iganga, their biggest romantic asset is not in their wallets but in their actions and words. Like Sam's romantic disappointment at the beginning of the book, there is often a fear among unemployed or underemployed young males from lower- and lower-middle-class families of losing their love interests to older and professional men. In the letter below, a nineteen-year-old girl reminds one of her unemployed suitors that she is in great demand by other men with money: "Let me assure that I have so many boys/men who are in need of me. Moreover they are reasonable, responsible and even snobs. . . . Do you know these days I am after somebody who is educated and also working?" (letter G:18). For younger adolescents, simply being educated or going to school is enough. As girls age and feel pressure to be with or marry a man who is a good provider, the characteristics of "working," "responsible," and upwardly mobile are added to the list of desirable characteristics for a suitor. According to the adolescent females I knew, money for hygiene products (such as sanitary napkins and soap) was among their greatest financial needs. The idea that men should provide women with money is often capitalized on in letters written by girls. For example, a girl promises to love the boy who "fulfills" her need: "Get for me six thousand [shillings ($3.5 USD)] and I pay the other man's money. I conclude by saying that my future is your future and if at all you handle me properly you will not hear anything bad about me and if 'u' fulfill all my needs please everything will be okay and if you do so your highly appreciated" (letter G:14). When facing fierce competition, some boys try to attract girls with the promise of gifts, money, and other financial gains. The next letter is from a boy who is trying to rekindle the interest of a girl. He writes:

> The major point is the way how you deceived me to come on Friday and you didn't come. . . . Last Saturday I had planned to show you I really love as I shown to your Namulondo. . . . I had budgeted for 80,000 shillings [$80] for that day but you disappointed me by not coming. . . . Am planning to take you

next month for an agriculture show in Jinja. . . . I am planning to spend at least 100,000 shillings [$100] for those functions. And I will be making you happy by giving you other programs after my mocks in June next term. And after the show next month, I will be shopping for you, very expensive clothes and shoes you will want. . . . Lastly, I request you to stop deceiving me or disappointing me because am going to plan for you more good things which will force you never to love any other guy. (letter B:25)

Through promises of gifts and commercial outings, this boy hopes to secure the love of the girl, even though it is unlikely that he can make good on his promises. The sexual script has changed from one of self-realization, flattery, and arranging secret meetings after school to the adult economies of love. "My love for you is as lasting as a gravity stone" loses its effectiveness over time, as girls and boys face the realities of economic responsibilities and social autonomy. Girls know that most boys do not have money and that the promises of gifts and commercial outings will go unmet.

This concept of money as a supposed motivator of love is explored in the Tamatave province of Madagascar by anthropologist Jennifer Cole, who observes that there exists a "sexual economy" that involves an intertwining of "material resources, emotional attachments, and social power" (2010:73). She observes, "All women must learn to navigate this economy in order to succeed in life" (ibid). Cole describes how *jeune* (from the French word meaning "young") is a term used to imply a young man or woman who is up-to-date on modernity (92). This means that female *jeunes* follow the fashions and have "lovers in addition to boyfriends," and also that they have "watched the latest porn videos and learned new sexual techniques—tabooed by the ancestors" and "know how to access abortion and birth control to avert an unwanted child and a truncated future" (93). As Cole observes, female *jeunes* can also be called "*vehivavy mietsiketsika* (girls who move)" when they "enter the sexual economy with an eye to earning a livelihood from men" (112). These desires are similar to those expressed in love letters by young girls in Iganga, who believe that men should provide them with gifts and money and seek out the ones who have the means (almost always older men). Unlike the tension between younger men and older men in Iganga as a result of this behavior, however, male *jeunes* in Tamatave actually acknowledge "that the only way to succeed is to become a more powerful man's dependent and client" (ibid). Also, a key distinction between the female *jeunes* in Madagascar and young girls in Uganda lies in the fact that girls in Tamatave are encouraged early on, even by their parents, to "exercise their powers of seduction" in order "to earn money and obtain resources" (79) and to "use their sexuality to achieve social success and social mobility" (113). This is not the view I have presented of Igangan parents, and I do not mean to imply that I believe this is the path that parents and children should take. Young women in Tamatave are not necessarily happier as a result of being encouraged to utilize their own sexuality. As Cole posits, "the futures they [*jeunes*] imagine and the ones they create are often in tension with each other, and the desired outcome uncertain" (151).

Conclusion

In this chapter, I have examined letters written in advanced stages of a relationships or after the affection between two sweethearts has already been established. Friedrich Engels's considerations of how capitalism shapes gender dynamics in intimate relationships is useful in thinking about the meanings and individual significance of struggles and competing interests emerging within relationships. Specifically, romantic relationships with peers (as opposed to the much-written-about young woman/older man liaisons) have the allure of flattening out gender hierarchies that young people see operating in the relationships of older people. However, wider social and economic uncertainties as well as systems of gender inequality make their romantic ideals difficult to achieve, for both parties. As illustrated in the previous chapter, in earlier stages of a relationship, adolescent males struggle to prove their sincere affection to their sweethearts through their eloquently written letters, and male dominance is temporarily suspended (rhetorically, at least). During this time, adolescent girls creatively invoke AIDS, sex education messages, and religious scriptures to provide themselves with moral authority, and they use powerful language to negotiate favorable terms for intimate relationships. We also see how boys use the same messages to deter their lovers from encouraging other suitors, and how they eventually become bolder and more confident, pressuring girls to have sex. Yet, as the relationship progresses, young males feel the strain of not having the finances needed to maintain and demonstrate the type of consumer-based notions of romance and affection that youth have come to associate with modern relationships. This consumption-based romance is not simply about leisure activities but in many ways is necessitated by a monetized economy in which most youth in Iganga spend much time struggling with ways to achieve their desired future status in society. Apart from future desires that motivate romantic visions and strategies, young people's quest for a good life also involves addressing everyday necessities such as health-related issues, family problems, and school expenses.

Herein lies a central cruelty of the intersection of gender ideologies, age, and class in the context of economic precarity: the ideology of man-as-provider works against young males, who risk their reputations by continuing relationships in which their sweethearts are constantly disappointed and might be finding other means of meeting their economic needs. Instead, young men attempt to avoid damage to their reputations by slowly bowing out and entering into newer relationships in which romantic capital, as opposed to economic capital, is more highly valued. In contrast, adolescent females must consider their reputational risk when deciding to end a relationship after their peer networks presume that they have been sexually active. Hence, while young men's reputations are improved by being able to start, exit, and enter into a new relationship, young women have an incentive to remain in existing ones and to maintain the public appearance of a mutually beneficial and harmonious relationship, for exiting it or revealing its difficulties may have the reverse effect on an adolescent female's status.

A context in which gender inequality travels alongside a high dependency ratio (that is, when a few earners support many older and younger dependents) has a vastly different impact on adolescent males and females. As young people progress through adolescence into young adulthood, or as their opportunities for schooling end, earlier ideals of romantic relationships become secondary to other concerns, such as holding on to boyfriends (for girls) or competing with working men (for boys). At this point, girls might turn to older men who can provide financial assistance and attention while simultaneously maintaining the hope of achieving a romantic life with a companionate mate. As one girl writes, "I'm confused because this older guy is trying to get serious" (letter G: 27). Is this evidence of cruel optimism, as suggested by Berlant? Or is it a dream deferred until a future date, with the possibility of transforming into something quite different that initially imagined?[1] Revealed in both perspectives is that sentiments of disappointment are not simply located within the intimate relationship or directed toward a slowly fading lover. Rather, the affective structure of disappointment reflects young people's dawning awareness of the limits of romantic relationships within the context of poverty and precarity, while at the same time their deep belief that their vision is within the realm of possible. The various and conflicting sexual moralities that became increasingly visible and motivated around 1981—HIV interventions, global youth popular culture, and the evangelical movement—all made promises about companionate relationships that could not be sustained given everyday realities and economic necessities. The freedom to choose a mate and women appearing to exert greater agency than the older generations run the risk of reinforcing gender inequalities, as Engels predicted long ago, while ever threatening to cast aside as socially disruptive *nakyewombekeire* the very women who come close to achieving the evolving public ideal but whose actions circumvent patriarchal protection and control. What makes youthful romance so powerful and such an intriguing site for analysis is that, despite the structures and interventions that produce frequent sentiments of disappointment, the sincere and heartfelt process of envisioning a better life offers unique insights into creative and uncharted ways in which the future may unfold. Beyond being visions of utopia, however, these imaginings also signal places in the social structures of inequalities that stubbornly resist change and that lead not to simply a gradual sedation of individual romantic imaginations but also to generational reproduction of the tension between hopeful desires and fearful protections.

CONCLUSION

Sam's Death and Refusals to Submit

In December 2005, while I was in the United States, I received an e-mail from a research assistant with the subject line "Death." The short message read: "Death occurred of Mukungu Sam. He was buried last week. Agnes is deeply grieving." Two weeks later, I received another e-mail with the news that Agnes had suffered an even greater tragedy. Her much-beloved lastborn child, thirteen-year-old Grace, was to be buried the week before Christmas. This woman, who had already lost her husband, now had to endure the pain of losing two of her children—her first and last born. I wondered why life had dealt such a bad hand to Agnes and the family.

I returned to Iganga the following summer and paid my respects to Agnes. I sat with her one afternoon as we caught up on life, but mostly there was silence between us as we gazed at the soil under our feet and the landscape around us, gently caressing each other's hands and breaking our meditation to greet neighbors who passed by. My suspicions were confirmed. Both Sam and Grace had died of AIDS-related illnesses—Sam most likely from HIV contracted through his sexual activities, and Grace likely through vertical transmission (i.e., mother-to-child transmission, or MTCT) passed along from Agnes. In their customary spirit of togetherness, community members were still displaying sympathy and compassion to Agnes, stopping her along the walkways to offer condolences and visiting in the evenings with foodstuffs and sometimes money to help offset the burden of her losses.

Over twenty-five years into the epidemic that disproportionately and violently took the lives of the community's most productive and reproductive members (young adults in their prime), parents burying their children is not unusual. However, the death of a child still garners collective community grieving and empathy. "The pain is no less. We have just learned to mourn more quietly and privately," explained an elder who had suffered his own series of losses.

Alongside this culture of compassion a parallel moral commentary exists. That commentary tied the family's dreadful fate to the legacy of a gradual weakening of their *máka*—the breakdown in and chaotic state of the moral and sexual regulation of its members who floated without a sense of belonging. To Iganga residents, the weakening affilial and affective ties of the *máka* leaves members floating, searching for a sense of belonging in other forms of social organizing in Uganda's civil society. Youthful bodies—particularly that of *nakyewombekeire*—frequently become the platform through which discourses about this floating caused by disrupters of historical moral regulation are understood.

I begin and end this book with the stories of Sam and Agnes as a way of exploring various ways in which the intersection of desire (for people or things), moral regulation (disciplinary regimes that tie people both to their community and to a cosmological belonging), and life strategies within the context of precarity plays itself out over a person's life cycle and across generations. Ultimately, my chronicling of the family's story is a way of advancing the critical analysis of interventions that has motivated this ethnography. This Conclusion builds on Part II of this book, in which I demonstrated how interventions that are generated in particular spaces (be they legal, biomedical, public health, religious, or related to popular culture) and with particular aims of shifting the direction and effects of desire and regulation in social life become folded into local landscapes with their own unique histories, tensions, and other particularities. I have critiqued the politics of intervention by examining how the medicomoral authority of Uganda's urgent HIV epidemic legitimized the emergence of a very visible sexual public sphere that soon after became populated with competing moral discourses, some more local, others initiated by the return of a young group of bentu (Chapter 1).

My analysis of interventions is multilevel, paying particular attention to not only the internal contentiousness and contradiction of each intervention project but also how it is refracted through local hierarchies and particular sets of moral anxieties in ways that produce outcomes that are unintended, different than expected, and sometimes directly counter to the stated intentions. For example, we see the use of a law intended to protect girls from sexually predatory older men by legally extending the category of innocent childhood to eighteen-years-old being used by desperate fathers of adolescent girls as a state-sanctioned tool to reclaim their weakened patriarchal authority, protect their public reputation, and prevent the financial burden of their daughter becoming impregnated by a poor man. In a context of increased moral anxiety about the threat that freely floating young *nakyewombekeire* pose to the community and their natal households, an unintended use of the age of consent law is the criminalization of youth sexual liaisons. Individual defilement cases have produced a police state that disciplines daughters for having sexual agency and punishes their boyfriends for defying the Basoga custom of obtaining the father's permission for sexual access to his daughter. At the same time, the collusion of state and community interests has allowed older sugar daddies who were the intended target of the law evade punishment precisely because the politics of respectability ties an individual's criminal culpability to his community status, access to resources, and perceived value in and contributions to society.

Shifting from legal interventions around the body to public health ones, this book also has traced how the Basoga ideology of sexuality in which risk and pleasure were intricately linked has become bifurcated as disparate discourses of sexuality are generated and circulated by public health (risk), popular culture (pleasure), and newer evangelical movements (immorality). As discourses of sexuality and regulation have been increasingly gone public, the historical sexuality educator of adolescent girls, the *ssenga* (paternal aunt), transforms from the private teacher of female sexuality and bedroom tricks to a public educator of sexually curious adults, leaving a void in the education of younger girls (Chapter 6).

Yet, alongside this dominant public sphere in which competing moral discourses about the regulation of contemporary sexuality circulate, young people create a counterpublic world in which they engage in youthful romance through the exchange of love letters, as I have explored in Part III of this book. We observe through their love letters how, far from simply recycling dominant discourses in developing romantic relationships with peers, youth actively envision and pursue their own versions of romance, desire, and hope as they imagine and attempt to begin forging their futures. These imaginations about future possibilities are constantly tempered by and revised given the reality of economic and social precarity and various regulatory interventions that often undermine opportunities for youthful explorations of romantic possibilities. Structures of gender inequalities (both ideologically and economically) combined with consumer-based notions of romance shape relationship trajectories. Adolescent girls may find themselves increasingly limited in their ability to negotiate the terms of a relationship but fearful of the reputational consequences of leaving it, and adolescent boys often feel the consequences of having limited or no access to producing the economically defined masculine demonstration of affect and care as expected both in Basoga convention and within the contemporary commercialization of love. Although youthful romance often seems to fade into what Lauren Berlant has called a "cruel optimism," young people's desires for and belief in a better life continue to be modified, suppressed, or completely thwarted.

I conclude this tale of regulations and romance with two aims. First, while anthropologists remain committed to the framework of structural violence in understanding the outcomes and experiences of the poor, how to operationalize interventions to address these "pie in the sky" notions of systemic inequalities continues to trouble and fuel debate among policy makers, practitioners, and social engineers (see Blankenship et al. 2006). Even if not explicitly named, two explanatory models tend to inform US domestic and international programs and policies designed to ameliorate the impact of poverty on individuals and communities—one explanation being the culture of poverty, and the other, fatalism. At the time of Sam's and Grace's deaths, antiretroviral therapy (ART) promised to extend the possibilities of life throughout the world, but as many have previously noted, the roll-out has been anything but consistent, reliable, and even, remaining particularly inaccessible to the poor and young such as Sam and Grace. Hence, using the stories of Agnes and her family, I demonstrate the analytic shortcomings of the two popular explanatory models. Second, I offer a counterexplanation of how to understand not only the place of cruel optimism in local situations of precarity but also how ethnography can reveal local acts of refusal to submit to (but also collude with) a position of subordination within the global economy and humanitarian philanthrocapitalism.

Poverty, Culture, and Fatalism

Sam predicted his death a decade before his passing. During one of our conversations after his breakup with Birungi in the mid-1990s, he stated that by the age of thirty he would be ready to die because he would have "already seen everything in life." A terrible numbness came over me as I listened to him elaborate. Both before his death and posthumously, I have reflected on Sam's sobering commentary on life and death. His statement could be dismissed as youthful reckless banter or juvenile myopia. Analytically, however, his resignation to an early death, combined with his insistence on engaging in what he knew to be medically risky behaviors of heavy drinking and sexual networking, could be explained as a manifestation of either the culture of poverty or fatalism. While the former attributes poor people's "misbehaving" to bad values that emerge out of contexts of economic depravity, the latter attempts to offer a corrective by shifting blame away from the poor and instead argues that the realization that one lacks power over external forces leads to behaviors that might be risky or to a disinclination to engage in risk reduction practices. I argue that both explanatory models, even if not explicitly named as such, still guide much thinking about actions of the poor and marginalized and perform an analytic violence by curtailing considerations of other ways of understanding.

The culture of poverty thesis can be traced to sociologist E. Franklin Frazier's (1932) study on poor blacks in Chicago and to anthropologist Oscar Lewis's (1959) comparative work on Mexican families, and was popularized in a report by Daniel Patrick Moynihan, the assistant secretary of labor for policy planning and research when he published "The Negro Family: The Case for National Action" (1965). Displaying a historical approach similar to that used by Moynihan's predecessors, the report argued that the history of slavery, the Jim Crow South, and the migration to northern cities lacking adequate jobs and support had left black communities "caught up in the tangle of pathology" that had negative consequences such as single-parenthood, crime, drugs, and generational poverty (30).

While the report had a generally warm reception among the liberal policy makers and planners with whom Moynihan was ideologically aligned, the thesis received scholarly criticism for its tendency to "blame the victim" (Ryan 1976), its theoretical inconsistencies (Valentine 1968), and its use as a convenient explanation that served the political purposes of the elite (Stack 1974). Despite these critiques, the connection between poverty and bad values drove social policy and programs during subsequent decades.

More recently, sociologists and anthropologists have called for reconsiderations of how the concept of "culture" refers to a wide range of social and institutional aspects of society—such as shared values, individual interpretive frames, coping strategies, symbolic boundaries, and the like—with the main emphasis on "meaning-making" from below (Small, Harding, Lamont 2010:20). The call for bringing lived experiences of coping, meaning-making, strategies, and contestations over community beliefs into focus under the rubric of "culture" has been made by others and the perspective that culture is both dynamic and contested is a perspective shared by this book. Nevertheless, the emphasis on cultural ways tends to locate the motives for people's (risky) behaviors in their immediate social environment and therefore often translates into interventions that are designed to solve community problems by introducing good values and stomping out bad or negative influences (see Nichter 2008). Focused on fixing what is perceived as bad cultural tendencies that lead to negative outcomes, these same interventions that are built on the neoliberal ideas of individual responsibility

and freedom inadequately address the contemporary manifestations of historically produced inequalities that continue to alienate poor communities from the wider labor
and consumer marketplaces and other regional centers of power and decision making.

A flip side to the culture of poverty thesis is fatalism, or the belief that one's life is
predetermined by external forces over which the person has little or no control. Earlier ruminations by Émile Durkheim describe fatalistic sentiment resulting from an
excessively regulated existence "with futures pitilessly blocked and passions violently
chocked by oppressive discipline" (1951:276). Recent uses of the concept of fatalism in
public health literature attempt to explain why marginalized groups do not do things
that they know promote good health, such as getting screened for cancer or following
through with a recommended treatment (Powe 1997; Gullatte et al. 2009), and why
they continue behaviors that are inimical to their health and well-being, such as engaging in risky sexual practices (Hess and McKinney 2007; Meyer-Weitz 2005). The
concept of fatalism is typically applied to lower socioeconomic groups or otherwise
marginalized people or lifestyles to describe a cognitive state in which they are resigned
to the idea of a predestined outcome that cannot be changed regardless of their actions.
People become fatalistic when faced with limited options. Hence, when gay men in
the United States continue to participate and create new avenues for engaging in unprotected sex, these risky actions read as evidence of their resignation to the inevitable
contraction of HIV. The concept of fatalism is intended to move beyond the theory of
irrationality in accounting for the results of people's entrapments and contradictions in
their actions. However, it inadequately considers the ways in which socially constructed
meanings, desires, and significance drive people's selected actions, the value of pleasures
received, and in which the absence of an identity or engagement that is so core to the
person's subjectivity can itself collapse into a state of existential crisis. Individuals priori-
tize pleasures and acts of belonging in ways that do not always conform with the utopic
goals of humanitarian, development, or social interventions.

A main analytic difference between the culture of poverty and fatalism lies in the
conceptualization of individual agency, or people's capacity to act independently and
to make their own free choices. Whereas the culture of poverty thesis foregrounds
communities and people as active agents in the selection and creation of practices,
meanings, and strategies (hence, policies that focus on revising behaviors—say, more so
than addressing structural factors), fatalism's focus on a person's sense of lack of control
and the internalization of external factors tends to obfuscate ways in which the person
may exhibit a form of agency. A challenge taken up in much anthropological and sociological work is to appreciate the dialectic that connects individual's actions to the
wider landscapes of opportunities and constraints, as discussed in the Introduction of
this book (Bourdieu 1977; Giddens 1984).

Considering Sam's desires *before* his heartbreak with Birungi, when he imagined
a life of love with his sweetheart, and *after* his realization of the romantic limits of his
family's decline into poverty, which led him to cycle through lovers while inebriated,
calls into question the limits of these theories and compels us to consider other explanations. Sam's devolution into a life of debauchery would not be read as evidence of a
culture of poverty (which might be suggested were we to analyze behavioral surveillance

surveys that tracked his sexual networking, concurrent partnerships, and condom use). Rather, when considering his trajectory, his road to Kasokoso can be understood as the *consequence* of his limited options for achieving competence in the hegemonic masculinity he so desired, given the realities of regional and global inequalities. The conditions do not necessarily mean a particular path is inevitable, as fatalism would suggest, for even though data may indicate the high likelihood of a consequence, there are other factors that determine which behavioral choices are made or other paths taken. And, even if Sam were fatalistically resigned to the fact that he would die young, given the limited opportunities and "oppressive discipline" that surrounded him, his decisions to live his life a certain way were a demonstration of his understanding of the possibilities for intimacy and economic progress available to him. He created alternate ways of forming and managing social relationships that had personal significance to him, such as the development of his social network in Kasokoso as a strategy to forge a community and attain masculinity. Unable to fulfill (his and the community's) expectations of masculinity, which tie wealth acquisition to manhood status, and discouraged by his inability to sustain an alternate form of masculinity (such as affiliation with one of the newer religious movements or solidifying his attachment to the police force), Sam took to drinking and womanizing as coping strategies, not only to deal with his disappointments but also as attempts to perform yet another alternative masculinity and pursuit of intimacy (see Hunter 2010; Bourgois 2002; Connell and Messerschmidt 2005; Campbell 1997; Connell 1987, 2003; Smith 2014). Sam's failed attempts during his youth to develop and nurture attachments to a community in ways that were meaningful and significant to him led him down several paths (often simultaneously), seeking to find connections in other ways. When Sam reflected on his limited opportunities and the plight of his family, he often invoked his father's name and story.

The Legacy of Mukungu

The legacy of Agnes's husband, Mukungu, has had an enduring impact on the family. Mukungu died in Buluba Hospital, or what residents refer to as a leprosy hospital, around 1994, a couple of years before I met Agnes. As others around that time, he presumably died from leprosy but most likely from HIV. His charisma and muscular physique earned him a high-ranking position in the local police office, and access to many women.

Mukungu's legacy of philandering would surface at his *okwabya lumbe*, the ceremony at which the will of the deceased is read and the property is divided.[1] During the distribution of his matrimonial property, three informal wives of Mukungu and their children, all previously unknown to Agnes, came forward with their children to claim their share of the deceased man's estate. Between the man's natal family reclaiming their portion of their clan property and Agnes's three co-wives demanding part of his pension to support their children, a mournful Agnes was left with little of their matrimonial wealth and property but with a cast of young dependents to support.

This set off the family's economic downward spiral. About seven years later, Agnes would again live in the shadow of Mukungu's legacy when she was admitted to the hospital "close to death," as I was informed, being diagnosed with AIDS. This was 2001. No one thought Agnes would survive, much less outlive her children. But she was a fighter and managed to emerge from the hospital, as if her will to live was motivated by her desire to support her younger children.[2]

I insert the legacy of Mukungu to demonstrate how one person's death has a ripple effect beyond their immediate social and kin network, affecting subsequent generations and their social relationships. Agnes was once active in village leadership roles as the women's representative elected to the village Local Council, but over time her days became consumed with "chasing money" to cover the costs of her illness and to support her children. Sam, the oldest child in the house, found himself without consistent access to school fees and with little chance of building a life with the lovely Birungi. Agnes was deeply regretful about Sam's decision to drop out of secondary school and her inability to provide for her children's economic and emotional needs as she had once envisioned. An evening drinking routine helped relieve her pain. I would sometimes accept her invitation to accompany her, but over the years I often declined: selfishly, I became uncomfortable watching her emotionally lubricate her pain, but I also had few viable suggestions of how she could manage the unfortunate series of events that kept confronting her family. As of 2015, Agnes remains alive and on ARVs.

"Dying like thunder": Bureaucratization, Dependency, and Acts of Refusal

The management of pain is a particularly complicated phenomenon. The introduction of antiretroviral therapy (ART) was intended to do just that—to manage the pain of individuals suffering from HIV as well as the burden on loved ones, households, and communities. At the time of Sam's and Grace's deaths ART was being aggressively advertised throughout much of Uganda and around the world as the answer to living longer with HIV and preventing its further spread, yet the pace of the scale-up was not keeping up with people's rapidly increasing knowledge of ART's magical powers, particularly in nonpriority places like Iganga and among people such as Sam who were seen as responsible for their infection and too irresponsible to adhere to therapy. While residents were generally delighted about the increased availability of ARVs (antiretrovirals, which refers to the actual drugs) in Iganga, the general sentiment was that enrollment was neither entirely transparent nor fair. Instead, the process was meditated by what scholars studying the rollout of ART have called forms of "social triage" that emerge when a system confronts a great imbalance between limited resources and large numbers of people in need. As a result of greater demand than supply, the agents in control of the distribution of ARVs made decisions about who to enroll based not solely on biomarkers such as CD4 count but also on socially determined notions of deservingness, ability to adhere, social worth, and the like, which turned each HIV center into "an operation that differentiates people into groups based on specific criteria" (Nguyen 2010:109). Patients were selected based on "their perceived value to organizations, communities, or programs" and their ability to tell their story to the gatekeepers of drugs or to serve as a face for the success of ART programs. Hence, Florence

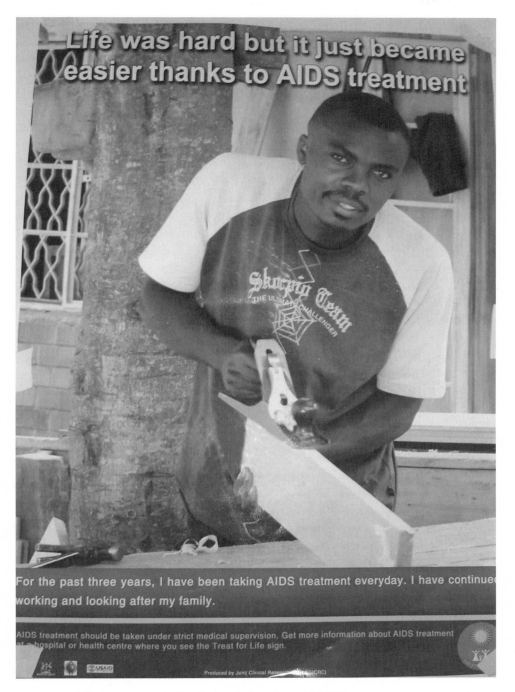

FIGURE 12.1. "Life became easier" antiretroviral poster, mid-2000s

Kumunu, the saint in Chapter 3 who spoke out publicly about her HIV status and ways to "live positively," was the model ART patient; Sam probably would not have been. As anthropologists studying the impact of medical advancements have argued, ART as an intervention designed to *combat* disease, suffering, and effects of marginality has also served to *exacerbate* existing inequalities and create new forms of stratification as the delivery of care effectively reaches and appeals to certain groups while alienating or failing to capture others (see Nguyen 2010; Petryna 2009; Biehl 2004, 2009; Rouse 2009; James 2010; Prince 2014; Fassin 2007b; Whyte et al. 2004).

Examining Agnes's interpretations of the deaths of her children offers insight into how residents understand their community's interaction with the commercialization and bureaucratization of living with HIV, a story that dovetails with my account of the evolution of biomedical and public health interventions in Iganga in Chapter 3. In addition to providing further insight into how ART programs reinforce inequalities, I offer an account of how we can understand collective community reactions to the continuation of death and suffering during the age of ART.

I reflect back to my research assistants' reactions to an announcement of the UNAIDS Drug Access Initiative introduced in Uganda in 1998 and subsequent pilot ART programs (see Okero et al. 2003). After sharing a newspaper article in 1999 about pilot ART projects, one assistant remarked, "This is just another way of getting us dependent on the West." The others chimed in with various statements that reflected a similar sentiment toward continued dependency on Western aid and support. Despite each of them having witnessed the extreme suffering of relatives in their short lifetimes and wishing that the suffering could stop, they were cautious about receiving Western aid to solve a problem that many in the community believed was started in or invented by the West.

Awareness of the systems of dependency that foreign aid causes and the realities of people continuing to die despite promises of ART were fueling new rumors of foul play and witchcraft. The analytic distinction between gossip and rumors becomes important in this discussion. L. C. Smith, Lucas, and Latkin (1998) argue that while sharing gossip is a form of building intimacy and control within a defined social group (Gluckman 1968), rumors are circulated more widely from person to person with unknown origins as a new social fact (Turner 1993). Agnes's different understandings of the death of her oldest and youngest highlight this point. A hospital worker suggested that Grace's cause was likely cryptococcal meningitis. Grace's final days were marked by what the grieving mother describes as a very painful, whitish mass that was "growing uncontrollably in her mouth" (most likely *oral candida*, thrush spreading on her tongue). The painful affliction left her daughter unable to eat, a situation that eventually overpowered the body of the fragile girl whose own growth had been greatly stunted since birth and who had endured unpredictable epileptic seizures at least since I first met her ten years earlier. Both conditions could have been the result of being born with HIV. Agnes's years of doting on and tender care of Grace may have been partly out of mother's guilt and partly wanting to provide her daughter the best life during what Agnes thought might be a short one, particularly, as I later found out, after her daughter was rejected from a treatment program. Agnes's struggling to find money to send Grace to an expensive boarding school and to buy her fine clothes during her last stage of life (to some extent at the expense of the needs of her other children) began to make sense. The system may have given up on innocent Grace, but her mother would not. Agnes held her daughter's hand as she departed to join the world of her ancestors.

Agnes also shared with me Sam's death certificate and the story of his death. His cause of death was listed as "PCP" (*Pneumocystis carinii* pneumonia), another AIDS-related opportunistic infection. Although Agnes was aware of the official diagnosis, she maintained that her son's death was not a result of AIDS. According to her, following a short struggle with "strange illness," Sam *yafuire kibwatukira* (literally "died with thunder," or abruptly). He had been bewitched, she insisted, because of his involvement in a police investigation in which a large sum of money mysteriously "went missing." Agnes was not denying that there was a good chance her son may have contracted the virus before he settled down with the mother of his child, during his hedonistic stage of drinking and networking with the town's *nakyewombekeire* in Kasokoso, or even after this phase. She had also heard the rumors about his various quests to obtain medicine for his condition and likely for his wife. Based on his physical appearance and weight, she had figured (and certainly hoped) that the treatment was working. His dying abruptly certainly was *related* to his HIV status but, according to Agnes, was not the actual *cause* of his death, as evidenced by his death certificate, which made no mention of HIV or AIDS. Rather, her interpretation was that her son's death was related to his actions of secretly chasing after miracle HIV pills produced by a global system of capitalist inequalities that required individuals to commit to the global pharmaceutical and information marketplace over moral structures that had kept communities bound together. She was not alone in this sentiment, this refusal to submit to global powers.

Central to Sam's and Grace's stories is how the introduction of foreign ARVs not only changed people's relationship to their communities but also changed the presentation of HIV-related dying. This new way of dying was likewise folded into local understandings about the relationship between their community and global markets. The ARVs' promises to extend life and keep people looking healthy faded into a confusing reality: not everyone had access to the magical pills, and even those who supposedly did were dying. But unlike the pre-ART days when people with HIV, rich or poor, slowly and painfully wasted away in a similar and predictable manner, people in the era of ART were "dying like thunder." After a rapid onset of extreme hysteria and hallucinations for a week or so, which often included vivid and fantastical dreams, the person would suddenly die. This rapid form of dying neither resembled the familiar death from untreated HIV nor was the way people on the magical ARVs were supposed to die, if they were to die at all. Hospital workers believed that the symptoms associated with the new dying like thunder were often the result of cryptococcal meningitis or, more broadly, a form of AIDS dementia. However, this biomedical explanation had not yet reached the general population in Iganga in 2006, and if it had, it had not yet been absorbed or fully accepted into the local understandings of HIV mortality.

For residents, the onset of a short period of delirium and sweats, followed by the death of an otherwise physically healthy-looking person (someone who had retained their normal body weight, rather than wasting away), had at least two immediate explanations.

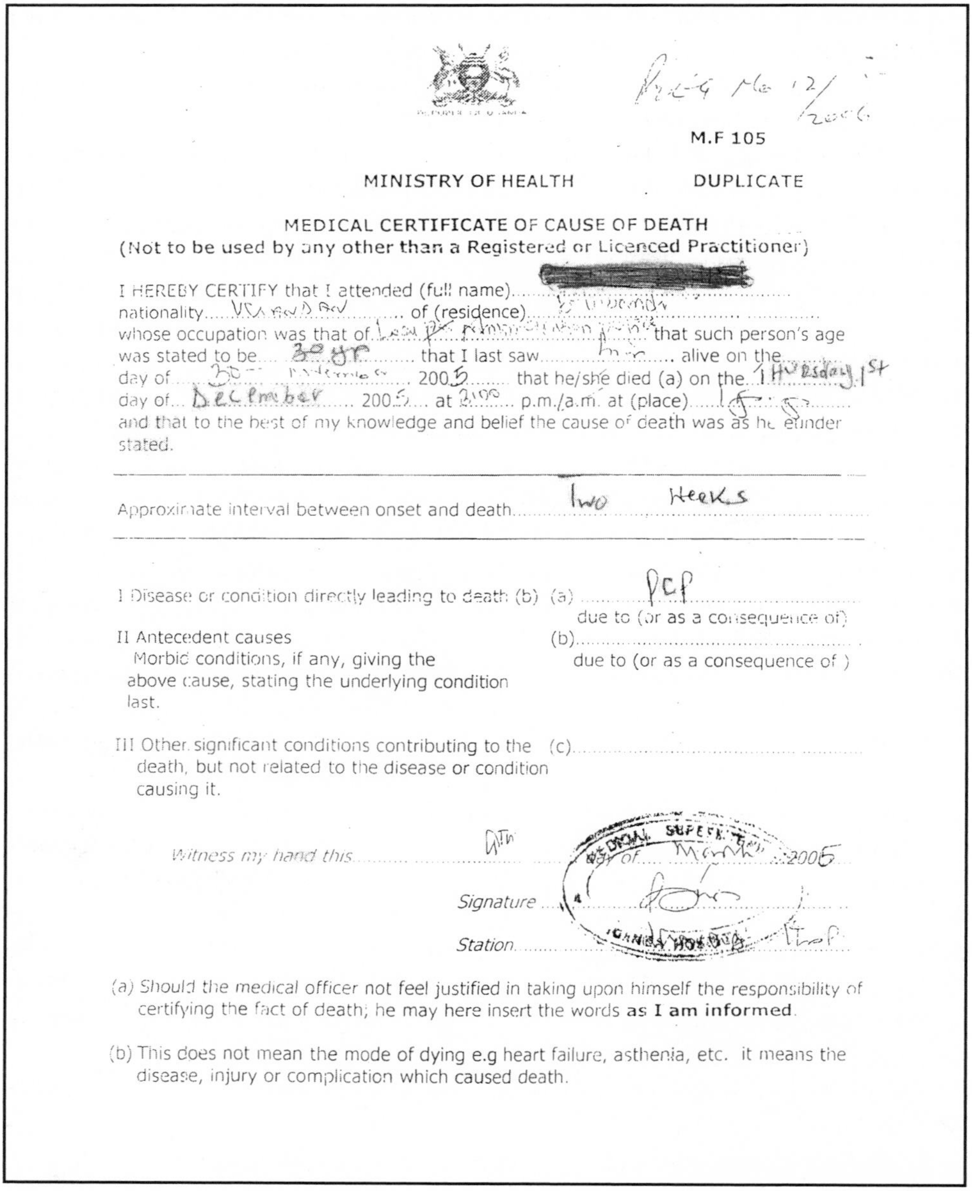

FIGURE 12.2. Sam's death certificate

In some cases residents called upon past understandings of the state of delirium as the soul moving from a diseased or dying body into the world of the ancestors—i.e., the separation of the body and soul, during which the soul begins its communication to the spirits of the dead. Stories about Grace's pre-dying state followed the narrative arc. Agnes's description of Grace's final moments fits into this interpretative framework: the young girl announced to the ancestors that she was coming home to her *máka*.

A second interpretation of delirium preceding death was dominant in cases in which the person's involvement in ART was the source of community gossip, such as Sam's. In these cases, the unexplained dying like thunder was the result of being bewitched or succumbing to other forms of intentional foul play, which Western researchers often lump under the term "witchcraft." When I began my research in 1996, I had rarely heard people associate contemporary cases of HIV with bewitching, but this new way of dying brought back these rumors, which had existed before Museveni started the country's aggressive HIV education campaign. But the unfolding of interventions in a local landscape is always an iterative process—a continually shifting dialectic between the penetration and scale-up of the intervention and a community's understandings and responses to it, creating a loop with one informing and shaping the other.

While initially residents were hopeful about ARVs, over the next few years they became disappointed and disillusioned as the number of available slots opened up at a slow pace. They became suspicious of relatives and neighbors who might be concealing their access to this valuable and scarce commodity. The knowledge of people's desire to conceal their access to ARVs, including the venue through which they acquired the drugs, led to rumors about who had special social and economic connections, and hence to suspicions about that person's loyalties and hidden networks and wealth. The contradictory but not wholly incompatible mix of desire for and suspicion of biomedical interventions converged with the fear of dependency, fueling rumors and prompting acts of refusal, where residents resisted completely and willingly submitting themselves to global forces over which they had little control (see, for example, Kroeger 2003; Butt 2005; Stadler and Saethre 2010; Niehaus 2005).

If Sam were indeed on some sort of HIV medicine, as neighbors and friends suspected, he could have been obtaining them through an official HIV center (though residents doubted he would have passed the criteria of being responsible or worthy) or through the commercial or black market, and the selfish and secret pursuit of any of these routes could have led to his death. If the drugs were obtained through an official HIV center such as a government program, a person likely was on what the World Health Organization calls the "first-line" combination, which includes only two drug classes, is not as effective in preventing resistance, and has documented chances of "treatment failure," as opposed to "second-line" therapy, which commonly includes one of the more effective drugs such as a protease inhibitor (PI) booster and is standard HIV care in wealthier countries (for ARV treatment guidelines, see WHO 2013). If Sam obtained treatment through the commercial or black market, it is possible that his access was not consistent or the regimen was incomplete (say, missing a critical drug) or included ineffective counterfeit drugs. Residents' suspicions that people in sub-Saharan Africa do not have access to drugs that were as efficacious as people in the global North further fueled lively rumors about the deadly consequences of secretly chasing after ARVs.

If a person was on a self-centered quest, death came either because of the ineffective or poisonous Western drugs themselves or through the retaliation of those cheated in that person's attempts to obtain resources necessary for the purchase of the drugs, which may have been the case with Sam. Secretly chasing after drugs became evidence that a person had sacrificed a connection to their *máka* or their kinship or social network to become a member of a larger system of self-serving greed (capitalism) in which the person was permanently suspended in an inferior status. Thus, in some ways Agnes was right: Sam's dying like thunder was not the result of HIV. Rather, his death had resulted from either a retaliation for his involvement in a wealth-acquiring quest to support his HIV care, or from his marginal position relative to a global system of medical powers that could have extended his life even further.

I argue that we can understand these tales about Sam's and others' deaths as "acts of refusal" to highlight how these emergent stories about HIV deaths during a time of ARV scale-up, like other local stories of illness and dying that came before, are not based on irrational or ill-informed beliefs, but rather reflect residents' keen awareness of their marginal place in the global marketplace, and their refusal to submit completely to a system of belief in which health, well-being, and healing are increasingly commercialized, exclusionary, and dependent on foreign interventions. Acts of refusal are interpretatively polysemous and contradictory. Refusals to submit are performed along with acts of collaborating with the oppressive system, and might be enacted with "subjective ambivalence," as Sherry Ortner (1995:175) writes in her call for greater ethnographic thickness in studies of resistance, which, she and others argue, lean toward ideologically romantic rather than strategically pragmatic readings of noncapitalist conforming acts among the marginalized. These new patterns of HIV death rumors, in one sense, can be understood as refusals to participate fully in the totalizing power of consuming a foreign fetish—in this case global pharmaceuticals and the specialized knowledge and technology needed to utilize them—that remains out of reach for most. Acts of refusal are disruptive. But often only temporarily disruptive, as acts of collaboration masquerade as advancement, subtly enticing the dispossessed to deeply hope that a better life or lesser suffering is the reward for believing.

Acts of refusal are also a direct commentary about the individual desire in places of poverty and marginality to move ahead or to imagine a possibility that defies the norm when the odds are stacked against the entire community, or the cruel optimism about which Berlant and others speak. Dying like thunder is a result of being anticollective within a marginal place, demonstrating the incompatibility of individualism within the context of marginalization from the global distribution of pharmaceuticals (see Biehl 2007). Acts of refusal may not lead to immediate changes to systems of oppression and might be combined with acts of collaborating with systems of oppression, but are both an expression of awareness of the global forces that shape the lives and deaths of the marginalized and also a form of disciplining community members who try to escape their marginal status by undermining others with whom they share a common social and moral landscape. Refusing to accept that ARVs are the panacea to Africa's problems and that a virus was the sole cause of death of a loved one highlights local responses to externally driven interventions that bring their already marginalized communities into global bureaucracies and philanthrocapital markets in ways that make power imbalances painfully clear while reproducing them.

I offer two other examples to illustrate this point about the contradictory relationship between refusal and collaboration. With the increased bureaucratization and medicalization of the global AIDS industry, over my years in Iganga I have witnessed the town's oldest HIV organization, IDAAC, and other CBOs get squeezed out of the allocation of resources such as the funding process, virtually unable to provide the flexible services they once did to hard-to-reach places and people. Without a link to the international community of donors and lacking the human and technical capacity required to compete in increasingly standardized foreign funding processes, many grass-roots agencies in HIV destigmatization movements, such as that led by Florence, now operate on a bare-bones budget. The top-down funding priorities set by international institutions, donors, and governments require that IDAAC fit its programs into pre-determined risk categories or behavioral change strategies (e.g., the ABC model) and into evaluation criteria that might not make sense in affected communities, and have essentially squeezed out the flexible agencies that emerged from the needs of these communities and were so instrumental in mobilizing them. Once nimble efforts that grew out of and shifted based on organic community needs, these organizations and initiatives exist in a world in which AIDS agencies are dependent on priorities, programs, and measurable outcomes determined in places that are often situated far away from affected communities. This is not an argument against the prevailing trend of evidence-based programs and need for evaluation, nor do I want to suggest that the initial HIV agencies were perfect and did not have internal problems or practice forms of corruption. Rather, I am interested in reflecting on what the processes of bureaucratization of interventions have meant when the quest for assistance (say, for one's HIV illness) has become an increasingly individualized effort in which people's relationships with institutions and agents of these institutions determine people's access to scarce and commodified resources, leading to what's been called "bio-legitimacy."

Rumors and other refusals to submit are not only local responses to being pulled into global economic markets in subordinate positions. But it is also resistance to and continued collaboration with entanglements with a network of international donor agencies and foreign governments who can decide the fate of Uganda and undermine the sovereignty and autonomy of poorer countries throughout the world to set their own agendas and priorities. Certainly, not all these rumors or acts of refusals are locally benign. We saw this in the case with reactions against women's rights and the defilement law being constructed as a war against men. More recently, Uganda's Anti-Homosexuality Bill got caught up in the politics of global intervention as neocolonialism.

Specifically, as donor countries such as the United Kingdom and the United States threatened to withhold aid if the Anti-Homosexuality Bill were not dropped and the state did not protect (or at least stop its own acts of hostility toward) sexual minorities from social and physical violence, Ugandan refusal to accept such threats escalated into a global culture war (Figure 12.3).[3] The demand for gay rights and the requisite visibility of queer subjects became the most recent symbol of Western penetration into Africa, prompting a counterresponse—a denial that same-sex desires were already being enacted in Africa. Socially conservative religious and political leaders as well as community members in Uganda responded to the Western act of domination by increasing their refusal to accept queer subjects, their historical realities within Africa, and the transformative power of alternatives to colonial-based missionary positions.

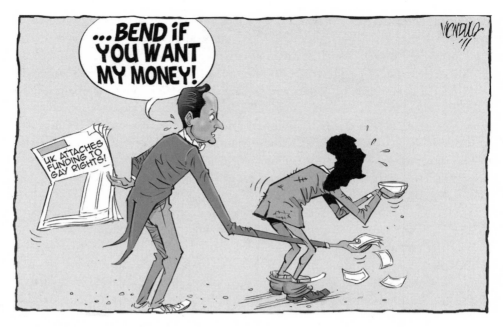

FIGURE 12.3. Cartoon satirizing Western imposition of gay rights in Africa, 2011

Gay rights and expressions of same-sex affection in Uganda, much like the previous foreign-funded liberating of the young female body, were constructed as a direct affront to the African patriarchy that was supposed to keep communities morally safe and socially reproductive, free from HIV and all the other diseases that had come with foreign contact. Like the earlier going public of the youthful body and premarital romance that had incited much anxiety, the demand to publicly name and make visible queerness in Uganda was taken by opponents as an attempt to further dismantle hetero-patriarchy, revealing the fragility of masculinity in postcolonial places subject to submission in neoliberal times (see Fanon 1967:35–36). As the antigay movement used the local tabloid media to increase its hostility and its policing of queer subjects, the gay movement shifted from relatively underground identity-based support to publicly challenging Uganda to embrace sexual and gender diversity and reject the imported homophobia of the West. In December 2014, a gay activist in Uganda, Kasha Jacqueline Nabagesera, released the first issue of *Bombastic*, a magazine dedicated to expressing the voices and stories of same-sex desire and transgender identity (France-Presse 2015). Nabagesera hand-delivered a copy of the seventy-two-page unapologetically nonheteronormative publication to the man who had spearheaded Uganda's Anti-Homosexuality Bill and who had played a large role in inviting foreign leaders of the global antigay movement into the country, Member of Parliament David Bahati. The gay activist remarked on the timing of her symbolic gesture: seven years earlier, Bahati said that his bill was a Christmas gift to the citizens of Uganda. Nabagesera too was delivering a queer holiday gift to the nation—an act of refusing to submit to the policing, silencing, and moral shaming of sexualities and expressions of desire in Uganda (ibid.).

Youthful Romantic Futures

For residents of Iganga, unfortunate and early deaths, such as those of Sam and Grace, are precisely manifestations of the external penetrations into their community that engendered the gradual breakdown of social conventions governing morality and belonging. The two most immediately visible manifestations of this breakdown—young people's individual pursuit of sexual freedom and pleasure (either as idle young men or freely floating *nakyewombekeire*), and HIV as the by-product of that freedom— remain inextricably linked in these and other sad stories about the consequences and generational legacies of sexual and moral transgressions. Sam's death represents a case of HIV transmitted through the youthful chasing of romance and escape; Grace's early death from vertically transmitted of HIV symbolized what residents see as an innocent death—a legacy of the freedom of the older generation, her parents. Hence, while health interventions are typically based on changing local notions and behaviors, for residents HIV is precisely the result of not holding onto local ways and conventions. External influences might help solve community problems, but those influences have also occasioned a cascade of changes that have disrupted things. Sexuality becomes a target of regulation from both external donors and policy makers as well as local stakeholders such as family, elders, leaders, and the like.

But the regulation of youth romance is not one thing. It is a constellation of various interventions that generally share the overall aims of protecting young people and their families from the reputational, economic, and health risks associated with their sexual bodies. This protecting translates into intense policing as legal, moral, and cultural regimes seek to monitor and limit their sexual experiences as well as their romantic imaginations that appear even more harmful (or anxiety-inducing) when mixed with gender inequalities and marginality from regional or global resources. For residents of Iganga, this chasing after an imagined good life that requires conditions other than those immediately available presents a cruel optimism that only intensifies demands to control it (Berlant 2011). The willfully stubborn dreams of romance that appear with each generation impair a person's judgment about what is doable without repercussions. Local precarity and global ideas of romance not only present an incompatible mix, but also represent the death of the youthful subject. These stubborn dreams also create opportunities for new routes of exploring future possibilities—some being risky and constructed as criminal, but others forging new pathways of expression and transgressive resistance.

One of Sam's younger sisters, Rose, represents an unexpected case. Agnes spent much time worrying about and policing Rose during her adolescence. Rose gave birth while still at her mother's house around the age of sixteen, and Agnes on several occasions threatened to bring defilement charges against the father of her child until Rose neared eighteen years old and the threat no longer worked. When Agnes found out that her daughter was about five months pregnant with her second child, Rose decided to leave the house and avoid further conflict and accusations of spoiling the younger girls. Rose then periodically disappeared for stretches of time, reappearing to check on her mother or to bring a newborn child for her mother's blessing. In their respectful, unspoken way, neighbors and family friends had written off Rose as a *nakyewombekeire* who would need to tap from many sources to support herself and her children.

About six months after the deaths of Sam and Grace, Rose brought her third child to meet her mother; Agnes did not inquire about the paternity of the child for fear of the answer. But Rose returned a few weeks later with her long-term boyfriend and his representative to deliver the customary Basoga letter, which signified his formal request to become engaged to Rose in a *kwandhula* ceremony. It had been a long time since I had seen Agnes that pleased. One of her burdens had been lifted.

Rose and her fiancé could have certainly continued their informal marriage with little risk to their social reputation where they lived. But something had changed. Their upcoming nuptials might be easily read as the effective penetration of messages asserting that monogamous marriage is a prophylaxis for STIs and HIV. It could also be evidence of the rapid spread of evangelical doctrines of public confession and conversion, their collaborating in regimes that sought to discipline the morality and sexuality of young people. However, interpreting Rose's story as a journey from sexually risky local ways to risk-reducing modernity eclipses how her desire to wed might indeed have been prompted by other subjective senses of self and changes in her and her boyfriend's life conditions. Her desire to wed emerged partly from a sense of obligation: Rose felt it was up to her to protect the social reproduction and reputation of her parents' *máka*, a concern that became more immediate after she witnessed the spiritual deterioration of her mother, and when the deaths of Sam and Grace meant that she, as the eldest offspring of her mother, would have to take on a larger role in the family.

Rose reminded me of a love letter I had discussed with her some years ago—a letter that she had given to me during one of our collection activities and that had gotten her and her young lover in trouble with her mother. In the letter, the man who would become her future husband spoke of his love for her, his struggles to provide for her during her pregnancy, his promises for a better future, and his fear that he could not achieve it. Unlike many other young people whose stories are in this book, Rose did not seem to fully buy into the romantic plot circulated through romance novels, songs, and even HIV campaigns, though she could have been being coy. But now she reflected on her long desire to be with him. Like Sam, her life and hopes with her lover had been deferred after the death of her father and the emergence of his other three informal households. As she told me of her upcoming *kwandhula*, it became clear that solemnizing her marriage had been for a long time part of the romantic future she had imagined for herself, and that it would be a reclaiming of her legitimacy as a daughter and a woman with ties to a *máka* that had been taken away with the death of her father and the family's dramatic reversal of wealth. While such youthful romantic dreams often go unrealized, they provide the space for imagining future possibilities that offer insight into how things could be, except for and on occasion despite the precarities of everyday life.

Notes

Introduction

1. "Sam" and "Birungi" are pseudonyms, as are the names of other Iganga residents mentioned in this book. To maintain confidentiality and protect the privacy of people's whose intimate stories I discuss, I have also tried to remove identifying characteristics unique to them.

2. "Basoga" (plural) refers to the people of this ethnic group; "Musoga" (singular) is one person. "Busoga" and "Busogaland" refer to a geographic location or state, as in the Busoga Kingdom, Busogaland, or Busoga District. "Lusoga" is the language. Similarly, for the neighboring ethnic group discussed in this book and to whom the Basoga are closely related, "Baganda" refers to the people and to their practices; "Muganda" to one person; "Buganda" to the region; and "Luganda" to the language.

   Following contemporary language use in Uganda, I also use "Basoga" as an adjective to refer to things, customs, and practices of this ethnic group, such as Basoga folktales or Basoga marriage customs. Some texts and documents use "Kisoga" as the adjective form; however, "Kisoga" is not part of the Lusoga lexicon. After consulting several African linguists and Lusoga teachers, I have decided to use "Basoga" as the adjective form, which corresponds to how it would be said in Lusoga. For example, wedding customs of the Basoga would be in Lusoga *obulombolombo bw' obufumbirwa mu Basoga* (literally "practices of getting married of the Basoga").

3. This book deals with heterosexual liaisons not because same-sex liaisons and desire do not exist in Uganda, for they do. Rather, for practical reasons, same-sex liaisons were not readily visible to me in Iganga during my research trips, and heterosexual marriage and reproduction are still the expected norms and duties of people regardless of their actual sexual desires, activities, or identity. Analytically, examining sexuality that transgresses the public norm requires a different set of tools and questions. Over the span of this project, I did come to know several same-sex social networks and gay rights groups in the capital, Kampala, where the social and physical geographies allowed for greater anonymity among individuals participating in nonconforming sexual activities. I did not learn, however, of any particular gay spaces or social networks in Iganga. I briefly return to debates about same-sex relationships in the Conclusion of this book with a short discussion of Uganda's 2009 Anti-Homosexuality Bill.

4. Carole Vance's seminal 1984 volume emerged out of a conference that was historically significant for feminism in the United States, "The Scholar and the Feminist IX: Towards a Politics of Sexuality," held at Barnard College on April 24, 1982. The long-standing conundrum of how to balance attention between sexual danger and sexual pleasure in the lives of women took center stage at the conference. At the time, the central debate in feminist arenas was whether pornography exploited women as sexual objects or reflected their ability to profit from their own sexuality.

5. For a discussion of why and how to include notions of desire and pleasure in research on sexual health, see also J. Holland et al. (1990, 1992); Higgins and Hirsch (2008); Philpott, Knerr, and Maher (2006); Padilla (2007); Carrillo (2001); Fullilove et al. (1990).

6. Uganda's HIV sentinel surveillance system was established in 1989 to gather information and data on HIV prevalence, incidence, and mortality. This information is used for strategic monitoring, evaluation, and planning, of AIDS control efforts. In Uganda, as in most countries with generalized epidemics (defined by UNAIDS as countries reporting HIV prevalence of 1 to 5 percent), the prevalence of HIV in selected antenatal (or prenatal) clinics (ANC) has provided the most important source of data for national HIV surveillance and monitoring, with STI testing centers providing sentinel data on higher-risk groups (see UNAIDS 2013 for a fuller discussion of the methodology used for obtaining HIV estimates). There were initially six ANC sentinel sites in Uganda, located mainly in urban or town areas. By the time the 2010 Epidemiological Surveillance Report was issued, there were thirty ANC and STI surveillance sites, including twenty-four located at antenatal clinics and one in an urban STI referral clinic. More recently, in addition to sentinel sites, the Ministry of Health expanded surveillance activities to include estimates and projections through modeling; special studies on topics such as most-at-risk-populations (MARPs); population-based HIV surveys; data from antiretroviral therapy (ART), voluntary counseling and testing (VCT), and prevention of mother-to-child transmission (PMTC) programs; and data from partner cohorts conducted by the Medical Research Council and the Rakai Health Sciences Program (MOH 2010).

   International bodies such as the Joint United Nations Programme on HIV/AIDS (UNAIDS), the World Health Organization (WHO), the World Bank, and UNICEF provide technical support for surveillance teams in countries throughout the world, and also compile, aggregate, and disseminate data and analysis with surveillance data from individual countries and regions.

7. For literature crediting President Yoweri Museveni for his role in the country's impressive HIV efforts, see, for example, Allen and Heald (2004); Parkhurst (2001). On the controversy about how to interpret Uganda's HIV data, see Parkhurst (2002); Singh, Darroch, and Bankole (2003); Stoneburner and Low-Beer (2004); Low-Beer and Stoneburner (2003). To obtain an overview of the primary two positions in the debate about Uganda's success, see Kilian et al. (1999) and Green et al. (2006) for analyses that credits the ABC approach for the decline, and Murphy, Greene, Mihailovic, and Olupot-Olupo (2006), Singh, Darroch and Bankole (2003), and Ntozi, Najjumba, Ahimbisibwe, et al. (2003) for overviews that question the extent to which the ABC approach can be credited without accounting for other changes. Researchers who question the role of the ABC approach have attributed some of Uganda's success to environmental and structural changes that began early in the epidemic, such as the end to civil conflict in the regions with the highest rates (Schoepf 2003; Gray et al. 2006), the natural life cycle of an epidemic or excess of mortality (Morgan et al. 2002; Wawer, Serwadda, et al. 1997), STD management initiatives (Korenromp et al. 2002), increases in condom use and the age of sexual debut (Asiimwe-Okiror, Opio, et al. 1997), and clean needles and the reduction in medical iatrogenic transmission (Brody 2004).

8. See also Farmer (1992); Hunter (2009); Stillwaggon (2005); Parker and Easton (1998); Singer (1997).

9. My approach to the critical analysis of intervention is informed by a growing body of anthropological and other scholarly literature interested in a deep understanding of the ideological and economic underpinnings and political impact of humanitarian and development efforts. These critiques emerge from various fields of inquiry, including feminist analyses of discourses of nation building, critiques of development projects and policies, and poststructural analyses of the discursive construction of subjects by NGOs' efforts. This

literature has made tremendous contributions in exposing how contemporary humanitarian and development efforts are not neutral but embedded in global politics and capital flows and ideologically driven ways of understanding suffering and those affected. Two of the seminal texts are James Ferguson's *The Anti-Politics Machine: Development, Depoliticization, and Bureaucratic Power in Lesotho* (1990) and Arturo Escobar's *Encountering Development: The Making and Unmaking of the Third World* (1995). Other excellent ethnographic studies of ideological constructions, global power dynamics, and unintended consequences of international interventions include Adams and Pigg (2005); M. Barnett and Weiss (2008); Bornstein (2001, 2005, 2010); Crane (2013); Fassin (2012); Elyachar (2005); Hannigan (2012); Herring and Swedlund (2010); Hyndman (2011); James (2010); Krause (2014); Livingston (2012); Nguyen (2010); Redfield (2010); Rivkin-Fish (2005); Scherz (2014); Schoen (2005); J. H. Smith (2008); Ticktin (2005).

10. Even in the places not immediately connected to MTV in the early 1980s, such as East Africa, sexually suggestive music videos would have a great moral and imaginative influence on youth sexual culture. In fact, when I first went to Kenya in 1990, music videos from Zaire and Kenya were a staple at discos, pool halls, and bars throughout the country, as were music videos from the United States and older and newer forms of Indian musical melodramas. Long before MTV launched a station in Uganda in 2006, music videos from other parts of Africa and overseas were being imported and played on television stations, and in nightclubs and sports bars.

11. Like others, I use the term "AIDS industry" to refer to the elaborate network of international, multifaceted, and politically, economically, and ideologically driven HIV control efforts and interventions. Since the early 1980s, enormous amounts of capital, information, and monitoring and surveillance tools have been generated, debated, and circulated through the international and national AIDS industries. The AIDS industry is neither homogenous nor hegemonic, but at any particular moment there does emerge a dominant ideology and set of lexicons. Global inequalities among wealthier donor countries and harder-hit, poorer recipient countries are reproduced through the politics of international humanitarian HIV-related efforts and philanthrocapitalism.

12. PEPFAR was authorized by the United States Leadership Against HIV/AIDS, Tuberculosis and Malaria Act of 2003 (Public Law 108-25). Phase 1 (2003–2007) included a $15 billion, five-year commitment included $5 billion for existing bilateral programs throughout the world, $1 billion for the UN fund ($200 million per year), and $9 billion for new programs. President George W. Bush named the following fourteen focus countries in 2003: Botswana, Cote d'Ivoire, Ethiopia, Guyana, Haiti, Kenya, Mozambique, Namibia, Nigeria, Rwanda, South Africa, Tanzania, Uganda, and Zambia. Vietnam was added as the fifteenth focus country in June 2004. In July 2008, the Reauthorizing Act was signed into law, authorizing up to $48 billion for PEPFAR's five-year phase 2 (2009–2013). As of 2015, sixty-five countries are considered PEPFAR bilateral partner countries. Of those, thirty-two countries that receive PEPFAR assistance are required to submit Country Operational Plans (COPs). The Caribbean, Central Asia, and Central America regions are also required to submit regional operational plans. Other recipients of PEPFAR funds are not required to submit tracking COPs.

13. In PEPFAR's original authorization, Congress required that 55 percent of funds be spent on treatment, 15 percent on palliative care, 20 percent on prevention (of which at least 33 percent was to be spent on abstinence-until-marriage programs), and 10 percent on orphans and vulnerable children.

14. The PEPFAR "ideology versus science" debate will be discussed later, but for a brief example of the debate see *Lancet* (2006) for an editorial critique of PEPFAR's focus on abstinence and monogamy, and see Kamwi, Kenyon, and Newton (2006) for a "country perspective" response to the *Lancet* critique and a defense of PEPFAR.

15. See also GAO (2006); J. Cohen and Tate (2005); S. A. Cohen (2006). For further analysis of the negative effects of PEPFAR's abstinence earmark, see CHANGE (2004); Jamison and Padian (2006); Kaiser Family Foundation (2008); Evertz (2010); J. Cohen and Tate (2005); Alrich (2007); Check (2007).

16. See also Muyiyi (2009); Nalugo (2009).

17. Fallers occupied what I call the analytically progressive branch of the structural functionalist school in anthropological inquiry. Like his intellectual contemporaries, such as Max Gluckman, Fallers believed that each aspect of the social and political system was interrelated and formed a unique cog in the large social system; he pursued an ethnographic project that presented a holistic picture of society. While some intellectual histories of anthropology criticize the structural functionalist period as being ahistorical for its inattention to local and precolonial histories, this gloss misses a major analytic advancement of Fallers and his contemporaries. They may have neglected explorations into local histories and the way in which it is a site for contestation and power—something that many anthropologists now pay special attention to (see Fox 1991; Vincent 1991)—but it cannot be said that they treated Africa as unchanging and as a series of isolated communities. In fact, Fallers was deeply concerned about understanding social change and modernity as brought on by colonialism, capitalism, urbanization, and newer forms of non-kin-based political power.

    In addition to conducting ethnographic research among the Basoga, Fallers is probably best known for his research from the 1940s to the 1960s among the then politically predominant Baganda ethnic group in central Uganda, to the south of Busogaland. The Buganda king played a particularly important role in the consolidation of British power and colonial rule in Uganda. The Baganda had a monarchical political system, which was organized under a king with royals and commoners. It was the similarity between the British monarchy and the Buganda political system that initially drew the two together as allies, for the British thought the Baganda were naturally more advanced than other African ethnic groups that lacked a centralized government, such as Nilotic groups in northern Uganda or other groups surrounding Lake Victoria in Kenya and Tanzania. The Baganda also drew the attention of anthropologists and other social scientists who were interested in understanding various types of African political systems. Lesser known was Fallers's work among the Basoga ethnic group, who could essentially be described as the historically and politically weaker cousins of the Baganda in terms of language, cultural practices, and kinship structure.

18. In Jane Collier's (1972) rereading of Fallers's court material, she writes that while sexual relations "may have been strained in Soga . . . the adultery cases and marital disputes which came to court did not arise directly out of this 'trouble spot.'" Rather, she suggests that the cases that made it to the native courts were ones filed "by men who were capitalizing on an available marital dispute to get money from an opponent" (857). I agree with Collier's critiques about the distinction between legal reasoning and economic motives. That critique withstanding, Fallers's work provides an interesting historical look at wider debates surrounding sexual relationships in the early 1950s.

    Colonial administrators and Christian missionaries were often at odds in how best to civilize Africans. The former focused on creating a disciplined labor force and consumer base, the latter on the Christian conversion of immoral black souls; however, they found common ground in the project of gender engineering that focused on controlling female sexuality to meet their respective agendas (see, for instance, Allman and Tashjian 2000; Peterson 2012; Burke 1996; Thomas 2003; Hunt 1997; Hodgson and McCurdy 2001).

19. For a useful discussion of problems with the term "female agency," see Holly Wardlow's *Wayward Women: Sexuality and Agency in a New Guinea Society* (2006:9–18). In her insightful reflection on "agency," Wardlow draws a distinction between "encompassed agency" and "negative agency." "Encompassed agency" refers to women's actions that primarily serve or benefit the wider social purpose—for example, the husband's clan. As such, encompassed agency recognizes women's ability to produce effect but reminds us that women's work is inferior to or valued less than men's, whereas negative agency is "the refusal to cooperate with others' projects" and "the refusal to be encompassed," such as a woman withdrawing her labor from her kin group or husband (14). With Wardlow's distinction in mind, in this book I appreciate both types of enacted agency: one works within the hegemonic system and the other operates outside with the intentional aim of not participating.

20. My use of the term "middle class" draws from historical work on the emergence of an elite group with access to regular cash income and advanced education during the colonial period (see West 2002; Mamdani 1976), political science work that examines the interaction of class formation with state and access to global networks in postcolonial Africa (Leys 1978; Kitching 1980; Kasfir 1983; Magubane 1976), and ethnographic work that considers local manifestations of the presentation and tensions of class-based expectations in everyday life (Ferguson 2006).

21. National Institutes of Health (NIH) R01 grant 41724-01A1, "Love, Marriage, and HIV: A Multisite Study of Gender and HIV Risk."

22. My use of generational cohorts to understand discursive and experiential shifts as occasioned by specific political and social transformations is inspired by Lisa Rofel's (1999) *Other Modernities: Gendered Yearnings in China after Socialism.*

23. See also Vansina's updated version (1985), published more than two decades after the original text (1961). Social histories that have cautioned about the ideological construction of life histories include Beidelman (1965), Barber and de Moraes Farias (1989), and White, Miescher, and Cohen (2001). Examples of uses of oral histories to demonstrate African acts of resistance and agency include Isaacman (1996), Comaroff (1985), and Feierman (1990).

24. Community-based participatory research (CBPR) and participatory action research (PAR) are based on the premise that communities should be actively involved and integrated into every stage of the research process, not just as informants, to ensure capacity building of local resources and sustainable programs. CBPR and PAR attempt to reframe the top-down or trickle-down approaches to development and rote teaching methods that dominated in the 1970s and 1980s. The participatory and community-based approaches take community members as "experts" and partners in the processes of determining the key research question, gathering and analyzing information about their own lives, and in determining strategies for problem solving. In other words, research and action should be done *by* the community and not *to* the community. This approach is widely advocated by the World Bank, other international agencies, and NGOs in Uganda supporting community-based development efforts. There are many versions and variations of these techniques, but the basic philosophy remains the same—community empowerment through active participation.

Practitioners of CBPR and PAR trace various lineages; however, most point to a set of common theorists whose ideas have been influential in developing the foundation of this approach, including Kurt Lewin (1946), Paulo Freire (1970), Orlando Fals Borda (1982),

Robert Chambers (1983), Stan Burkey (1993), and Budd Hall (1975), as well as the authors of Clark University (1990). For recent discussions and uses, see B. L. Hall (2005), Minkler and Wallerstein (2008), Trickett et al. (2011), and Reinharz (1992).

   While I find participatory techniques a useful community development tool for getting residents involved, they are unable to address the larger structural problems that undergird many issues faced by poor communities and that emerge as a result of larger inequalities between the global North and South, rich and poor, men and women. However, according to Brazilian activist and theorist of critical pedagogy Paulo Freire, if the process is implemented over an extended period of time, it should lead to the development of critical consciousness, or *conscientization*, of the peasantry or the marginalized and eventually lead to mass mobilization for change.

25. See also Schoepf (1993); Park (1993).

26. See also Washington (2006); Rothman (2000); Angell (1997); Lurie and Wolfe (1997).

27. In theory, the entire process of participatory research takes a long period of time. It begins with a community identifying its resources and problems, and eventually designing projects to solve its problems. I used a much-abbreviated version during research, and because of my own project goals, as well as financial and time constraints, I did not apply the techniques to their full potential. However, I do believe that the participatory activities I used provided a forum for people to discuss common issues and reflect on their lives. This building of communication is of utmost importance in Uganda, since the postcolonial political unrest and economic stratification have left scars of distrust among neighbors.

Chapter 1

1. See Introduction, Note 9, for literature on unintended consequences of international interventions.

2. Gupta and Ferguson (1997:5) argue that analytic approaches to contemporary processes of globalization should not assume that global flows are imposed on or unquestionably accepted by local cultures. Rather, they argue for analyses that focus on how "dominant cultural forms may be picked up and used—and significantly transformed—in the midst of the field of power relations that links localities to a wider world."

3. See also Campbell (2003); Stillwaggon (2005); Thornton (2008); Susser (2009); Simpson (2009); Hunter (2010); Fuller (2008); Fassin (2007a); Nguyen (2010); Rödlach (2006); D. J. Smith (2006); Kalipeni et al. (2003); Farmer (2004).

4. See also Gagnon and Parker (1994); Wardlow and Hirsch (2006); Padilla et al. (2007); Padilla (2007); Hunter (2010); J. S. Hirsch, Wardlow, Smith, et al. (2010).

5. Two other works similarly criticized for being ahistorical and emphasizing notions of universality over specificities in how emotion evolves in particular settings were de Munck (1998) and Jankowiak (1995). For instance, the edited volume by William Jankowiak, *Romantic Passion: A Universal Experience?* was influential in studies around affect and romance in non-Western settings. While particular articles provide in-depth analysis, scholars found problematic the overarching goal of proving the universality of romance, and the general social evolutionary framework proposed in the introduction was criticized for relying too heavily on a unilinear approach to the development of love and not taking into account the context that shapes the shifting configurations.

Chapter 2

1. Many elders in Iganga associate the plague with the cotton industry; however, a study by G. H. E. Hopkins and R. S. F. Hennessey (1938) did not find evidence to support this connection. Hopkins and Hennessey correlated data from the hospital with cotton production and storage data and found that the plague was neither more prevalent in areas with high cotton storage nor less prevalent in regions without high cotton storage (1938:245). It is important to note that, at the time of the study, Hennessey was employed by the colonial government and was later the director of medical services. I have spoken with enough people in Iganga who believe that there was a connection between the expansion of the railroad in Uganda and the rats that carried the plague. Imagined or not, it is worth mentioning, for it has become part of elders' historical memory of disease, change, and modernization. This collective understanding of the negative impact of external intervention on their communities emerges regularly when speaking with both older and younger residents about recent changes and social problems, such as in local interpretations of the arrival of HIV. But residents also collaborate with and often welcome these external interventions, as well as efforts to incorporate their communities into the global economy, in spite of their collective memories and regardless of their subordinate position in global networks. As a Marxist analysis suggests, this is the dilemma of capitalism for the poor.

2. Elders also talked about the past through the lens of famines. During the first half of the twentieth century, these included the *bukala* (blackjack weed) and *soya* (soy beans) famines; both were named after the food people ate to survive the excessive drought. The second half of the century was marked by the *bikutiya* (gunny sack) famines, and in the 1980s the *chwada* (ground cassava) famine, which was on the periphery of what became the internationally known East African famine. When I was conducting research, the floods caused by the 1997–1998 *El Niño* raged and caused further food shortages.

3. For a useful historical analysis of the roots of Uganda's political turbulence since independence, see Mutibwa (1992).

4. For background on Uganda's history of postcolonial economic and social turmoil see articles in volumes edited by H. B. Hansen and Twaddle (1988, 1991, 1995, and 1998).

5. My use of community and social mapping blends various approaches to mapping. Applied geographers use community-mapping techniques to involve community members in the process of natural resource management and in designing community projects (see Clark University 1990). Social geographers, such as David Harvey (1989), use mapping as a framework for analyzing the connections between social and political processes. Anthropologists have also borrowed mapping metaphors to explain mobility and flows, such as Appadurai's (1990) notion of ethnoscape. I find anthropologist Kate Crehan's (1997) use of the mapping framework to be particularly useful. Using layers of a map, Crehan examines how people in rural northwestern Zambia were located within the larger economic and political order before the collapse of the one-party state in the late 1980s.

6. Unless otherwise noted, all current demographic data on Bulubandi was collected in 1998 by me and my research assistants. When historical comparisons are made, data comes from the work of Lloyd Fallers. Fallers (1965) presented the numeric data from his three research villages in Nakigo Subcounty in aggregate. To get the average per village, I have divided his figures by three. Throughout this chapter, I use Fallers's 1950–1952 demographic data as my historic baseline. I refer only to his data from the Busambira area of Nakigo Subcounty, which is near Bulubandi, and not to his data from the northern area of the district.

I use data from Uganda's National Population and Household Census for national comparisons. Uganda has conducted ten National Population Censuses, of which three were conducted during the British colonial period (in 1911, 1921, and 1931), two during the pre-independence period (in 1948 and 1951), and five post-independence (in 1969, 1980, 1991, 2002, and 2014). For a discussion of the survey methodology, see UBOS (2014:1–5).

7. In the early 1950s, the three villages in Nakigo Subcounty in which Fallers conducted research had an average of 80 households per village, and an average population of 360 people per village, or an average of 4.5 residents in each household.

8. Residents' beliefs in and practice of rituals surrounding *lubaale* (the local god) are held simultaneously with the beliefs and rituals in Christianity or Islam. In this system of plurality, in which beliefs in a world religion and in *lubaale* are held simultaneously, the former tends to be a person's a public identity while the latter is mainly followed for clan or more intimate purposes. However, the blending of two belief systems is being increasingly challenged by some of the fundamentalist groups, such as the born-agains. It is also causing conflict within families where some members believe it is important to perform certain ceremonies, such as those surrounding the naming of twins, while other family members might oppose the practice, claiming that it is against modern religion.

9. The 2002 national population survey was the first time that Pentecostalism was included in the survey, which is conducted every ten years. As of the writing of this manuscript, the data on the distribution of religion from the 2013-2014 survey was not yet released.

10. Mahmood Mamdani's *Politics and Class Formation in Uganda* (1976) remains an important work on the history of class formation in Uganda.

11. Much has been written on economic strategies of Africa's poor in the context of repressive state regimes, civil wars, inflation, international trade imbalances, weak financial institutions, currency instability, and historical changes in land and labor. For literature on Uganda, see Brett (1993); Jamal (1998); Obbo (1991); and H. B. Hansen and Twaddle (1998). For work on Africa in general, see Berry (1993); Guyer (1994).

12. The average number of household residents in Bulubandi is close to the national average and has slightly increased from the 1950s average of 4.45 in Fallers's research (1965:73). The average household size in Uganda has been increasing slightly over the past two decades, from 4.9 residents per household in the 2002–2003 national survey to 5.2 in the 2005–2006 survey and to 6.2 in the 2009–2010 survey (UBOS 2010: 9). This slight and steady increase in household size reflects not only a general growth in population but also an increase in the number of dependents in households partially as a result of children being absorbed into relatives' households because of AIDS-related deaths or the labor-migration of their parents.

Chapter 3

1. For overviews of anthropological approaches to marriage in Africa see Burnham (1987); Parkin and Nyamwaya (1987); Guyer (1994); Feldman-Savelsberg (1995).

2. Regardless of its scale, the *kwandhula* ceremony is a staged and highly dramatic visit and negotiation between the families of the bride and groom. The bride's side is seated in one area, and across from them and facing them are people from the groom's side. With the bride's side seated, the groom's side enters with a procession of gifts, some of which are the bridewealth and others simply gifts to show their status and appreciation. In an attempt to position themselves above the groom's family, the bride's family might complain about the

paltriness of the offerings and pretend to be insulted that the groom's family thinks their daughter is worth so little. Central to the *kwandhula* is the idea of two subclans coming together through marriage. Unlike Christian weddings in Iganga, in which couples stand in front of the congregation, the focus of the *kwandhula* is on the extended families.

3. These visions would include attire made from expensive fabrics, including *gomesis* (also *gomasis* and *busuutis*), colorful floor-length dresses with full skirts and pointed shoulders, which were introduced by British missionaries but are now considered traditional dress, as well as elaborate Western wedding dresses.

4. See also Mann (1994); Musisi (1991); Obbo (1987).

Chapter 4

1. See also Serwadda, Wawer, et al. (1992); Garrett (1994); Hooper (1999). The initial *MMWR* documented five young gay men in Los Angeles who were diagnosed with a rare lung infection, *Pneumocystis carinii* pneumonia, or PCP (CDC 1981). A second *MMWR* published on July 3 documented twenty-six similar cases of young gay men (twenty in New York City and six in California) being diagnosed with PCP and/or Kaposi's sarcoma (KS), a rare form of a relatively benign cancer that typically occurs in central European Jews or in older men of Mediterranean descent. The Associated Press, the *New York Times*, the *Washington Post*, National Public Radio, and CNN soon followed with stories of the mysterious illness (for example, see Altman 1981; Hilts 1981). By the end of the first decade of the epidemic, it was clear that the deadly virus was disproportionately infecting resource-poor regions and marginalized populations, such as sexual and ethnic minorities, migrants, prisoners, and women (see Farmer 2001; Parker 2001; Piot, Greener, and Russell 2007; T. Barnett and Whiteside 2006).

Although the June 1981 *MMWR* publication is recognized as the first report in the medical literature that alerted the world to this new immunodeficiency syndrome, molecular and evolutionary biologists suggest that SIV_{cpz} (simian immunodeficiency virus) in primates mutated to HIV-1 in humans early in the twentieth century through human contact with bush meat. Ongoing research led by evolutionary biologist Michael Worobey and microbiologist Beatrice Hahn reconstructs the emergence of HIV-1 in central Africa using viral fossils of lymph node tissue samples collected between 1958 and 1962 in a hospital in Kinshasa. Based on genome sequencing they estimate that HIV-1 first emerged in colonial west central Africa anywhere between 1884 and 1924 through zoonotic mutation of a naturally occurring virus in primates (SIV_{cpz}) to a virus in humans (Worobey et al. 2008; Sharp and Hahn 2011). They argue that the development of and populating of cities under Belgian colonial rule, combined with the harsh conditions of forced labor-migration, facilitated the explosion of diseases among Africans in the 1960s, including the spread of the new virus within west central Africa in what was then the Leopoldville/Kinshasa region (Worobey et al. 2008; see also J. Cohen 2007).

Similarly, investigative science journalist Edward Hooper has examined medical cases and anecdotal evidence and suggests that HIV may have been spread around the same time period, but identifies the epicenter of explosion at a location further east and argues that it was facilitated by the movement of refugees from Rwanda and Burundi into Uganda and Tanzania during civil conflicts (1999:764, 282, 248). While Hooper's findings also suggest that HIV mutated from SIV found in chimpanzees, he believes that the origin of HIV is connected to the testing of the oral polio vaccine (OPV). The OPV origin theory has received great criticism from the mainstream scientific community. Hooper and the proponents of the OPV theory argue that the vaccine was prepared in chimpanzee cells and administered orally to almost one million Africans during vaccine trials, facilitating the spread of the virus from primates to humans. For an overview of the HIV origin debate, see J. Cohen 2000.

2. HIV-related opportunistic infections (OIs) occur in people with a severe immunodeficiency because their weakened immune system is unable to fight off infections. In areas where antibody testing is not easily accessible, OIs are often the first signs that someone might have HIV. People with a healthy immune system can be exposed to certain viruses, bacteria, parasites, or fungus and have little or no reaction to them. However, people with a weakened immune system lack white cells needed to fight off infection, hence the infections "opportunistically" take advantage of a weakened immune system. People are infected with OIs often before their HIV progresses to AIDS. Common OIs in Africa in early HIV disease include tuberculosis, herpes zoster, bacterial pneumonia, and skin infections. In advanced HIV or AIDS, pneumocystis carinii pneumonia (PCP), toxoplasmosis, and cryptococcosis are common.

Chapter 5

1. Social historians of Africa have shown that morality and sexuality education have been the objects of study, evaluation, profit, and public scrutiny since colonial public health campaigns, the introduction of birthing and other medical practices, and Christian missionizing. In the process, the existing moral economy has been infused with new and competing sets of moralities and meanings. From the 1910s to the 1950s, in an attempt to control syphilis and infertility in East Africa, colonial missionaries, physicians, and government officials introduced policies and programs that tended to tighten the regulation of female sexuality through religious discourses, reproductive policies, physical exams, laws, and domesticity programs (see Ahlberg 1991; P. J. Davis 2000; K. T. Hansen 1992; Lyons 1999; Musisi 2002; Vaughan 1991). Other social historians interested in gender or sexuality have written about the medicalization of childbirth practices and reproduction (Hunt 1999; Thomas 2003), religious and legal discourses on sexual immorality (Comaroff and Comaroff 1991; McCulloch 2000; Jeater 1993), and the anxiety surrounding youth sexuality in coed schools (Stambach 2000; Summers 2002).

2. *Sôngá* is the Lusoga spelling of "paternal aunt." The Luganda spelling, *ssenga*, is more commonly recognized in Uganda today because of the dominance of the Baganda ethnic group and language in the media. Throughout this chapter, I use the term *sôngá* when referring to the Basoga kinship term and *ssenga* when referring to today's popular concept of the traditional sex educator.

3. Notions of risk and pleasure were intertwined in many historical contexts in sub-Saharan Africa (Ahlberg 1994; Jeater 1993). However, there are some exceptions. For example, in his well-known article on rape among the Gusii in Kenya, Robert LeVine argues that "normal forms of sexual intercourse among the Gusii involve male force and female resistance with an emphasis on the pain inflicted by the male on the female" (1959:986). More recently, Philip Setel (1999) argues that Chagga in northern Tanzania "appear never to have had a positive cultural emphasis on sexual pleasure. . . . None of the accounts of male initiation speak of teaching that husbands were entitled to sexual pleasure or that wives experienced desire" (92). The idea of female pain during intercourse or discouraging female pleasure as a cultural convention does not appear to be the case among the elder men and women I interviewed. Instead, their historical narratives reflect the importance of female sexual pleasure, though the demonstration of it was to be modest and cloaked.

4. Of the 260 students, 150 were primary school students (ages nine to sixteen) and 110 were secondary school students (ages fourteen to twenty).

5. The students were asked to state their number one fear, but some listed more than one, hence the total percentage is more than 100 percent. Other fears about sex included friends finding out (4.6 percent), nothing (2 percent), and parents finding out (1 percent); others listed by less than 1 percent of respondents were becoming addicted to sex, receiving a punishment from God, being too young, getting tired during sex, being arrested, and wanting to avoid the financial expense of sex.

   An important note: the significantly disproportionate mention of fear of HIV (87 percent) over pregnancy (10 percent) draws attention to Uganda's recent history with national development priorities and flows of international funding. Unlike the neighboring countries of Kenya and Tanzania, which have had continuous and internationally funded family planning campaigns throughout the 1980s and 1990s, Uganda's sexual health efforts since 1986 have focused primarily on HIV reduction. This is in large part because national development programs and international funding almost completely ceased during Uganda's internal insecurity (see Chapter 2 on the Obote and Amin regimes). Hence, when the country emerged from civil war in 1986, Uganda's new and politically astute president, Yoweri Museveni, welcomed economic aid and human resources from international agencies that were eager to situate themselves at the "epicenter" of the AIDS epidemic. This brought in a flood of foreign donors, development workers, and public health specialists (see Bond and Vincent 1997; Lyons 1997).

6. "Who Should Teach Our Children about Sex?" was the title of one of the many articles on sex education and young people that appeared in the daily newspapers during the late 1990s. The debate continues to receive considerable public attention, and there is little consensus about how to educate young people about sex and what constitutes sexuality education.

7. My description of the Basoga sex education system comes not only from elders' and adults' experiences but also from what younger adults remember learning about their older kin's experiences. The ideal Basoga system has been gradually changing and I certainly found variations in how people experienced it, but in general most people who actually went through the system described a very similar pattern. Similar sexual education systems in Southern Africa are detailed by Diane Jeater (1993). Previous ethnographic work among the Basoga of Iganga undertaken by anthropologist Lloyd Fallers in the 1950s (1957, 1965, and 1969) and early descriptive accounts by missionary John Roscoe (1911 and 1915), based in Uganda from 1893 to 1911, form important historical baselines through which I interpret and understand elders' narratives of sexual learning in the recent past.

8. Groups that have male coming-of-age practices at adolescence that often involve circumcision include the Maasi, Luhya, Kisii, and Kikuyu in Kenya; the Bagisu, Sebei, Baamba, and Bakonzo of Uganda; the Sotho, Tswana, Xhosa, and Zulu of Southern Africa; and the Kurya in northeastern Tanzania. For anthropological literature on circumcision among the Ugandan Bagisu see La Fontaine (1977) and Heald (1999).

9. Fallers (1969:96) recorded that 30 percent of the cases brought to the subcounty court involved disagreements among males over female sexuality. These included alleged violations against the owner of a female's sexuality (e.g., adultery), disputes about the proper owner of a female's sexuality, or charges against a father "harboring" a daughter for whom another man had given bridewealth.

10. It is worth noting that turn-of-the-century colonial observer, missionary, and explorer John Roscoe incorrectly assumed that the twin-naming songs represented and confirmed

"licentious" tendencies of Africans (see Roscoe 1911:72), but elders and later ethnographic accounts are clear that the sexually explicit nature of songs during ceremonies are indeed particular to these social spaces and in other contexts would be considered an impropriety.

11. On the practice of elongating the labia minora, see Grassivaro Gallo and Villa 2006; Khau 2009; Martínez Pérez and Namulondo 2011; Muyinda et al. 2003; Mwenda 2006; Parikh 2005; Tamale 2006.

12. Fallers writes little about the period between the introduction and wedding ceremonies. He writes, "The bride is secluded until the wedding under the care of an elderly woman, who bathes and anoints her and teaches her wifely duties" (1957:112). During this period of seclusion, the girl should have limited interaction with her future husband and other people. In reality, however, this period could extend for an indefinite duration because of difficulties the groom faced in securing the agreed bridewealth and other prerequisites such as completing his home or paying off debts.

13. Waist beads are ten strands of colorful plastic beads (before the introduction of plastic beads, dyed seeds were used) joined at the ends and tied loosely around the waist.

14. In his study of the history of the commodification of cleanliness in Zimbabwe, Timothy Burke (1996:29) writes that the historical accuracy of the practice of a wife washing her husband after sex is "a subject of considerable debate and ambiguity among women and men today." He found that while men "enthusiastically supported the practice," women held a variety of opinions about it. I did not encounter any outright debate about the practice of washing, and it seemed to be a fairly accepted and noncontroversial idea.

15. Dorothy L. Hodgson and Sheryl A. McCurdy (2001:1) observed in sub-Saharan Africa that " 'vagabond, 'prostitute,' 'wayward, 'unruly' and 'immoral' are just a few terms used to label and stigmatize women whose behavior in some way threatens other people's expectations of 'the way things ought to be.' " As the articles in their edited volume illustrate, women who challenge the "boundaries of 'acceptable' behavior" by surviving without the assistance of kin or husbands often get cast as sexually immoral. For a historical perspective in Uganda, see P. J. Davis (2000).

Similarly, for residents of Iganga, the term "prostitute" (or the KiSwahili word *malaya*) serves as a method of controlling the actions of women by stigmatizing certain behaviors and characteristics (such as dress, physical mobility, and comportment) and normalizing others. It is a powerful category often invoked when people discuss the moral decline of young people and females in particular. Even if a female does not engage in direct acts of commercial sex work, she may be labeled as a "prostitute" by merely appearing to have unrestricted physical mobility and acting in ways that defy normative notions of female propriety.

16. There is a methodological lesson here. In an article I published on data collected between 1996 and 1998 (Parikh 2005), I wrote, "It is commonly agreed that most girls in Iganga today do not pull, and I did not meet a female under the age of thirty-five who told me that she had." In subsequent trips, I realized that I was wrong and that adolescent girls in villages around Iganga still practiced pulling, though I cannot tell how widespread it was. My initially faulty data was the result of a question to older women who were in the category of *sôngá*: "Do *sôngá*s today teach girls how to pull?" The women frequently replied that *sôngá*s today did not instruct on pulling. When I asked adolescent girls, they responded with embarrassment or giggles, leading me as a new researcher to back off from the question. What I later came to realize is that while *sôngá*s might not be the instructors, older adolescent girls were teaching younger ones.

17. When I was in Iganga, no church or mosque had a sexuality education program for youth. Two visible programs did exist in Kampala, the Baptist program "True Love Waits" and the Catholic program "Youth Alive." Both programs focus on abstinence by offering young people alternative activities (such as worship, skill training, or planning for the future) to divert their attention away from sexual activity.

18. For a similar debate in Nepal, see Pigg (2002).

19. I use the term "cultural scripts" to refer to patterned behavior that youth invoked when describing various sexualized interactions between men and women (see also Gagnon 1990). Scripts are significant in that they become a gendered and cultural toolkit of acceptable or possible behaviors that young people might draw upon when they encounter a new sexual situation.

Chapter 6

1. Defilement is one of five capital offenses, the others being murder, rape, robbery, and treason. No one has been sentenced to death by hanging for defilement. In 2007, the legislature amended the Penal Code, abolishing corporal punishment, making punishments harsher if the perpetrator has HIV, and expanding the offence to include sex acts with males under the age of eighteen (the Uganda Penal Code [Amendment] Act, 2007 Supplement No. 4, August 17, 2007).

2. For relevant scholarship on the legal regulation of the sexuality of adolescent girls in the United States and Europe see, for example, Cocca (2002); Hollenberg (1999); Odem (1995); Olsen (1984); S. Robertson (2002a, 2002b). A useful study for this chapter is the work of historian Mary Odem (1995), who explores how moral reform and social purity campaigns of the late nineteenth and early twentieth centuries in the United States were used to discipline daughters who had brought shame to the family, either through premarital pregnancy or reprobate behaviors.

3. This regulation of young men is tied to the marriage system, as described earlier in this ethnography, which is based upon men in two patrilineages agreeing upon terms (often in the form of bridewealth) that would give a man access to a female from the other patrilineage. On this, see Evans-Pritchard (1951); Radcliffe-Brown and Forde (1950); Fortes (1962); and Schapera (1941).

4. My theoretical framework for this chapter is informed by recent critical legal scholarship as influenced by Michel Foucault's theory of power (Foucault 1990). This literature highlights how institutions that generate and circulate discourses of rights—the mass media, legal aid agencies, law enforcement, and other arbitration venues—act as powerful mechanisms through which global and national ideologies are negotiated, contested, and adapted at local and national levels (Goodale 2006a, 2006b; Cowan 2006; Merry 2001, 2006; Shell-Duncan 2008; Messer 1997). When applied to laws governing sexuality, these interlocutors play a crucial role in authorizing, legitimizing, and normalizing certain types of sexual relationships while simultaneously criminalizing, marginalizing, and pathologizing others through continual surveillance and censure (S. Hirsch 1998; Lazarus-Black 2001; Stephen 1999). I push Foucault's idea of the normalization of categories and ideologies further by building on a long-standing anthropological appreciation of law not as a static rule imposed from above but as a process of creative interpretation and manipulation, suggesting that individual cases brought into the judicial system and various agents' attempts to push their version as the "correct" or "true" version creates various narratives of ideal social, moral, or economic order (Comaroff and Roberts 1981; Moore 1986).

5. These international forums included the World Summit for Children (1990), the World Conference on Education for All (1990), the World Conference on Human Rights (1993), the World Summit for Social Development (1995), and the Fourth World Conference on Women (1995).

6. Historically, pedophilia has been considered an egregious social transgression—a violation of the social, cosmological, and moral orders. Given that this chapter is mainly concerned with cases involving adolescent girls, the reasons why pedophilia gets resolved outside the court system fall outside its scope.

Chapter 7

1. All names of letter writers have been changed and identifying indicators removed. I obtained permission to use all the letters contained in this book as well as the stories around them, including this story. I use the terms "adolescent female," "adolescent girl," and "girl" interchangeably throughout the second part of this book. I do the same for boys. I will make it clear to the reader if I am referring to a young girl (say, between seven and eleven years old) or an adolescent girl (above twelve years old). In Lusoga there is no linguistic distinction between a young girl and an adolescent girl. The term for both is *omúghalá*, which generally refers to a girl who does not have children, is not married, and is roughly below the age of twenty-five. For a young or adolescent boy, the term is *omúlénzí*.

2. As an example of the importance of education in public policy and the country's future security, both the 1996 "Educate the Girl Child" campaign and the 1997 Universal Primary Education (UPE) initiative promoted the notion that schooling leads to more opportunities for youth and enables them to make better life decisions. The girl child campaign further suggested that educating girls enables them to make judicious sexual decisions, such as delaying marriage and pregnancy, by exposing them to different options. Both campaigns had widespread appeal and success.

3. Virginity testing in KwaZulu/Natal in South Africa is based on a similar disciplining or monitoring of girls' sexual activity (Leclerc-Madlala 2001; Scorgie 2002; Daley 1999). The practice has been brought back as a local attempt to control the spread of HIV and counter other negative social effects of modernity. Women who support the practice hope that by "going back to the old ways," girls will be discouraged from engaging in premarital sex, and those who are thought to be sexually active can be tested for HIV and other STDs. Women's rights activists criticize the practice, arguing that it is an invasion of the girls' privacy and causes distress. In Iganga I did not hear about any similar past practice of testing adolescent girls' virginity, except to look for a bloodied sheet on the wedding night.

4. Historian David Cohen suggests that the resemblance of this story to that of Adam and Eve might be a more recent transformation (1972:84). While most versions of this story I heard had a similarly gendered Adam and Eve story line, there are alternative narratives in which Nambi's disobedience is less emphasized or is not featured as the central cause of earth's misfortune. Cohen also documents this legend as it appears in Sir Apolo Kaggwa's (1953) text. Cohen's rendition does not detail the opening courtship portion that is shown here. In his version, Kintu is the grandchild of God and is already married to Nambi; it is God who sends Kintu to earth with Nambi to produce children (1972:84). A play in 1997 that was written and produced by Namasagoli, the headmaster of the secondary school, stimulated discussion on the radio and in newspapers. The controversial British headmaster of the school, Father Damian Grimes (headmaster between 1967 and 2000), drew attention when he took the male-oriented version of the Genesis tale and transformed it into a

feminist tale for the school's annual musical. The play was entitled *In the Beginning God Was a Female*. Defending his play, Father Grimes said in an interview, "I have never believed in ideological theatre but theatre for entertainment. That is what underlies this play" (*Monitor*, July 17, 1998). Although his plays caused much controversy, newspapers never fail to run a full-page spread of photographs of his scantily dressed female dancers.

Chapter 9

1. As elsewhere in sub-Saharan Africa, in Iganga the development of the orthography of local languages corresponded with the translation of the Bible. The Bible was not translated into Lusoga, so Basoga youth learned from it at missionary schools in Luganda instead. From what I learned, the first comprehensive Lusoga dictionary and the development of a standardized orthography was done in 1998 by the (Basoga) Cultural Research Centre in Jinja. There are many debates about Lusoga orthography and the written language.

2. I would like to acknowledge Professor Harold Scheffler for the concept of the grand effect.

3. It is difficult to determine how romance novels inform youth's (mainly girls') *ideas* of romance and love, apart from a few words and grand effects. When I asked youth about romance novels, I received an assortment of responses: they enjoyed reading about foreign places and people; the novels did not relate to their worlds; they learned about love and sex; and simply, "the novels are interesting." I found few answers that supported many of the academic theories on romance novels. Among the most influential works on romance novels is Janice Radway's *Reading the Romance* (1984), in which she argues that middle-class women, whether married or unmarried, read romance novels because they get from them the nurturing, understanding, and love that they are not getting in their lives. Other authors disagree with Radway's hero-as-mother-figure thesis. For example, in *The Romantic Fiction of Mills and Boon, 1909–1995*, Jay Dixon (1999:30) posits that the hero is not mothering the heroine but rather that "he is showing that he cares for her; that he is capable of sharing her concerns." Once a copyeditor for Mills and Boon, Dixon argues that in order to "capture the readers, the hero has to be socialized into the heroine's world—becoming more like her" (33).

Chapter 10

1. Laura Ahearn (1998, 2001) found similar connections between love and success while analyzing love letters from young people in a Nepalese village. She writes that today, "Love is increasingly associated with being 'developed' and successful, and it is more and more associated with independence and the ability to overcome all obstacles in life" (1998:14). She further suggests that the ideological messages in written primary school textbooks and national development campaigns have partially informed changing and intertwined notions of love and success.

Chapter 11

1. "A dream deferred" alludes to "Harlem," a poem by Langston Hughes.

Conclusion

1. A married man historically had two successors: the *musika ow'enkoba* (the heir of the belt), and the *musika ow'embisi* (the heir of the property). The "heir of the belt" was often a younger brother of the deceased and he became the guardian of the man's wife and children via levirate marriage. The "heir of the property," generally the oldest son of the deceased, was responsible for overseeing the property, including land, cattle, and other goods (see D.

W. Cohen 1972:10 and Fallers 1965:90–92). Fallers suggests that prior to the introduction of cash crops there was only the "heir of the belt" since property was held in lineages, and that estates became divided between two heirs after the monetization of the economy. He proposes that "perhaps in such situations individuals felt it desirable to preserve control of the new wealth within the direct line of descent rather than to see it dispersed throughout the wider lineage" (1965:92).

The past thirty years of widespread AIDS deaths have further complicated the Basoga inheritance and succession system. First, it is not uncommon for a man's lineage to claim the property, arguing that the sons will move away and that the wife will soon die from HIV or will remarry and the land will be passed outside the deceased man's lineage. Second, widow inheritance has drastically changed. While a brother might symbolically inherit his deceased brother's wife, he will not have sexual relations with her for fear that she has HIV. Among other groups in sub-Saharan Africa, most notably the Luo in Kenya, widow inheritance continues and is thought to contribute to the spread of HIV in that region (for a compelling overview of the ethnocentric constructions of the role of widow inheritance and the spread of HIV see Agot 2008).

2. Readers familiar with the progression of HIV will recognize that this timeline for the husband's death (circa 1994), Agnes's AIDS diagnosis (circa 2001), Grace's vertical transmission death (circa 2005), and Agnes's continued survival defies what has become standard scientific knowledge, even if we take into account varying progression rates. I have no explanation for this, nor do residents believe that HIV takes the same path in everyone.

3. The antigay movement in Uganda has gained increasing legislative momentum and grassroots support since I began research. In 2005, Uganda became the first country in the world to state in its constitution that marriage is only between heterosexual couples. The amendment states that "marriage is lawful only if entered into between a man and a woman" and "it is unlawful for same-sex couples to marry." The genesis of the 2009 Anti-Homosexuality Bill is well known. After a speaking tour in Uganda by a three-person antigay delegation from the United States (including well-known antigay crusader Scott Lively), newly elected member of Parliament David Bahati introduced the Anti-Homosexuality Bill. The bill proposed some of the harshest punishments for same-sex activities, including death by hanging for "aggravated homosexuality" (Gettleman 2010). The bill sparked immediate global criticism and national debate, with the antigay movement within Uganda growing broader and more hostile and the gay rights side forming and finding international alliances. In 2014, the bill finally passed Parliament, only to be overturned by Uganda's Constitutional Court for not having the required quorum (Kalinaki 2014; Gettleman 2014).

Over the past few decades, there have been regular debates about homosexuality in Uganda's media, religious institutions, and political bodies. The dominant arguments against same-sex sexual acts include the belief that they are a Western import, that they are a sin, that they were absent from "traditional" Africa, and that they promote the sexual exploitation of boys (see also Murray and Roscoe 1998 for similar arguments elsewhere in Africa).

Despite or perhaps because of legislative and public conservatism surrounding same-sex liaisons, there has been greater gay and lesbian organizing in Kampala than in other parts of the country. Legal scholar Sylvia Tamale notes that gay organizing initially began in the form of support groups that have sustained their membership mainly through cyberspace, where "the anonymous involvement and communication that many organizations afford also proves safe when individuals, especially those in socially esteemed professions or high office, need to preserve the mainstream sexual identity" (2007:21).

Bibliography

ABC (Australian Broadcasting Corporation). (2005). Uganda rejects condom shortage claims. *ABC News*, August 30. *www.abc.net.au*.

Abu-Lughod, L. (1986). *Veiled Sentiments: Honor and Poetry in a Bedouin Society*. Berkeley: University of California Press.

———. (1995). Movie stars and Islamic moralism in Egypt. *Social Text* 42 (1): 53–67. Reprinted in Lancaster and Leonardo 1997:502–12.

Adams, V. (1998). Suffering the winds of Lhasa: Politicized bodies, human rights, cultural difference, and humanism in Tibet. *Medical Anthropology Quarterly* 12 (1): 74–102.

Adams, V., and S. L. Pigg, eds. (2005). *Sex in Development: Science, Sexuality, and Morality in Global Perspective*. Durham, NC: Duke University Press.

Adenaike, C. K., and J. Vansina, eds. (1996). *In Pursuit of History: Fieldwork in Africa*. Portsmouth, NH: Heinemann Press.

Adrian, B. (2003). *Framing the Bride: Globalizing Beauty and Romance in Taiwan's Bridal Industry*. Berkeley: University of California Press.

Agot, K. (2007). HIV/AIDS interventions and the politics of the African woman's body. In *A Companion to Feminist Geography*, edited by L. Nelson and J. Seager, 363–78. Oxford: Blackwell.

———. (2008). Women, culture, and HIV/AIDS in sub-Saharan Africa: What does the empowerment discourse leave out? In *Global Empowerment of Women: Responses to Globalization and Politicized Religions*, edited by C. M. Elliott, 287–302. New York: Routledge.

Ahearn, L. M. (1998). "Love keeps afflicting me": Agentive discourse in Nepali love letters. Paper presented at the American Anthropological Association annual meeting, Philadelphia, December 4.

———. (2001). *Invitations to Love: Literacy, Love Letters, and Social Change in Nepal*. Ann Arbor: University of Michigan Press.

Ahlberg, B. M. (1991). *Women, Sexuality, and the Changing Social Order: The Impact of Government Policies on Reproductive Behavior in Kenya*. Philadelphia: Gordon and Breach.

———. (1994). Is there a distinct African sexuality? A critical response to Caldwell et al. *Africa* 64 (2): 220–42.

Akumu, P. (2013). Marriage bill: Beyond property. *The Observer* [Kampala, Uganda], March 22. *www.observer.ug*.

Allen, T., and S. Heald. (2004). HIV/AIDS policy in Africa: What has worked in Uganda and what has failed in Botswana? *Journal of International Development* 16:1141–54.

Allman, J., and V. Tashjian. (2000). *"I Will Not Eat Stone": A Women's History of Colonial Asante*. Portsmouth, NH: Heinemann Press.

Alrich, C. (2007). Institute of Medicine: Abstinence education spending requirement hinders international response to HIV/AIDS. *Guttmacher Policy Review* 10 (2): 20.

Altman, L. K. (1981). Rare cancer seen in 41 homosexuals. *New York Times*, July 3.

———. (2005). U.S. blamed for condom shortage in fighting AIDS in Uganda. *New York Times*, August 30.

AMICAALL (Alliance of Mayors and Municipal Leaders on HIV/AIDS in Africa). (2004). *Iganga Municipality Profile*. Kampala, Uganda: AMICAALL. *www.amicaall.org*.

Amit-Talai, V., and H. Wulff, eds. (1995). *Youth Cultures: A Cross-Cultural Perspective*. New York: Routledge.

Anderson, A. (2004). African Pentecostalism and "spirit" churches. In *An Introduction to Pentecostalism: Global Charismatic Christianity*, edited by A. Anderson, 103–22. New York: Cambridge University Press.

Angell, M. (1997). The ethics of clinical research in the Third World. *New England Journal of Medicine* 337 (12): 847–49.

Ankrah, E. M. (1991). AIDS and the social side of health. *Social Science and Medicine* 32 (9): 967–80.

Appadurai, A. (1990). Disjunctures and difference in the global cultural economy. *Public Culture* 2 (2): 1–24.

———. (1996). *Modernity at Large: Cultural Dimensions of Globalization*. Minneapolis: University of Minnesota Press.

Ashe, R. P. (1890). *Chronicles of Uganda*. New York: Randolph Press.

Asiimwe-Okiror, G., J. Musinguzi, and E. Madraa. (1996). *A Report on the Declining Trends in HIV Infection Rates in Sentinel Surveillance Sites in Uganda*. Kampala, Uganda: STD/AIDS Control Programme, Ministry of Health.

Asiimwe-Okiror, G., A. A. Opio, J. Musinguzi, E. Madraa, G. Tembo, and M. Cara. (1997). Change in sexual behaviour and decline in HIV infection among young pregnant women in urban Uganda. *AIDS* 11: 1757–63.

Bailey, B. L. (1988). *From Front Porch to Back Seat: Courtship in Twentieth-Century America*. Baltimore: Johns Hopkins University Press.

Barber, K. (1997). Introduction. In *Readings in African Popular Culture*, edited by K. Barber, 1–11. Bloomington: Indiana University Press.

Barber, K., and P. F. de Moraes Farias, eds. (1989). *Discourse and Its Disguises: The Interpretation of African Oral Texts*. Birmingham, UK: Birmingham University African Studies Series 1.

Barnett, M., and T. G. Weiss. (2008). *Humanitarianism in Question: Politics, Power, Ethics*. Ithaca, NY: Cornell University Press.

Barnett, T., and A. Whiteside. (2002). *AIDS in the Twenty-First Century*. New York: Palgrave Macmillan.

———. (2006). *AIDS in the Twenty-First Century: Disease and Globalization*. New York: Palgrave Macmillan.

Bass, E. (2005). Fighting to close the condom gap in Uganda. *Lancet* 365 (9465): 1127–28.

Bastian, M. L. (2001). Acadas and fertilizer girls: Young Nigerian women and the romance of middle-class modernity. In *Gendered Modernities: Ethnographic Perspectives*, edited by D. L. Hodgson, 53–76. New York: Palgrave Macmillan.

Baxter, P. T. W., and U. Almagor. (1978). Introduction. In *Age Generation and Time: Some Features of East African Age Organisations*, edited by P. T. W. Baxter and U. Almagor, 1–35. London: Hurst.

BBC (British Broadcasting Corporation). (2004a). Fine for Ugandan radio gay show. October 3. *news.bbc.co.uk*.

———. (2004b). Uganda to run short of condoms. December 13. *news.bbc.co.uk*.

Beauvoir, S. (1953). *The Second Sex*. Translated by H. M. Parshley. New York: Knopf.

Beidelman, T. O. (1965). Myth, legend, and oral history: A Kaguru traditional text. *Anthropos* 65:74–97.

———. (1997). *The Cool Knife: Imagery of Gender, Sexuality, and Moral Education in Kaguru Initiation Ritual*. Washington, DC: Smithsonian Institution Press.

Berlant, L. (1997). *The Queen of America Goes to Washington City: Essays on Sex and Citizenship*. Durham, NC: Duke University Press.

———. (2011). *Cruel Optimism*. Durham, NC: Duke University Press.

Berlant, L., and M. Warner. (1998). Sex in public. *Critical Inquiry* 24 (2): 547–66.

Berry, S. (1993). *No Condition Is Permanent: The Social Dynamics of Agrarian Change in Sub-Saharan Africa*. Madison: University of Wisconsin Press.

Besnier, N. (1995). *Literacy, Emotion, and Authority: Reading and Writing on a Polynesian Atoll*. Cambridge: Cambridge University Press.

Biehl, J. (2004). The activist state: Global pharmaceuticals, AIDS, and citizenship in Brazil. *Social Text* 22 (3): 105–32.

———. (2007). Pharmaceuticalization: AIDS treatment and global health politics. *Anthropological Quarterly* 80 (4): 1083–26.

———. (2009). *Will to Live: AIDS Therapies and the Politics of Survival*. Princeton, NJ: Princeton University Press.

Biehl, J., and A. Petryna, eds. (2013). *When People Come First: Critical Studies in Global Health*. Princeton, NJ: Princeton University Press.

Birken, L. (1988). *Consuming Desire: Sexual Science and the Emergence of a Culture of Abundance*. Ithaca, NY: Cornell University Press.

Blankenship, K. M., S. R. Friedman, S. Dworkin, and J. E. Mantell. (2006). Structural interventions: Concepts, challenges and opportunities for research. *Journal of Urban Health: Bulletin of the New York Academy of Medicine* 83 (1): 59–72.

Bledsoe, C. (1990). Transformations in sub-Saharan African marriage and fertility. *Annals of the American Academy of Political and Social Science* 510:115–25.

Bledsoe, C., and G. Pison, eds. (1994). *Nuptiality in Sub-Saharan Africa: Contemporary Anthropological and Demographic Perspectives*. New York: Oxford University Press.

Boden, S. (2003). *Consumerism, Romance, and the Wedding Experience*. New York: Palgrave Macmillan.

Bond, G. C., J. Kreniske, and I. Susser. (1997). The anthropology of AIDS in Africa and the Caribbean. In Bond, Kreniske, Susser, and Vincent 1997:3–9.

Bond, G. C., J. Kreniske, I. Susser, and J. Vincent, eds. (1997). *AIDS in Africa and the Caribbean*. Boulder, CO: Westview Press.

Bond, G. C., and J. Vincent. (1991). Living on the edge: Changing social structures in the context of AIDS. In Hansen and Twaddle 1991:113–30.

———. (1997). AIDS in Uganda: The first decade. In Bond, Kreniske, Susser, and Vincent 1997: 85–98.

Booth, K. (2004). *Local Women, Global Science: Fighting AIDS in Kenya*. Bloomington: Indiana University Press.

Bornstein, E. (2001). Child sponsorship, evangelism, and belonging in the work of World Vision Zimbabwe. *American Ethnologist* 28 (3): 595–622.

———. (2005). *The Spirit of Development: Protestant NGOs, Morality, and Economics in Zimbabwe*. Stanford, CA: Stanford University Press.

———. (2010). *Forces of Compassion: Humanitarianism between Ethics and Politics*. Santa Fe, NM: School for Advanced Research, 2010.

Boseley, S. (2005). Uganda's AIDS programme faces crisis. *Guardian*, August 29.

Bourdieu, P. (1977). *Outline of a Theory of Practice*. New York: Cambridge University Press.

Bourgois, P. (2002). *In Search of Respect: Selling Crack in El Barrio*. New York: Cambridge University Press.

Boyd, R. E. (1989). Empowerment of women in Uganda: Real or symbolic? *Review of African Political Economy* 16 (45–46): 106–17.

Brennan, D. (2004). *What's Love Got To Do with It? Transnational Desires and Sex Tourism in the Dominican Republic*. Durham, NC: Duke University Press.

Brett, E. A. (1993). Voluntary agencies as development organizations: Theorizing the problem of efficiency and accountability. *Development and Change* 24 (2): 269–304.

Brody, S. (2004). Declining HIV rates in Uganda: Due to cleaner needles, not abstinence or condoms. *International Journal of STD and AIDS* 15 (7): 440–41.

Brummelhuis, H., and Herdt, G. (1995). *Culture and Sexual Risk*. Amsterdam: Overseas Publishers Association.

Bucholtz, M. (2002). Youth and cultural practice. *Annual Review of Anthropology* 31:525–52.

Burke, T. (1996). *Lifebuoy Men, Lux Women: Commodification, Consumption, and Cleanliness in Modern Zimbabwe*. Durham, NC: Duke University Press.

Burkey, S. (1993). *People First: A Guide to Self-Reliant Participatory Rural Development*. Atlantic Highlands, NJ: Zed Books.

Burnham, P. (1987). Changing themes in the analysis of African marriage. In *Transformations of African Marriage*, edited by D. Parkin and D. Nyamwaya, 37–53. Manchester, UK: Manchester University Press.

Butt, L. (2005). "Lipstick girls" and "fallen women": AIDS and conspiratorial thinking in Papua, Indonesia. *Cultural Anthropology* 20(3): 412–41.

Caldwell, J. C., P. Caldwell, and P. Quiggin. (1989). The social context of AIDS in sub-Saharan Africa. *Population and Development Review* 13:409–37.

Calhoun, C., ed. (1992). *Habermas and the Public Sphere*. Cambridge, MA: MIT Press.

Campbell, C. (1997). Migrancy, masculine identities and AIDS: The psychosocial context of HIV transmission on the South African gold mines. *Social Science and Medicine* 45 (2): 273–81.

———. (2003). *Letting Them Die: Why HIV/AIDS Intervention Programmes Fail*. Bloomington: Indiana University Press.

Cancian, F. M. (1986). The feminization of love signs. *Signs* 11 (4): 692–709.

Carrillo, H. (2001). *The Night Is Young: Sexuality in Mexico in the Time of AIDS*. Chicago: University of Chicago Press.

Casco, J. A. S. (2006). The language of the young people: Rap, urban culture and protest in Tanzania. *Journal of Asian and African Studies* 41 (3): 229–48.

CDC (Centers for Disease Control and Prevention). (1981). Pneumocystis pneumonia—Los Angeles. *Morbidity and Mortality Weekly Report* 30 (21): 1–3.

Chambers, R. (1983). *Rural Development: Putting the Last First*. London: Longman.

CHANGE (Center for Health and Gender Equity). (2004). *Debunking the Myths in the U.S. Global AIDS Strategy: An Evidence-Based Analysis*. Takoma Park, MD: CHANGE. *www.iswface.org/CHGE-DEBUNK.PDF* .

———. (2005). Condom crisis deepens in Uganda shortages spread to other countries US policies undermine HIV prevention programs. Press release, August 6, available at *www.genderhealth.org/pubs/PR20050826.pdf*.

Check, E. (2007). Criticism swells against AIDS program's abstinence policy. *Nature Medicine* 13 (5): 516.

Chic Magazine. (1997). Ladies: To pull or not to pull is the question. *Chic Magazine* 1 (2): 21–27.

Clark University. (1990). *Participatory Rural Appraisal Handbook*. Washington, DC: World Resources Institute.

Cocca, C. E. (2002). The politics of statutory rape laws: Adoption and reinvention of morality policy in the States, 1971–1999. *Polity* 35 (1): 51–72.

Coeytaux, F. M. (1988). Induced abortion in sub-Saharan Africa: What we do and do not know. *Studies in Family Planning* 19 (3): 186–90.

Cohen, C. (2009). Black sexuality, indigenous moral panics and respectability: From Bill Cosby to the "Down-Low." In *Moral Panics and Sexual Rights*, edited by G. Herdt, 104–29. New York: New York University Press.

Cohen, D. W. (1972). *The Historical Tradition of Busoga, Mukama and Kintu*. Oxford: Clarendon Press.

———. (1977). *Womunafu's Bunafu: A Study of Authority in a Nineteenth-Century African Community*. Princeton, NJ: Princeton University Press.

———. (1986). *Towards a Reconstructed Past: Historical Texts from Busoga, Uganda*. Oxford: Oxford University Press.

Cohen, J. (1986). The hunt for the origin of AIDS. *Atlantic*, October.

———. (2007). Bush boosts AIDS relief: Cause for applause and pause. *Science* 316 (5831): 1552.

Cohen, J., and T. Tate. (2005). *The Less They Know, the Better: Abstinence-Only HIV/AIDS Programs in Uganda*. London: Human Rights Watch.

Cohen, S. A. (2006). GAO Report: Global AIDS law's "abstinence-until-marriage" earmark shortchanges other key prevention strategies. *Guttmacher Policy Review* 9 (2): 19–20.

Cole, J. (2004). Fresh contact in Tamatave, Madagascar: Sex, money, and intergenerational transformation. *American Ethnologist* 31 (4): 573–88.

———. (2010). *Sex and Salvation: Imagining the Future in Madagascar*. Chicago: University of Chicago Press.

Cole, J., and D. Durham. (2006). Introduction: Age, regeneration, and the intimate politics of globalization. In *Generations and Globalization: Youth, Age, and Family in the New World Economy*, edited by J. Cole and D. Durham, 1–28. Bloomington: Indiana University Press.

Cole, J., and L. M. Thomas. (2009). *Love in Africa*. Chicago: University of Chicago Press.

Collier, J. (1972). Review of *Law without Precedent: Legal Ideas in Action in the Courts of Colonial Busoga*, by L. A. Fallers. *American Anthropologist* 74 (4): 854–58.

———. (1997). *From Duty to Desire: Remaking Families in a Spanish Village*. Princeton, NJ: Princeton University Press.

Comaroff, J. (1985). *Body of Power, Spirit of Resistance: The Culture and History of a South African People*. Chicago: University of Chicago Press.

Comaroff, J., and J. Comaroff. (1991). *Of Revelation and Revolution: Christianity, Colonialism, and Consciousness in South Africa*. Chicago: University of Chicago Press.

Comaroff, J., and S. Roberts. (1981). *Rules and Processes: The Cultural Logic of Dispute in an African Context*. Chicago: University of Chicago Press.

Connell, R. W. (1987). *Gender and Power: Society, the Person, and Sexual Politics*. Stanford: Stanford University Press.

———. (2003). Masculinities, change, and conflict in global society: Thinking about the future of men's studies. *Journal of Men's Studies* 11 (3): 249–67.

Connell, R. W., and J. Messerschmidt. (2005). Hegemonic masculinity: Rethinking the concept. *Gender and Society* 19 (6): 829–59.

Constable, N. (2003). *Romance on a Global Stage: Pen Pals, Virtual Ethnography, and "Mail-Order" Marriages*. Berkeley: University of California Press.

Cooper, B. M. (1997). *Marriage in Maradi: Gender and Culture in a Hausa Society in Niger, 1900–1989.* Portsmouth, NH: Heinemann Press.

Cowan, J. K. (2006). Culture and rights after "culture and rights." *American Anthropologist* 108 (1): 9–24.

Craddock, S. (2004). Beyond epidemiology: Locating AIDS in Africa. In *HIV and AIDS in Africa: Beyond Epidemiology*, edited by S. Craddock and J. Ghosh, 1–10. Malden, MA: Blackwell.

Crane, J. T. (2013). *Scrambling for Africa: AIDS, Expertise, and the Rise of American Global Health Science.* Ithaca, NY: Cornell University Press.

Crehan, K. A. F. (1997). *The Fractured Community: Landscapes of Power and Gender in Rural Zambia.* Berkeley: University of California Press.

Cultural Research Centre. (1998). *Folklore Pamphlet.* Jinja, Uganda: Basoga Diocese of Jinja.

Daley, S. (1999). Screening girls for abstinence in South Africa. *New York Times*, August 17.

Das, P. (2005). Condom crisis in Uganda. *Lancet Infectious Diseases* 5 (10): 601–2.

Davis, P. J. (2000). On the sexuality of "town women" in Kampala. *Africa Today* 47 (3–4): 29–60.

D'Emilio, J., and E. B. Freedman. (1988). *Intimate Matters: A History of Sexuality in America.* Chicago: University of Chicago Press.

de Munck, V. C. (1998). *Romantic Love and Sexual Behavior: Perspectives from the Social Sciences.* Westport, CT: Praeger.

Dilger, H. (2003). Sexuality, AIDS, and the lures of modernity: Reflexivity and morality among young people in rural Tanzania. *Medical Anthropology* 22 (1): 23–52.

Dinan, C. (1983). Sugar daddies and gold-diggers: The white-collar single women in Accra. In *Female and Male in West Africa*, edited by C. Oppong, 31–48. London: George, Allen, and Unwin.

Diouf, M. (2003). Engaging postcolonial cultures: African youth and public space. *African Studies Review* 46 (2): 1–12.

Dixon, J. (1999). *The Romantic Fiction of Mills and Boon, 1909–1995.* London: University College London Press.

Dolby, N. E. (2006). Popular culture and public space in Africa: The possibilities of cultural citizenship. *African Studies Review* 49 (3): 31–47.

Durham, D. (2000). Youth and the social imagination in Africa: Introduction to parts 1 and 2. *Anthropological Quarterly* 73 (3): 113–20.

———. (2004). Disappearing youth: Youth as a social shifter in Botswana. *American Ethnologist* 31 (4): 589–605.

Durkheim, E. (1951). *Suicide: A Study in Sociology.* Glencoe, IL: Free Press. First published in 1897.

Elyachar, J. (2005). *Markets of Dispossession: NGOs, Economic Development, and the State in Cairo.* Durham, NC: Duke University Press.

Engels, F. (1884). *The Origin of the Family, Private Property, and the State.* Translated by E. Untermann (1902). Chicago: C.H. Kerr.

Englund, H. (2011). Introduction: Rethinking African Christianities beyond the religion-politics conundrum. In *Christianity and Public Culture in Africa*, edited by H. Englund, 1–24. Athens: Ohio University Press.

Epstein, H. (2005). God and the fight against AIDS. *New York Review of Books*, April 28.

———. (2007). *The Invisible Cure: Why We Are Losing the Fight Against AIDS in Africa.* New York: Farrar, Straus and Giroux.

Erikson, E. H. (1968). *Identity, Youth, and Crisis.* New York: Norton.

———. (1970). Reflections on the dissent of contemporary youth. *International Journal of Psychoanalysis* 51:11–22.

Escobar, A. (1995). *Encountering Development: The Making and Unmaking of the Third World.* Princeton, NJ: Princeton University Press.

Evans-Pritchard, E. E. (1940). The Nuer of the southern Sudan. In Fortes and Evans-Pritchard 1940, 249–66.

———. (1951). *Kinship and Marriage among the Nuer.* Oxford: Clarendon Press.

Evertz, Scott. (2010). *How Ideology Trumped Science: Why PEPFAR has Failed to Meet Its Potential.* Washington, DC: Center for American Progress and The Council for Global Equality.

Fabian, J. (1978). Popular culture in Africa: Findings and conjectures. *Africa* 48 (4): 315–34.

———. (1998). *Moments of Freedom: Anthropology and Popular Culture.* Charlottesville, VA: University Press of Virginia.

Fallers, L. A. (1957). Some determinants of marriage stability in Basoga: A reformulation of Gluckman's hypothesis. *Africa: Journal of the International African Institute* 27 (2): 106–23.

———. (1964). *The King's Men: Leadership and Status in Buganda on the Eve of Independence.* London: Oxford University Press.

———. (1965). *Bantu Bureaucracy: A Century of Political Evolution among the Basoga of Uganda.* Chicago: University of Chicago Press.

———. (1969). *Law without Precedent: Legal Ideas in Action in the Courts of Colonial Busoga.* Chicago: University of Chicago Press.

Fallers, L. A., and C. Fallers. (1960). Homicide and suicide in Busoga. In *African Homicide and Suicide,* edited by P. Bohannen, 65–93. Princeton, NJ: Princeton University Press.

Fals Borda, O. (1982). Participatory research and rural social change. *Journal of Rural Cooperation* 10 (1): 25–39.

Fanon, F. (1967). *Black Skin, White Masks.* Translated by C. L. Markmann. London: Pluto Press.

Farmer, P. (1992). *AIDS and Accusation: Haiti and the Geography of Blame.* Berkeley: University of California Press.

———. (2001). *Infections and Inequalities: The Modern Plagues.* Berkeley: University of California Press.

———. (2004). *Pathologies of Power: Health, Human Rights, and the New War on the Poor.* Berkeley: University of California Press.

Farmer, P., M. Connors, and J. Simmons, eds. (1996). *Women, Poverty, and AIDS: Sex, Drugs, and Structural Violence.* Monroe, ME: Common Courage Press.

Fassin, D. (2007a). *When Bodies Remember: Experiences and Politics of AIDS in South Africa.* Berkeley: University of California Press.

———. (2007b). Humanitarianism as a politics of life. *Public Culture* 19 (3): 499–520.

———. (2012). Humanitarian Reason: A Moral History of the Present. Translated by Rachel Gomme. Berkeley: University of California Press.

Feierman, Steven. (1990). *Peasant Intellectuals: Anthropology and History in Tanzania.* Madison: University of Wisconsin Press.

Feldman-Savelsberg, P. (1995). Cooking inside: Kinship and gender in Bangangté; Idioms of marriage and procreation. *American Ethnologist* 22 (3): 483–501.

———. (1999). *Plundered Kitchens, Empty Wombs: Threatened Reproduction and Identity in the Cameroon Grasslands.* Ann Arbor: University of Michigan Press.

Ferguson, J. (1990). *The Anti-Politics Machine: Development, Depoliticization, and Bureaucratic Power in Lesotho*. New York: Cambridge University Press.

———. (1999). *Expectations of Modernity: Myths and Meanings of Urban Life on the Zambian Copperbelt*. Berkeley: University of California Press.

———. (2006). *Global Shadows: Africa in the Neoliberal World Order*. Durham, NC: Duke University Press.

Fèvre, E. M., P. G. Coleman, S. C. Welburn, and I. Maudlin. (2004). Reanalyzing the 1900–1920 sleeping sickness epidemic in Uganda. *Emerging Infectious Diseases* 10 (4): 567–73.

Fine, M. (1988). Sexuality, schooling and adolescent females: The missing discourse of desire. *Harvard Educational Review* 58 (1): 29–53.

———. (1992). *Disruptive Voices: The Possibilities of Feminist Research*. Ann Arbor: University of Michigan Press.

Fortes, M. (1962). *Marriage in Tribal Societies*. Cambridge: Cambridge University Press.

Fortes, M., and E. E. Evans-Pritchard, eds. (1940). *African Political Systems*. London: Oxford University Press.

Foucault, M. (1990). *History of Sexuality: An Introduction*. Vol. 1. Translated by R. Hurley. New York: Vintage.

Fox, R. G. (1991). Introduction: Working in the present. In *Recapturing Anthropology: Working in the Present*, edited by R. G. Fox, 1–16. Santa Fe, NM: School of American Research Press.

France-Presse, A. (2015). Gay Ugandans hope new magazine will rewrite wrongs by tackling homophobia. *Guardian*, February 9.

Fraser, N. (1990). Rethinking the public sphere: A contribution to the critique of actually existing democracy. *Social Text* 25–26:56–80.

Frazier, E. F. (1932). *The Negro Family in Chicago*. Chicago: University of Chicago Press.

Frederiksen, B. F. (2000). Popular culture, gender relations and the democratization of everyday life in Kenya. *Journal of Southern African Studies* 26 (2): 209–22.

Freeman, C. (2007). Neoliberalism and the marriage of reputation and respectability: Entrepreneurship and the Barbadian middle class. In *Love and Globalization: Transformations of Intimacy in the Contemporary World*, edited by M. B. Padilla, J. Hirsch, M. Munoz-Labov, R. Sember, and R. G. Parker, 3–37. Nashville: Vanderbilt University Press.

Freire, P. (1970). *Pedagogy of the Oppressed*. New York: Herder and Herder.

Fritz, K. (1998). *Women, Power, and HIV Risk in Rural Mbale District, Uganda*. PhD diss., Yale University.

Fuglesang, M. (1994). *Veils and Videos: Female Youth Culture on the Kenyan Coast*. Stockholm, Sweden: Stockholm University Press.

Fuller, L. K. (2008). *African Women's Unique Vulnerabilities to HIV/AIDS: Communication Perspectives and Promises*. New York: Palgrave Macmillan.

Fullilove, M. T., R. E. Fullilove, K. Haynes, and S. Gross. (1990). Black women and AIDS prevention: A view towards understanding the gender rules. *Journal of Sex Research*, 27 (1): 47–64.

Gable, E. (2000). The culture development club: Youth, neo-tradition, and the construction of society in Guinea-Bissau. *Anthropological Quarterly* 73 (4): 195–203.

Gagnon, J. H. (1990). The implicit and explicit use of the scripting perspective in sex research. *Annual Review of Sex Research* 1:1–43.

Gagnon, J. H., and R. G. Parker. (1994). Introduction: Conceiving sexuality. G. Parker and J. H. Gagnon, 3–19. New York: Routledge.

GAO (Government Accountability Office). (2006). *Global Health: Spending Requirement Presents Challenges for Allocating Prevention Funding under the President's Emergency Plan for AIDS Relief.* Report to Congressional Committees, April. GAO-06-395.

Garrett, L. (1994). *The Coming Plague: Newly Emerging Diseases in a World out of Balance.* New York: Farrar, Straus and Giroux.

Gettleman, J. (2010). Americans' role seen in Uganda anti-gay push. *New York Times*, January 3. *www.nytimes.com.*

———. (2014). Uganda anti-gay law struck down by court. *New York Times*, August 1. *www.nytimes.com.*

Giblin, J. (1999). Family life, indigenous culture, and Christianity in colonial Njombe. In *East African Expressions of Christianity*, edited by T. Spear and I. N. Kimambo, 309–23. Athens: Ohio University Press.

Giddens, A. (1984). *The Constitution of Society: Outline of the Theory of Structuration.* Cambridge: Polity Press.

———. (1992). *The Transformation of Intimacy: Sexuality, Love and Eroticism in Modern Societies.* Cambridge: Polity Press.

Gifford, P. (1998). *African Christianity: Its Public Role.* Bloomington: Indiana University Press.

Girard, F. (2004). *Global Implications of U.S. Domestic and International Policies on Sexuality.* New York: The International Working Group on Sexuality and Social Policy.

Gluckman, M. (1963). Papers in honor of Melville J. Herskovits: Gossip and scandal. *Current Anthropology* 4 (3): 307–16.

———. (1968). Psychological, sociological and anthropological explanations of witchcraft and gossip: A clarification. *Man* 3 (1): 20–34.

Goffman, E. (1959). *The Presentation of Self in Everyday Life.* New York: Overlook Press.

Goodale, M. (2006a). Introduction to "Anthropology and human rights in a new key." *American Anthropology* 108 (1): 1–8.

———. (2006b). Toward a critical anthropology of human rights. *Current Anthropology* 47 (3): 485–511.

Goody, J. (1973). Bridewealth and dowry in Africa and Eurasia. In *Bridewealth and Dowry*, edited by J. Goody and S. Tambiah, 1–59. Cambridge: Cambridge University Press.

———. (1998). *Food and Love: A Cultural History of East and West.* New York: Verso.

Gordon, L. (1990). Introduction. In *Women, The State, and Welfare*, edited by L. Gordon, 3–8. Madison: University of Wisconsin Press.

———. (1995). Putting children first: Women, maternalism, and welfare in the early twentieth century. In Kerber, Kessler-Harris, and Sklar 1995:63–86.

Grassivaro Gallo, P., and E. Villa. (2006). Ritual labia minora elongation among the Baganda women of Uganda. *Psychopathologie Africaine* 33:213–36.

Gray, R. H., D. Serwadda, G. Kigozi, F. Nalugoda, and M. J. Wawer. (2006). Uganda's HIV prevention success: The role of sexual behavior change and the national response. Commentary on Green et al., 2006. *AIDS and Behavior* 10 (4): 347–50.

Green, E. C., D. T. Halperin, V. Nantulya, and J. A. Hogle. (2006). Uganda's HIV prevention success: The role of sexual behavior change and the national response. *AIDS and Behavior* 10 (4): 335–46.

Gullatte, M. M., O. Brawley, A. Kinney, B. Powe, and K. Mooney. (2009). Religiosity, spirituality, and cancer fatalism beliefs on delay in breast cancer diagnosis in African American women. *Journal of Religion and Health* 49 (1): 62–72.

Gupta, A., and J. Ferguson. (1997). Culture, power, place: Ethnography at the end of an era. In *Culture, Power, Place: Explorations in Critical Anthropology*, edited by A. Gupta and J. Ferguson, 1–33. Durham, NC: Duke University Press.

Guyer, J. (1994). Lineal identities and lateral networks: The logic of polyandrous motherhood. In Bledsoe and Pison 1994, 231–52.

Habermas, J. (1991). *The Structural Transformation of the Public Sphere*. Translated by T. Burger and F. Lawrence. Cambridge, MA: MIT Press.

Hahn, R. A., and K. W. Harris, eds. (1999). *Anthropology in Public Health: Bridging Differences in Culture and Society*. New York: Oxford University Press.

Hall, B. L. (1975). Participatory research: An approach for change. *Convergence* 8 (2): 24–32.

———. (2005). In from the cold: Reflections on participatory action research from 1970–2005. *Convergence* 38 (1): 5–24.

Hall, E. T. (1976). *Beyond Culture*. Garden City, NY: Anchor.

Hall, S., and T. Jefferson, eds. (1976). *Resistance through Rituals: Youth Subcultures in Post-War Britain*. London: Hutchinson.

Halperin, D., and H. Epstein. (2004). Concurrent sexual partnerships help to explain Africa's high HIV prevalence: Implications for prevention. *Lancet* 364 (9428): 4–6.

Halperin, D. T., M. J. Steiner, M. M. Cassell, E. C. Green, N. Hearst, D. Kirby, H. D. Gayle, and W. Cates. (2004). The time has come for common ground on preventing sexual transmission of HIV. *Lancet* 364 (9449): 1913–15.

Hannigan, J. A. (2012). *Disasters without Borders: The International Politics of Natural Disasters*. Cambridge: Polity.

Hansen, H. B., and M. Twaddle, eds. (1988). *Uganda Now: Between Decay and Development*. Athens: Ohio University Press.

———. (1991). *Changing Uganda: The Dilemmas of Structural Adjustment and Revolutionary Change*. Athens: Ohio University Press.

———. (1995). *Religion and Politics in East Africa: The Period since Independence*. Athens: Ohio University Press.

———. (1998). *Developing Uganda*. Athens: Ohio University Press.

Hansen, K. T. (1992). Introduction: Domesticity in Africa. In *African Encounters with Domesticity*, edited by K. T. Hansen, 1–36. New Brunswick, NJ: Rutgers University Press.

———. (2000). Gender and difference: Youth, bodies, and clothing in Zambia. In *Gender, Agency, and Change: Anthropological Perspectives*, edited by V. A. Goddard, 32–56. London: Routledge.

Haram, L. (2005). "Eyes have no curtains": The moral economy of secrecy in managing love affairs among adolescents in northern Tanzania in the time of AIDS. *Africa Today* 51(4): 57–73.

Harrison, A. (2008). Hidden love: Sexual ideologies and relationship ideals among rural South African adolescents in the context of HIV/AIDS. *Culture, Health, and Sexuality* 10 (2): 175–89.

Harvey, D. (1989). *The Condition of Postmodernity: An Enquiry into the Origins of Cultural Change*. Cambridge, MA: Blackwell.

Haugerud, A. (1995). *The Culture of Politics in Modern Kenya*. Cambridge: Cambridge University Press.

Heald, S. (1995). The power of sex: Some reflections on the Caldwells' "African sexuality" thesis. *Africa* 65 (4): 489–505.

————. (1999). *Manhood and Morality: Sex, Violence, and Ritual in Gisu Society*. New York: Routledge.

Hebdige, D. (1979). *Subculture: The Meaning of Style*. London: Methuen.

Herdt, G. H. (1981). *Guardians of the Flutes: Idioms of Masculinity*. Chicago: McGraw-Hill.

Herdt, G. H., and S. Lindenbaum. (1992). *The Time of AIDS: Social Analysis, Theory, and Method*. Thousand Oaks, CA: Sage.

Herring, D. A., and A. C. Swedlund. (2010). *Plagues and Epidemics: Infected Spaces Past and Present*. Oxford: Berg.

Hess, R. F., and D. E. McKinney. (2007). Fatalism and HIV/AIDS beliefs in rural Mali, West Africa. *Journal of Nursing Scholarship* 39 (2): 113–18.

Higgins, J., and J. Hirsch. (2008). Pleasure, power, and inequality: Incorporating sexuality into research on contraceptive use. *American Journal of Public Health* 98 (10): 1803–13.

Hilts, P. J. (1981). 2 mysterious diseases killing homosexuals. *Washington Post*, August 30.

Hirsch, J. S., and H. Wardlow, eds. (2006). *Modern Loves: The Anthropology of Romantic Love and Companionate Marriage*. Ann Arbor: University of Michigan Press.

Hirsch, J. S., S. Meneses, B. Thompson, M. Negroni, B. Pelcastre, and C. del Rio. (2007). The inevitability of infidelity: Sexual reputation, social geographies, and marital HIV risk in rural Mexico. *American Journal of Public Health* 97 (6): 986–96.

Hirsch, J. S., H. Wardlow, D. J. Smith, H. M. Phinney, S. Parikh, and C. A. Nathanson (2010). *The Secret: Love, Marriage, and HIV*. Nashville: Vanderbilt University Press.

Hirsch, S. F. (1998). *Pronouncing and Persevering: Gender and the Discourses of Disputing in an African Islamic Court*. Chicago: University of Chicago Press.

Hodgson, D. L. (1996). "My daughter belongs to the government now": Marriage, maasai, and the Tanzanian state. *Canadian Journal of African Studies* 30 (1): 106–23.

Hodgson, D. L., and S. A. McCurdy, eds. (2001). *"Wicked" Women and the Reconfiguration of Gender in Africa*. Portsmouth, NH: Heinemann Press.

Hogle, J. A., ed. (2002). *What Happened in Uganda? Declining HIV Prevalence, Behavior Change, and the National Response*. Washington, DC: USAID.

Holland, D. C., and M. A. Eisenhart. (1992). *Educated in Romance: Women, Achievement, and College Culture*. Chicago: University of Chicago Press.

Holland, J., C. Ramazanoglu, S. Scott, S. Sharpe, and R. Thompson. (1990). Sex, gender and power: Young women's sexuality in the shadow of AIDS. *Sociology of Health and Illness* 12 (3): 336–50.

————. (1992). Risk, power and the possibility of pleasure: Young women and safer sex. *AIDS Care* 4:273–83.

Hollenberg, E. (1999). The criminalization of teenage sex: Statutory rape and the politics of teenage motherhood. *Stanford Law and Policy Review* 10:267–87.

Honwana, A., and F. De Boeck, eds. (2005). *Makers and Breakers: Children and Youth in Postcolonial Africa*. Trenton, NJ: Africa World Press.

Hooper, E. (1999). *The River: A Journey Back to the Source of HIV and AIDS*. London: Allen Lane.

Hopkins, G. H. E., and R. S. F. Hennessey. (1938). Cotton and plague in Uganda. *Journal of Hygiene* 38 (2): 233–47.

Hunt, N. R. (1997). Introduction. In *Gendered Colonialisms in African History*, edited by N. R. Hunt, T. P. Liu, and J. Quataert, 1–16. Malden, MA: Blackwell.

————. (1999). *A Colonial Lexicon of Birth Ritual, Medicalization, and Mobility in the Congo*. Durham, NC: Duke University Press.

Hunter, M. (2009). Providing love: Sex and exchange in twentieth-century South Africa. In Cole and Thomas 2009:135–57.

———. (2010). *Love in the Time of AIDS: Inequality, Gender, and Rights in South Africa*. Bloomington: Indiana University Press.

Hutchinson, S. (1996). *Nuer Dilemmas: Coping with Money, War, and the State*. Berkeley: University of California Press.

Hyndman, J. (2011). *Dual Disasters: Humanitarian Aid after the 2004 Tsunami*. Sterling, VA: Kumarian Press.

Illouz, E. (1997). *Consuming the Romantic Utopia: Love and the Cultural Contradictions of Capitalism*. Berkeley: University of California Press.

IOM (Institute of Medicine of the National Academies). (2007). *PEPFAR Implementation: Progress and Promise*. Washington, DC: National Academies Press.

Irvine, J. M. (1999). *Talk about Sex: The Battles over Sex Education in the United States*. Berkeley: University of California Press.

Isaacman, A. F. (1996). *Cotton Is the Mother of Poverty: Peasants, Work, and Rural Struggle in Colonial Mozambique, 1938–1961*. Portsmouth, NH: Heinemann Press.

Jackson, L. (2005). *Surfacing Up: Psychiatry and Social Order in Colonial Zimbabwe, 1908–1968*. Ithaca, NY: Cornell Press.

Jamal, V. (1998). Changes in poverty patterns in Uganda. In Hansen and Twaddle 1998:73–97.

James, E. C. (2010). *Democratic Insecurities: Violence, Trauma, and Intervention in Haiti*. Berkeley: University of California Press.

Jamison, D., and N. Padian. (2006). Where AIDS funding should go. *Washington Post*, May 20.

Jankowiak, W. (1995). Introduction. In *Romantic Passion: A Universal Experience?*, edited by W. Jankowiak, 1–21. New York: Columbia University Press.

Jeater, D. (1993). *Marriage, Perversion, and Power: The Construction of Moral Discourse in Southern Rhodesia, 1894–1930*. Oxford: Oxford University Press.

Johnson-Hanks, J. (2002). On the limits of life stages in ethnography: Toward a theory of vital conjunctures. *American Anthropologist* 104 (3): 865–80.

———. (2006). *Uncertain Honor: Modern Motherhood in an African Crisis*. Chicago: University of Chicago Press.

———. (2007). Women on the market: Marriage, consumption, and the Internet in urban Cameroon. *American Ethnologist* 34 (4): 642–58.

Kaiser Family Foundation. (2008). *Reauthorization of PEPFAR, The United States Global Leadership against HIV/AIDS, Tuberculosis and Malaria Act: A Side-by-Side Comparison to Prior Law*. Menlo Park, CA: Kaiser Foundation. *kaiserfamilyfoundation.files.wordpress.com/2013/01/7799.pdf*.

Kalema Commission. (1965). *Report of the Commission on Marriage, Divorce and the Status of Women*. Entebbe, Uganda: Government Printer.

Kalinaki, D. (2014). The death of the anti-gay law was expected, so why are we surprised? *Daily Monitor* [Kampala, Uganda], March 2.

Kalipeni, E., S. Craddock, J. R. Oppong, and J. Ghosh, eds. (2004). *HIV and AIDS in Africa: Beyond Epidemiology*. Malden, MA: Wiley-Blackwell.

Kalu, O. (2008). *African Pentecostalism: An Introduction*. New York: Oxford University Press.

Kamali, A., L. M. Carpenter, J. Whitworth, R. Pool, A. Ruberantwari, and A. Ojwiya. (2000). Seven-year trends in HIV-1 infection rates, and changes in sexual behaviour, among adults in rural Uganda. *AIDS* 14:427–34.

Kamwi, R., T. Kenyon, and G. Newton. (2006). PEPFAR and HIV prevention in Africa. *Lancet* 367 (9527): 1978–79.

Kane, S. (1993). National discourse and the dynamics of risk: Ethnography and AIDS intervention. *Human Organization* 52 (2): 224–28.

Kaoma, K. (2009/2010). The U.S. Christian Right and the attack on gays in Africa. *Public Eye*, Winter–Spring. *www.publiceye.org.*

Karanja, W. W. (1987). "Outside wives" and "inside wives" in Nigeria: A study of changing perceptions in marriage. In *Transformations of African Marriage*, edited by D. Parkin and D. Nyamwaya, 247–61. Manchester, UK: Manchester University Press.

Kasfir, N., ed. (1983). *State and Class in Africa*. London: Frank Cass.

Kasyate, S. (2010). Sexual network ad grating on nerves. *The Observer* [Kampala, Uganda], January 24. *www.observer.ug.*

Kayunga, S. S. (1994). Islamic fundamentalism in Uganda: A case study of the Tabligh youth movement. In *Uganda: Studies in Living Conditions, Popular Movements, and Constitutionalism*, edited by M. Mamdani and J. Oloka-Onyango, 319–63. Kampala, Uganda: Centre for Basic Research.

Kendall, L. (1996). *Getting Married in Korea: Of Gender, Morality, and Modernity*. Berkeley: University of California Press.

Kerber, L. K., A. Kessler-Harris, and K. K. Sklar, eds. (1995). *U.S. History as Women's History: New Feminist Essays*. Chapel Hill: University of North Carolina Press.

Khau, M. (2009). Exploring sexual customs: Girls and the politics of elongating the inner labia. *Agenda: Empowering Women for Gender Equity* 23 (79): 30–37.

Khiddu-Makubuya, E. (1991). The rule of law and human rights in Uganda: The missing link. In Hansen and Twaddle 1991:217–23.

Kilian, A. H. D., S. Gregson, B. Ndyanabangi, K. Walusaga, W. Kipp, G. Sahlmüller, G. P. Garnett, G. Asiimwe-Okiror, G. Kabagambe, P. Weis, and F. von Sonnenburg. (1999). Reductions in risk behaviour provide the most consistent explanation for declining HIV-1 prevalence in Uganda. *AIDS* 13 (3): 391–98.

Kinsman, J. (2010). *AIDS Policy in Uganda: Evidence, Ideology and the Making of an African Success Story*. New York: Palgrave Macmillan.

Kinsman, J., S. Nyanzi, and R. Pool. (2000). Socializing influences and the value of sex: The experience of adolescent school girls in rural Masaka, Uganda. *Culture of Health and Sexuality* 2 (2): 151–66.

Kleinman, A. (1988). *The Illness Narratives: Suffering, Healing, and the Human Condition*. New York: Basic Books.

Kitching, G. (1980). *Class and Economic Change in Kenya*. New Haven, CT: Yale University Press.

Kinyanda, E., S. Hoskins, J. Nakku, S. Nawaz, and V. Patel. (2001). Prevalence and risk factors of major depressive disorder in HIV/AIDS as seen in semi-urban Entebbe District, Uganda. *BMC Psychiatry* 11:205.

Kohn, David. (2005). More HIV funds to promote abstinence: Researchers call policy misguided. *Baltimore Sun*, December 10.

Konde-Lule, J. K. (1995). The declining HIV seroprevalence in Uganda: What evidence? *Health Transition Review* 5 (Supplement): 27–33.

Konde-Lule, J. K., M. Musagara, and S. Musgrave. (1993). Focus group interviews about AIDS in Rakai District of Uganda. *Social Science Medical Journal* 37 (5): 679–84.

Konde-Lule, J. K., and A. J. Sebina. (1993). The impact of AIDS in a rural Ugandan community. *East African Medical Journal* 70 (11): 725–29.

Konde-Lule, J. K., N. Sewankambo, and M. Morris. (1997). Adolescent sexual networking and HIV transmission in rural Uganda. *Health Transit Rev.* 7 Supplement: 89–100.

Konde-Lule, J. K., M. N. Tumwesigye, and R. G. Lubanga. (1997). Trends in attitudes and behavior relevant to AIDS in Ugandan community. *East African Medical Journal* 74 (7): 406–10.

Konde-Lule, J. K., M. J. Wawer, N. K. Sewankambo, D. Serwadda, R. Kelly, C. Li, R. H. Gray, and D. Kigongo. (1997). Adolescents, sexual behaviour and HIV-1 in rural Rakai district, Uganda. *AIDS* 11 (6): 791–99.

Korenromp, E. L., R. Bakker, R. Gray, M. J. Wawer, D. Serwadda, and J. D. F. Habbema. (2002). The effect of HIV, behavioural change, and STD syndromic management on STD epidemiology in sub-Saharan Africa: Simulations of Uganda. *Sexually Transmitted Infections* 78:55–63.

Koven, S., and S. Michel, eds. (1993). *Mothers of a New World: Maternalist Politics and the Origins of Welfare States*. New York: Routledge.

Krause, M. (2014). *The Good Project: Humanitarian Relief, NGOs, and the Fragmentation of Reason*. Chicago: University of Chicago Press.

Kroeger, K. (2003). AIDS rumors, imaginary enemies, and the body politic in Indonesia. *American Ethnologist* 30 (2): 243–57.

Kuhanen, J. (2008). The historiography of HIV and AIDS in Uganda. *History in Africa* 35:301–25.

La Fontaine, J. S. (1974). The free women of Kinshasa: Prostitution in a city of Zaire. In *Choice and Change: Essays in Honour of Lucy Mair*, edited by J. Davis, 89–113. Athlone, NY: Humanities Press.

———. (1977). The power of rights. *Man* 12 (3–4): 421–37.

Lancaster, R. N. (2011). *Sex Panic and the Punitive State*. Berkeley: University of California Press.

Lancaster, R. N., and M. di Leonardo, eds. (1997). *The Gender/Sexuality Reader: Culture, History, Political Economy*. New York: Routledge.

Lancet. (2006). Editorial: HIV prevention policy needs an urgent cure. *Lancet* 367 (9518): 1213.

Larimore, A. E. (1959). *The Alien Town: Patterns of Settlement in Busoga, Uganda*. Chicago: University of Chicago Press.

Larkin, B. (1997). Indian films and Nigerian lovers: Media and the creation of parallel modernities. *Africa* 67 (3): 406–39.

Lazarus-Black, M. (2001). Law and the pragmatics of inclusion: Governing domestic violence in Trinidad and Tobago. *American Ethnologist* 28 (2): 388–416.

Le Blanc, M.-N., D. Meintel, and V. Piché. (1991). The African sexual system: Comment on Caldwell et al. *Population and Development Review* 17 (3): 497–505.

Leclerc-Madlala, S. (2001). Virginity testing: Managing sexuality in a maturing HIV/AIDS epidemic. *Medical Anthropology Quarterly* 15 (4): 533–52.

Lees, S. (1989). Learning to love: Sexual reputation, morality, and the social control of girls. In *Growing Up Good: Policing the Behavior of Girls in Europe*, edited by M. Cain, 19–37. London: Sage.

——. (1993). *Sugar and Spice: Sexuality and Adolescent Girls*. London: Penguin.

LeVine, R. A. (1959). Gusii sex offences: A study in social control. *American Anthropologist* 61 (6): 965–90.

LeVine, R. A., and W. H. Sangree. (1962). The diffusion of age-group organization in East Africa: A controlled comparison. *Africa* 32 (2): 97–110.

Lévi-Strauss, C. (1969). *The Elementary Structures of Kinship*. London: Eyre and Spottiswoode. First published in 1949.

Levy, R. (1984). Emotion, knowing, and culture. In *Culture Theory: Essays on Mind, Self, and Emotion*, edited by R. A. Shweder and R. A. LeVine, 214–37. Cambridge: Cambridge University Press.

Lewin, K. (1946). Action research and minority problems. *Journal of Social Issues* 2 (4): 34–46.

Lewis, O. (1959). *Five Families: Mexican Case Studies in the Culture of Poverty*. New York: New American Library.

Lewontin, R. C. (1995). Sex, lies, and social science. *New York Review of Books* 42:24–29.

Leys, C. (1978). Capital accumulation, class formation and dependency: The significance of the Kenya case. *Socialist Register* 15:241–66.

Lively, S. (2009). Comments about March 3–9 pro-family mission to Uganda. *Pro-Family Resource Center of Aiding Truth Ministries. www.defendthefamily.com*.

Livingston, J. (2012). *Improvising Medicine: An African Oncology Ward in an Emerging Cancer Epidemic*. Durham, NC: Duke University Press.

Low-Beer, D., and R. L. Stoneburner. (2003). Behavior and communication change in reducing HIV: Is Uganda unique? *African Journal of AIDS Research* 2 (1): 9–21.

Lubulwa, H. (2014). Wife case: Bukenya admits paying Shs110m. *Daily Monitor* [Kampala, Uganda], June 19.

Lurie, M. N., and S. Rosenthal. (2010). Concurrent partnerships as a driver of the HIV epidemic in sub-Saharan Africa? The evidence is limited. *AIDS and Behavior* 14 (1): 17–24.

Lurie, P., and S. M. Wolfe. (1997). Unethical trials of interventions to reduce perinatal transmission of the human immunodeficiency virus in developing countries. *New England Journal of Medicine* 337 (12): 853–56.

Lutz, C. A. (1988). *Unnatural Emotions: Everyday Sentiments on a Micronesian Atoll and Their Challenge to Western Theory*. Chicago: University of Chicago Press.

Lutz, C. A., and L. Abu-Lughod, eds. (1990). *Language and the Politics of Emotion*. Cambridge: Cambridge University Press.

Lyons, M. (1997). Point of view: Perspectives on AIDS in Uganda. In Bond, Kreniske, Susser, and Vincent 1997:131–48.

———. (1999). Medicine and morality: A review of responses to sexually transmitted diseases in Uganda in the twentieth century. In Setel, Lewis, and Lyons 1999:97–118.

Lystra, K. (1989). *Searching the Heart: Women, Men, and Romantic Love in Nineteenth-Century America*. New York: Oxford University Press.

Magubane, B. (1976). The evolution of the class structure in Africa. In *The Political Economy of Contemporary Africa*, edited by Peter C. W. Gutkind and Immanuel Wallerstein, 173–75. Beverly Hills, CA: Sage.

Mah, T. K., and D. T. Halperin. (2008). Concurrent sexual partnerships and the HIV epidemics in Africa: Evidence to move forward. *AIDS and Behavior* 14 (1): 11–16.

Mair, L. P. (1969). *African Marriage and Social Change*. London: Frank Cass.

Malinowski, B. (1922). *Argonauts of the Western Pacific: An Account of Native Enterprise and Adventure in the Archipelagoes of Melanesian New Guinea*. New York: Dutton.

———. (1929). *The Sexual Life of Savages in North-Western Melanesia: An Ethnographic Account of Courtship, Marriage and Family Life among the Natives of the Trobriand Islands, British New Guinea*. New York: Halcyon House.

Malkki, L. H. (1995). *Purity and Exile: Violence, Memory, and National Cosmology among Hutu Refugees in Tanzania.* Chicago: University of Chicago Press.

Mamdani, M. (1976). *Politics and Class Formation in Uganda.* New York: Monthly Review Press.

Mann, K. (1994). The historical roots and cultural logics of outside marriage in colonial Lagos. In Bledsoe and Pison 1994, 167–93.

Martínez Pérez, G., and H. Namulondo. (2011). Elongation of labia minora in Uganda: Including Baganda men in a risk reduction education programme. *Culture, Health & Sexuality* 13 (1): 45–57.

Mbire-Barungi, B. (1999). Ugandan feminism: Political rhetoric or reality? *Women's Studies International Forum* 22 (4): 435–39.

Mbiti, J. S. (1973). *Love and Marriage in Africa.* London: Longman.

Mbulaiteye, S., C. Mahe, J. Whitworth, A. Ruberantwari, J. Nakiyingi, A. Ojwiya, and A. Kamali. (2002). Declining HIV-1 incidence and associated prevalence over ten years in a rural population in south-west Uganda: A cohort study. *Lancet* 360:41–46.

McCulloch, J. (2000). *Black Peril, White Virtue: Sexual Crime in Southern Rhodesia, 1902–1935.* Bloomington: Indiana University Press.

McGrath, J. W., C. B. Rwabukwali, D. A. Schumann, J. Pearson-Marks, S. Nakayima, B. Namande, L. Nakyobe, and R. Makusa. (1993). Anthropology and AIDS: The cultural context of sexual risk behaviour among urban Baganda women in Kampala, Uganda. *Social Science and Medicine* 36 (4): 429–39.

Mead, M. (1928). *Coming of Age in Samoa: a Psychological Study of Primitive Youth for Western Civilization.* New York: Morrow.

Meillassoux, C. (1981). *Maidens, Meal, and Money: Capitalism and the Domestic Community.* Cambridge: Cambridge University Press.

Merry, S. E. (2001). Spatial governmentality and the new urban social order: Controlling gender violence through law. *American Anthropologist* 103 (1): 16–29.

———. (2006). Transnational human rights and local activism: Mapping the middle. *American Anthropologist* 108 (1): 38–51.

Messer, E. (1997). Pluralist approaches to human rights. *Journal of Anthropological Research* 53 (3): 293–317.

Meyer-Weitz, A. (2005). Understanding fatalism in HIV/AIDS protection: The individual in dialogue with contextual factors. *African Journal of AIDS Research* 4 (2): 75–82.

Mills, D., and R. Ssewakiryanga. (2005). "No romance without finance": Commodities, masculinities, and relationships amongst Kampalan students. In *Readings in Gender in Africa,* edited by A. Cornwall, 90–95. Bloomington, IN: International African Institute, Indiana University Press.

Ministry of Health (MOH) [Uganda]. (2010). *The Status of the HIV/AIDS Epidemic in Uganda: The HIV/AIDS Epidemiological Surveillance Report, 2010.* Kampala, Uganda: Ministry of Health.

Ministry of Health (MOH) [Uganda] and ORC Macro. (2006). *Uganda HIV/AIDS Sero-behavioural Survey, 2004–2005.* Calverton, MD: Ministry of Health and ORC Macro.

Minkler, M., and N. Wallerstein, eds. (2008). *Community-Based Participatory Research for Health: From Process to Outcomes.* San Francisco: Jossey-Bass.

Mogwanja, M. (2005). *The Condom Shortage in Uganda: Statement by the Chair of the United Nations Theme Group on HIV/AIDS.* Kampala, Uganda: United Nations.

Moore, S. F. (1986). *Social Facts and Fabrication: "Customary" Law on Kilimanjaro, 1880–1980.* Cambridge: Cambridge University Press.

————. (1994). The ethnography of the present and the analysis of process. In *Assessing Cultural Anthropology*, edited by R. Borofsky, 362–76. New York: McGraw-Hill.

Morgan, D., C. Mahe, B. Mayanja, J. M. Okongo, R. Lubega, and J. A. Whitworth. (2002). HIV-1 infection in rural Africa: Is there a difference in median time to AIDS and survival compared with that in industrialized countries? *AIDS* 16(4):597-603.

Morris, H. F. (1967). Marriage law in Uganda: Sixty years of attempted reform. In *Family Law in Asia and Africa*, edited J. N. D. Anderson, 34–48. New York: Praeger.

Moynihan, D. P. (1965). *The Negro Family: The Case for National Action*. Washington, DC: US Department of Labor, Office of Policy Planning and Research.

MSF (Médecins Sans Frontiéres, or Doctors without Borders). (2005). Briefing note: The Second wave of the access crisis: Unaffordable AIDS drug prices again. *Doctors without Borders*, December 10. *www.doctorswithoutborders.org.*

Mudoola, D. M. (1974). *Chiefs and Political Action: The Case of the Busoga, 1900–1962*. PhD diss., Makerere University.

Mugyenyi, M. R. (1998). Towards the empowerment of women: A critique of NRM policies and programs. In Hansen and Twaddle 1998:133–44.

Muhangi, J. (1991). Women demand castration for men over sex abuse. *New Vision*, December 18.

Murphy, E. M., M. E. Greene, A. Mihailovic, and P. Olupot-Olupot. (2006). Was the "ABC" approach (abstinence, being faithful, using condoms) responsible for Uganda's decline in HIV? *PLoS Medicine* 3 (9): 1443–47.

Murray, S. O., and W. Roscoe, eds. (1998). *Boy-Wives and Female Husbands: Studies of African Homosexualities*. New York: St. Martin's Press.

Musere, J. (1990). *African Sleeping Sickness: Political Ecology, Colonialism, and Control in Uganda*. Lewiston, NY: Mellen Press.

Museveni, Y. (1992). *What Is Africa's Problem? Speeches and Writings on Africa*. Kampala, Uganda: MRM Publications.

————. (1995). Opening speech at the Ninth International Conference on AIDS and STDs in Africa, Kampala, Uganda, December.

Musiga, A., and A. Okanya. (2010). Activists challenge polygamy in court. *New Vision*, February 18. *www.newvision.co.ug.*

Musisi, N. B. (1991). Women, "elite polygyny," and Buganda state formation. *Signs* 16 (4): 757–86.

————. (2002). Politics of perception or perception as politics? Colonial and missionary representations of Baganda women, 1900–1945. In *Women in African Colonial Histories*, edited by J. Allman, S. Geiger, and N. Musisi, 95–115. Bloomington: University of Indiana Press.

Mutibwa, P. M. (1992). *Uganda since Independence: A Story of Unfulfilled Hopes*. New York: Africa World Press.

Mutongi, K. (2000). "Dear Dolly's" advice: Representations of youth, courtship, and sexualities in Africa, 1960–1980. *International Journal of African Historical Studies* 33 (1): 1–25.

Mutunga, K. (2012). When marriage issues breed national political debate. *Daily Monitor* [Kampala, Uganda], December 9. *www.monitor.co.ug.*

Muyinda, H., J. Nakuya, R. Pool, and J. Whitworth. (2003). Harnessing the *senga* institution of adolescent sex education for the control of HIV and STDs in rural Uganda. *AIDS Care: Psychological and Socio-medical Aspects of AIDS/HIV* 15 (2): 159–67.

Muyiyi, S. (2009). UNICEF book supports teen homosexuality. *New Vision* [Kampala, Uganda], April 5. *www.newvision.co.ug.*

Mwenda, K. K. (2006). Labia elongation under African customary law: A violation of women's rights? *International Journal of Human Rights* 10 (4): 341–57.

Nabwiso-Bulima, W. F. (1967). The evolution of the Kyabazingaship of Busoga. *Uganda Journal* 31 (1): 89–99.

Nalugo, M. (2009). Homosexuality threat to Ugandans—activists. *Daily Monitor* [Kampala, Uganda], April 24.

Namubiru, L. (2013). You can get off that sexual network. *New Vision* [Kampala, Uganda], February 25. *www.newvision.co.ug.*

Nayenga, P. F. B. (1976). *An Economic History of the Lacustrine States of Basoga, Uganda, 1750–1939.* PhD diss., University of Michigan.

Neema, S., N. Musisi, and R. Kibombo. (2004). *Adolescent Sexual and Reproductive Health in Uganda: A Synthesis of Research Evidence.* Occasional Report 14. New York: Guttmacher Institute.

New Vision. (2008). New domestic relations bill is acceptable to most Ugandans. *New Vision,* July 13. *www.newvision.co.ug.*

Ngokwey, N. (1988). Pluralistic etiological systems in their social context: A Brazilian case study; In memory of James S. Coleman. *Social Science and Medicine* 26 (8): 793–802.

Nguyen, V.-K. (2004). Antiretroviral globalism, bio-politics, and therapeutic citizenship. In Ong and Collier 2004, 124–44.

———. (2010). *The Republic of Therapy: Triage and Sovereignty in West Africa's Time of AIDS.* Durham, NC: Duke University Press.

Nichter, M. (2008). *Global Health: Why Cultural Perceptions, Social Representations, and Bio-politics Matter.* Tucson: University of Arizona Press.

Niehaus, I. (2005). Malicious whites, greedy women, and virtuous volunteers: Negotiating social relations through clinical trial narratives in South Africa. *Medical Anthropology Quarterly* 27 (1): 103–20.

Ntozi, J. P., I. Najjumba, F. Ahimbisibwe, N. Ayiga, and J. Odwee. (2003). Has the HIV/AIDS epidemic changed sexual behaviour of high risk groups in Uganda? *African Health Sciences* 3:107–16.

Obbo, C. (1980). *African Women: Their Struggle for Economic Independence.* London: Zed Press.

———. (1987). The old and the new in East African elite marriages. In *Transformations of African Marriage,* edited by D. Parkin and D. Nyamwaya, 263–80. Manchester, UK: Manchester University Press.

———. (1991). Women, children and a "living age." In Hansen and Twaddle 1991:98–113.

———. (1993). HIV transmission through social and geographical networks in Uganda. *Social Science and Medicine* 36 (7): 949–55.

———. (1995). Gender, age and class: Discourses on HIV transmission and control in Uganda. In ten Brummelhuis and G. Herdt 1995:79–96.

Oberman, M. (2001). Girls in the master's house: Of protection, patriarchy and the potential for using the master's tools to reconfigure statutory rape law. *DePaul Law Review* 50:799–826.

Odem, M. E. (1995). *Delinquent Daughters: Protecting and Policing Adolescent Female Sexuality in the United States, 1885–1920.* Chapel Hill: University of North Carolina Press.

Okero, F. A., E. Aceng, E. Madraa, E. Namagala, and J. Serutoke. (2003). *Scaling Up Antiretroviral Therapy: Experience in Uganda.* Geneva, Switzerland: World Health Organization.

Okurut, M. K. (1998). Matembe: "Castration brigade" takes charge. *Daily Monitor* [Kampala, Uganda], July 31.

Olsen, F. (1984). Statutory rape: A feminist critique of rights analysis. *Texas Law Review* 63:387–432.

Ong, A., and S. J. Collier. (2004). *Global Assemblages: Technology, Politics, and Ethics as Anthropological Problems*. Malden, MA: Blackwell.

Oppong, J., and E. Kalipeni. (2004). Perceptions and misperceptions of AIDS in Africa. In Kalipeni, Craddock, Oppong, and Ghosh 2004, 47–57.

Orley, J. H. (1970). *Culture and Mental Illness: A Study from Uganda*. Nairobi, Kenya: East African Publishing House.

Ortner, S. (1984). Theory in anthropology since the sixties. *Comparative Studies in Society and History* 26 (1): 126–66.

———. (1995). Resistance and the problem of ethnographic refusal. *Comparative Studies in Society and History* 37 (1): 173–93.

Packard, R. M., and P. Epstein. (1991). Epidemiologists, social scientists, and the structure of medical research on AIDS in Africa. *Social Science and Medicine* 33 (7): 771–94.

Padilla, M. (2007). *Caribbean Pleasure Industry: Tourism, Sexuality, and AIDS in the Dominican Republic*. Chicago: University of Chicago Press.

Padilla, M., J. S. Hirsch, M. Muñoz-Laboy, R. E. Sember, and R. G. Parker, eds. (2007). *Love and Globalization: Transformations of Intimacy in the Contemporary World*. Nashville: Vanderbilt University Press.

Parikh, S. (2004). Sugar daddies and sexual citizenship in Uganda: Rethinking third-wave feminism. *Black Renaissance/Renaissance Noir* 6 (1): 82–107.

———. (2005). From auntie to disco: The bifurcation of risk and pleasure in sex education in Uganda. In *Sex in Development: Science, Sexuality, and Morality in Global Perspective*, edited by V. Adams and S. L. Pigg, 125–58. Durham, NC: Duke University Press.

———. (2007). The political economy of marriage and HIV: The ABC approach, "safe infidelity," and managing moral risk in Uganda. *American Journal of Public Health* 97 (7): 1198–1208.

———. (2009). Going public: Modern wives, men's infidelity, and marriage in East-Central Uganda. In *The Secret: Love, Marriage, and HIV*, by J. S. Hirsch, H. Wardlow, D. J. Smith, H. M. Phinney, S. Parikh, and C. A. Nathanson, 168–96. Nashville: Vanderbilt University Press.

Park, P. (1993). What is participatory research? A theoretical and methodological perspective. In *Voices of Change: Participatory Research in Canada and the United States*, edited by P. Park, M. Brydon-Miller, B. Hall, and T. Jackson, 1–20. Toronto: Ontario Institute for Studies in Education.

Parker, R. G. (2001). Sexuality, culture, and power in HIV/AIDS research. *Annual Review of Anthropology* 30: 163–79.

———. (2002). The Global HIV/AIDS pandemic, structural inequalities and the politics of international health. *American Journal of Public Health* 92 (3): 343–47.

Parker R. G., and P. Aggleton. (2003). HIV and AIDS-related stigma and discrimination: A conceptual framework and implications for action. *Social Science and Medicine* 57:13–24.

Parker R. G., G. Herdt, and M. Carballo. (1991). Sexual culture, HIV transmission, and AIDS research. *Journal of Sex Research* 28 (1): 77–98.

Parker, R. G., and D. Easton. (1998). Sexuality, culture, and political economy: Recent developments in anthropological and cross-cultural sex research. *Annual Review of Sex Research* 9 (1): 1–19.

Parker, R. G., D. Easton, and C. H. Klein. (2000). Structural barriers and facilitators in HIV prevention: A review of international research. *AIDS* 14:S22–S32.

Parker, R. G., and J. H. Gagnon, eds. (1995). *Conceiving Sexuality: Approaches to Sex Research in a Postmodern World*. New York: Routledge.

Parker R. G., G. Herdt, and M. Carballo. (1991). Sexual culture, HIV transmission, and AIDS research. *Journal of Sex Research* 28 (1): 77–98.

Parkhurst, J. O. (2001). The crisis of AIDS and the politics of response: The case of Uganda. *International Relations* 15 (6): 69–87.

———. (2002). The Ugandan success story? Evidence and claims of HIV-1 prevention. *Lancet* 360 (9326): 78–80.

Parkin, D., and D. Nyamwaya, eds. (1987). *Transformations of African Marriage*. Manchester, UK: Manchester University Press.

Parsons, T. (1999). *The African Rank-and-File*. Portsmouth, NH: Heinemann.

Patton, C. (1990). *Inventing AIDS*. New York: Routledge.

———. (1996). *Fatal Advice: How Safe-Sex Education Went Wrong*. Durham, NC: Duke University Press.

———. (1997). From nation to family: Containing African AIDS. In Lancaster and di Leonardo 1997:279–90.

———. (2002). *Globalizing AIDS*. Minneapolis: University of Minnesota Press.

Paxson, H. (2002). Rationalizing sex: Family planning and the making of modern lovers in urban Greece. *American Ethnologist* 29 (2): 307–34.

Peterson, D. R. (2006). Morality plays: Marriage, church courts, and colonial agency in central Tanganyika, ca. 1876–1928. *American Historical Review* 111 (4): 983–1010.

———. (2012). *Ethnic Patriotism and the East African Revival: A History of Dissent, c. 1935–1972*. Cambridge: Cambridge University Press.

Petryna, A. (2002). *Life Exposed: Biological Citizens after Chernobyl*. Princeton, NJ: Princeton University Press.

———. (2009). *When Experiments Travel: Clinical Trials and the Global Search for Human Subjects*. Princeton, NJ: Princeton University Press.

Pfeiffer, J. (2004). Condom social marketing, Pentecostalism, and structural adjustment in Mozambique: A clash of AIDS prevention messages. *Medical Anthropology Quarterly* 18 (1): 77–103.

Phillips, A., ed. (1953). *Survey of African Marriage and Family Life*. New York: Oxford University Press.

Philpott, A., W. Knerr, and D. Maher. (2006). Promoting protection and pleasure: Amplifying the effectiveness of barriers against sexually transmitted infections and pregnancy. *Lancet* 368 (9551): 2028–31.

Phinney, H. (2008). "Rice is essential but tiresome; you should get some noodles": Doi Moi and the political economy of men's extramarital sexual relations and marital HIV risk in Hanoi, Vietnam. *American Journal of Public Health* 98 (4): 650–60.

Pickering, H., M. Okongo, K. Bwanika, B. Nnalusiba, and J. Whitworth. (1996). Sexual mixing patterns in Uganda: Small-time urban/rural traders. *AIDS* 10 (5): 533–36.

———. (1997). Sexual networks in Uganda: Casual and commercial sex in a trading town. *AIDS Care* 9 (2): 199–208.

Pigg, S. L. (2002). Too bold, too hot: Crossing "culture" in AIDS prevention in Nepal. In *New Horizons in Medical Anthropology: Essays in Honour of Charles Leslie*, edited by M. Nichter and M. Lock, 58–80. New York: Routledge.

Piot, C. (1999). *Remotely Global: Village Modernity in West Africa*. Chicago: University of Chicago Press.

Piot, P., R. Greener, and S. Russell. (2007). Squaring the circle: AIDS, poverty, and human development. *PLoS Medicine* 4 (10): e314.

Pirouet, M. L. (1991). Human rights issues in Museveni's Uganda. In Hansen and Twaddle 1992:197–207.

PlusNews. (2010). Uganda: Challenging culture in HIV campaigns. *PlusNews*, June 30. *www.plusnews.org*.

Population Reference Bureau. (2007). *2007 World Population Data Sheet*. Washington, DC: Population Reference Bureau. *www.prb.org*.

Porter, L., H. Lingxin, D. Bishai, D. Serwadda, M. J. Wawer, T. Lutalo, R. Gray, and the Rakai Project Team. (2004). HIV status and union dissolution in sub-Saharan Africa: The case of Rakai, Uganda. *Demography* 41 (3): 465–82.

Povinelli, E. A. (2006). *The Empire of Love: Toward a Theory of Intimacy, Genealogy, and Carnality*. Durham, NC: Duke University Press.

Powe, B. (1997). Cancer fatalism: Spiritual perspectives. *Journal of Religion and Health* 36 (2): 135–44.

Prince, R. J. (2014). Situating health and the public in Africa: Historical and anthropological perspectives. In *Making and Unmaking Public Health in Africa: Ethnographic and Historical Perspectives*, edited by R. J. Prince and R. Marsland. Athens: Ohio University Press.

Putzel, J. (2004). The politics of action on AIDS: A case study of Uganda. *Public Administration and Development* 24 (1): 19–30.

Radcliffe-Brown, A. R., and D. Forde, eds. (1950). *African Systems of Kinship and Marriage*. London: Oxford University Press.

Radway, J. A. (1984). *Reading Romance: Women, Patriarchy, and Popular Literature*. Chapel Hill: University of North Carolina Press.

Ranger, T. (1983). The invention of tradition in colonial Africa. In *The Invention of Tradition*, edited by E. Hobsbawm and T. Ranger, 211–61. New York: Cambridge University Press.

Rebhun, L. A. (1999). *The Heart Is Unknown Country: Love in the Changing Economy of Northeast Brazil*. Stanford, CA: Stanford University Press.

Redfield, P. (2010). The verge of crisis: Doctors Without Borders in Uganda. In *Contemporary States of Emergency: The Politics of Military and Humanitarian Interventions*, edited by D. Fassin and M. Pandolfi, 173–95. Brooklyn, NY: Zone Books.

Reinharz, S. (1992). *Feminist Methods in Social Research*. New York: Oxford University Press, New York.

Rice, Xan. (2011). Death by tabloid: Uganda's most infamous journalist makes no apologies. *Atlantic*, April 26, 18–20.

Richards, A. I. (1956). *Chisungu: A Girl's Initiation Ceremony among the Bemba of Northern Rhodesia*. London: Faber and Faber.

Rivkin-Fish, M. R. (2005). *Women's Health in Post-Soviet Russia: The Politics of Intervention*. Bloomington: Indiana University Press.

Robertson, A. F. (1978). *Community of Strangers: A Journal of Discovery in Uganda*. London: Scholar Press.

Robertson, S. (2002a). Age of consent law and the making of modern childhood in New York City, 1886–1921. *Journal of Social History* 35 (4): 781–98.

———. (2002b). Making right a girl's ruin: Working-class legal cultures and forced marriage in New York City, 1890–1950. *Journal of American Studies* 36 (2): 199–230.

Rödlach, A. (2006). *Witches, Westerners, and HIV: AIDS and Cultures of Blame in Africa*. Walnut Creek, CA: Left Coast Press.

Rofel, L. (1999). *Other Modernities: Gendered Yearnings in China after Socialism*. Berkeley: University of California Press.

Roscoe, J. (1911). *The Baganda: An Account of Their Native Customs and Beliefs*. London: Macmillan.

———. (1915). *The Northern Bantu, an Account of Some Central African Tribes of the Uganda Protectorate*. London: F. Cass.

———. (1922). *The Soul of Central Africa: A General Account of the Mackie Ethnological Expedition*. London: Cassell.

Rose, N., and C. Novas. (2004). Biological citizenship. In Ong and Collier 2004, 439–63.

Rose, T. (1994). *Black Noise: Rap Music and Black Culture in Contemporary America*. Hanover, NH: Wesleyan University Press.

Roseberry, W. (1988). Political economy. *Annual Review of Anthropology* 17:161–85.

Rothman, D. J. (2000). The shame of medical research. *New York Review of Books* 47 (19): 60–64.

Rouse, C. (2009). *Uncertain Suffering: Racial Health Care Disparities and Sickle Cell Disease*. Berkeley: University of California Press.

Rubin, G. (1992). Thinking sex: Notes for a radical theory of the politics of sexuality. In *Pleasure and Danger: Exploring Female Sexuality*, 2nd ed., edited by C. S. Vance, 267–93. London: Pandora.

Rushing, W. A. (1995). *The AIDS Epidemic: Social Dimensions of an Infectious Disease*. Boulder, CO: Westview Press.

Ryan, W. (1976). *Blaming the Victim*. New York: Vintage.

Sacks, K. (1974). Engels revisited: Women, the organization of production, and private property. In *Woman, Culture and Society*, edited by M. Z. Rosaldo and L. Lamphere, 201–22. Stanford, CA: Stanford University Press.

Schapera, I. (1941). *Married Life in an African Tribe*. New York: Sheridan House.

Scheier, R. (2003). Teaching safe sex, Ugandan-style: "Aunts" who used to join couples on their wedding nights, now dispense health advice. *Boston Globe*, October 28. *www.boston.com*.

Scheper-Hughes, N. (1994). An essay: AIDS and the social body. *Social Science and Medicine* 39 (7): 991–1003.

Scherz, C. (2014). *Having People, Having Heart: Charity, Sustainable Development, and Problems of Dependence in Central Uganda*. Chicago: University of Chicago Press.

Schlegel, A, and R. Eloul. (1988). Marriage transactions: Labor, property, status. *American Anthropologist* 90:291–309.

Schmidt, E. (1990). Negotiated spaces and contested terrain: Men, women and the law in colonial Zimbabwe, 1890–1939. *Journal of Southern African Studies* 14 (4): 622–48.

Schoen, J. (2005). *Choice and Coercion: Birth Control, Sterilization, and Abortion in Public Health and Welfare*. Chapel Hill: University of North Carolina Press.

Schoepf, B. G. (1988). Women, AIDS, and economic crisis in central Africa. *Canadian Journal of African Studies* 22 (3): 625–44.

———. (1992). Women at risk: Case studies from Zaire. In Herdt and Lindenbaum 1992:259–86.

———. (1993). AIDS action-research with women in Kinshasa, Zaire. *Social Science and Medicine* 37 (11): 1401–13.

———. (1995). Culture, sex research and AIDS prevention in Africa. In ten Brummelhuis and Herdt 1995:29–52.

————. (1997). AIDS, gender, and sexuality during Africa's economic crisis. In *African Feminism: The Politics of Survival in Sub-Saharan Africa*, edited by G. Mikell, 310–32. Philadelphia: University of Pennsylvania Press.

————. (2003). Uganda: Lessons for AIDS control in Africa. *Review of African Political Economy* 30:553–72.

Scorgie, F. (2002). Virginity testing and the politics of sexual responsibility: Implications for AIDS intervention. *African Studies* 61 (1): 55–75.

Scott, J. C. (1985). *Weapons of the Weak: Everyday Forms of Peasant Resistance*. New Haven, CT: Yale University Press.

Serwadda, D., R. Mugerwa, N. K. Sewankambo, A. Lwegaba, J. W. Carswell, G. B. Kirya, et al. (1985). "Slim disease": A new disease in Uganda and its association with HTLV-III infection. *Lancet* 2 (8460): 849–52.

Serwadda, D., M. J. Wawer, S. D. Musgrave, N. K. Sewankambo, J. E. Kaplan, and R. Gray. (1992). HIV risk factors in three geographic strata of rural Rakai District, Uganda. *AIDS* 6: 983–89.

Setel, P. W. (1999). *A Plague of Paradoxes: AIDS, Culture, and Demography in Northern Tanzania*. Chicago: University of Chicago Press.

Setel, P. W., M. Lewis, and M. Lyons (1999). *Histories of Sexually Transmitted Diseases and HIV/AIDS in Sub-Saharan Africa*. Westport, CT: Greenwood Press.

Shafer, L. A., S. Biraro, J. Nakiyingi-Miiro, A. Kamali, D. Ssematimba, J. Ouma, et al. (2008). HIV prevalence and incidence are no longer falling in southwest Uganda: Evidence from a rural population cohort, 1989–2005. *AIDS* 22 (13): 1641–49.

Sharp, P., and B. Hahn. (2011). Origins of HIV and the AIDS pandemic. *Cold Spring Harbor Perspectives in Medicine* 1 (1): 1–22.

Shell-Duncan, B. (2008). From health to human rights: Female genital cutting and the politics of intervention. *American Anthropologist* 110 (2): 225–63.

Shuman, A. (1986). *Storytelling Rights: The Uses of Oral and Written Texts by Urban Adolescents*. Cambridge: Cambridge University Press.

Silberschmidt, M., and V. Rasch. (2000). Adolescent girls with illegally induced abortions in Dar es Salaam: The discrepancy between sexual behaviour and lack of access to contraception. *Reproductive Health Matters* 8 (15): 52–62.

Simmons, C. (1979). Companionate marriage and the lesbian threat. *Frontiers* 4 (3): 54–59.

Simpson, V. L. (2009). Africa-bound pope says condoms increase AIDS. *San Francisco Chronicle*, March 18. *www.sfgate.com*.

Singer, M. (1997). Forging a political economy of AIDS. In *The Political Economy of AIDS*, edited by M. Singer, 131–48. Amityville, NY: Baywood Publishing.

Singh, S., J. E. Darroch, and A. Bankole. (2003). *A, B and C in Uganda: The Roles of Abstinence, Monogamy and Condom Use in HIV Decline*. Occasional Report 9. New York: Guttmacher Institute.

Skolnik, A. (1991). *Embattled Paradise: The American Family in an Age of Uncertainty*. New York: Basic Books.

Slutkin, G., J. Chin, D. Tarantola, and J. Man. (1988). *Sentinel Surveillance for HIV Infection: A Method to Monitor HIV Infection Trends in Population Groups*. WHO/GPA/DIR/88.8. Geneva: World Health Organization.

Small, M. L., D. J. Harding, and M. Lamont. (2010). Reconsidering culture and poverty. *Annals of the Academy of Political and Social Science* 629 (1): 6–27.

Smith, D. J. (2006). Cell phones, social inequality, and contemporary culture in southeastern Nigeria. *Canadian Journal of African Studies* 40 (3): 496–523.

———. (2007). Modern marriage, extramarital sex, and HIV risk in southeastern Nigeria. *American Journal of Public Health* 97 (6): 997–1005.

———. (2014). *AIDS Doesn't Show Its Face: Inequality, Morality, and Social Change in Nigeria.* Chicago: University of Chicago Press.

Smith, J. H. (2008). *Bewitching Development: Witchcraft and the Reinvention of Development in Neoliberal Kenya.* Chicago: University of Chicago Press.

Smith, L. C., K. Lucas, and C. Latkin. (1999). Rumor and gossip: Social discourse on HIV and AIDS. *Anthropology & Medicine* 6 (1): 121–31.

Sobo, E. J. (1995). *Choosing Unsafe Sex: AIDS-Risk Denial among Disadvantaged Women.* Philadelphia: University of Pennsylvania Press.

Sontag, S. (1988). *AIDS and Its Metaphors.* New York: Farrar, Straus and Giroux.

Spear, T., and I. N. Kimambo, eds. (1999). *East African Expressions of Christianity.* Athens: Ohio University Press.

Speke, J. H. (1863). *Journal of the Discovery of the Source of the Nile.* Edinburgh: Blackwood.

Spivak, G. (1988). Can the subaltern speak? In *Marxism and the Interpretation of Culture,* edited by C. Nelson and L. Grossberg, 271–13. Champaign: University of Illinois Press.

Ssejoba, E. (2004). Museveni condemns condom distribution to pupils. *New Vision* [Kampala, Uganda]. May 17.

Stack, C. (1974). *All Our Kin.* New York: Harper and Row.

Stadler, J., and E. Saethre. (2010). Rumours about blood and reimbursements in a microbicide gel trial. *African Journal of AIDS Research* 9 (4): 345–53.

Stambach, A. (2000). *Lessons from Mount Kilimanjaro: Schooling, Community, and Gender in East Africa.* New York: Routledge.

Stephen, L. (1999). The construction of indigenous suspects: Militarization and the gendered and ethnic dynamics of human rights abuses in Southern Mexico. *American Ethnologist* 26 (4): 822–42.

Stewart, K. (2000). Toward a historical perspective on sexuality in Uganda: The reproductive lifeline technique for grandmothers and their daughters. *Africa Today* 47 (3–4): 123–48.

Stillwaggon, E. (2005). *AIDS and the Ecology of Poverty.* New York: Oxford University Press.

Stoeltje, B. J. (2002). Introduction to women, language, and law in Africa II: Gender and relations of power. *Africa Today* 49 (2): vii–xiv.

Stoneburner, R. L., and D. Low-Beer. (2004). Population-level HIV declines and behavioral risk avoidance in Uganda. *Science* 302:714–18.

Summers, C. (2000). Whips and women: Forcing change in eastern Uganda during the 1920s. Paper presented in the "Development and Change in East Africa" seminar, University of Nairobi, Kenya.

———. (2002). *Colonial Lessons: Africans' Education in Southern Rhodesia, 1918–1940.* Portsmouth, NH: Heinemann Press.

Susser, I. (2009). *AIDS, Sex, and Culture: Global Politics and Survival in Southern Africa.* Malden, MA: Wiley-Blackwell.

Tamale, S. (1999). *When Hens Begin to Crow: Gender and Parliamentary Politics in Uganda.* Boulder, CO: Westview Press.

———. (2001). How old is old enough? Defilement law and the age of consent in Uganda. *East African Journal of Peace and Human Rights* 7 (1): 82–101.

———. (2006). Eroticism, sensuality and "women's secrets" among the Baganda: A critical analysis. *IDS Bulletin* 37 (5): 89–97.

———. (2007). Out of the closet: Unveiling sexuality discourses in Uganda. In *Africa after Gender?*, edited by C. M. Cole, T. Manuh, and S. F. Miescher, 17–29. Bloomington: Indiana University Press.

Taussig, M. (1999). *Defacement: Public Secrecy and the Labor of the Negative.* Stanford, CA: Stanford University Press.

Thomas, L. M. (2003). *Politics of the Womb: Women, Reproduction, and the State in Kenya.* Berkeley: University of California Press.

Thomas, L. M., and J. Cole. (2009). Introduction: Thinking through love in Africa. In Cole and Thomas 2009:1–30.

Thompson, S. (1984). Search for tomorrow: On feminism and the reconstruction of teen romance. In Vance 1992:350–85.

———. (1995). *Going All the Way: Teenage Girls' Tales of Sex, Romance, and Pregnancy.* New York: Hill and Wang.

Thornton, R. J. (2008). *Unimagined Community: Sex, Networks, and AIDS in Uganda and South Africa.* Berkeley: University of California Press.

Ticktin, M. (2005). Policing and humanitarianism in France: Immigration and the turn to law as state of exception. *Interventions: International Journal of Postcolonial Studies* 7 (3) 2005: 347–68.

Tolman, D. L. (1994). Doing desire: Adolescent girls' struggles with/for sexuality. *Gender & Society* 8 (3): 324–42.

Treichler, P. A. (1987). AIDS, homophobia and biomedical discourse: An epidemic of signification. *Cultural Studies* 1 (3): 263–305.

———. (1999). *How to Have Theory in an Epidemic: Cultural Chronicles of AIDS.* Durham, NC: Duke University Press.

Trickett, E., S. Beehler, C. Deutsch, L. W. Green, P. Hawe, K. McLeroy, et al. (2011). Advancing the science of community-level interventions. *American Journal of Public Health* 101 (8): 1410–19.

Tripp, A. M. (1994). Gender, political participation and the transformation of associational life in Uganda and Tanzania. *African Studies Review* 37 (1): 107–21.

———. (2000). *Women and Politics in Uganda.* Madison: University of Wisconsin Press.

Tuma, T. (1980). *Building a Ugandan Church: African Participation in Church Growth and Expansion in Busoga, 1891–1940.* Nairobi: Kenya Literature Bureau.

Turner, P. A. (1993). *I Heard It through the Grapevine: Rumor in African-American Culture.* Berkeley: University of California Press.

Twaddle, M. (1993). *Kakungulu and the Creation of Uganda, 1868–1928.* Athens: Ohio University Press.

UAC (Uganda AIDS Commission). (1993). The multi-sectoral approach to AIDS control in Uganda: Executive summary. Kampala: UAC. *hivhealthclearinghouse.unesco.org.*

———. (1996). 1996 annual report. Kampala: UAC.

———. (2012). *Global AIDS Response Progress Report: Country Progress Report, Uganda.* Kampala: UAC. *www.unaids.org.*

———. (2014). *HIV and AIDS Uganda Country Progress Report; 2013.* Kampala: UAC. *www.unaids.org.*

UBOS (Uganda Bureau of Statistics). (1996). *Uganda—Demographic and Health Survey 1995.* Kampala: UBOS. *www.ubos.org.*

————. (2006). *2002 Uganda Population and Housing Census, Analytic Report.* Kampala: UBOS. *www.ubos.org.*

————. (2010). *Uganda National Household Survey 2009/2010.* Kampala: UBOS *www.ubos. org.*

————. (2014). *National Population and Housing Census 2014.* Kampala: UBOS. *www.ubos. org.*

UBOS and ICF International. (2012). *Uganda Demographic and Health Survey 2011.* Kampala: UBS; Calverton, MD: ICF International. *www.ubos.org.*

UNAIDS. (2008). *Report on the Global AIDS Epidemic: Executive Summary.* Geneva: Joint United Nations Programme on HIV/AIDS (UNAIDS). *www.unaids.org.*

————. (2012). *Global Report: UNAIDS Report on the Global Aids Epidemic 2012.* Geneva: Joint United Nations Programme on HIV/AIDS (UNAIDS). *www.unaids.org.*

————. (2013). *Methodology: Understanding the HIV Estimates.* Geneva: Joint United Nations Programme on HIV/AIDS (UNAIDS). *www.unaids.org.*

Valentine, C. A. (1968). *Culture and Poverty: Critique and Counter-Proposals.* Chicago: University of Chicago Press.

Vance, C. S. (1984a). Introduction. In Vance 1984b:1–27.

————, ed. (1984b). *Pleasure and Danger: Exploring Female Sexuality.* Boston: Routledge and Kegan Paul.

Vansina, J. (1961). *Oral Tradition: A Study in Historical Methodology.* London: Routledge and Kegan Paul.

————. (1985). *Oral Tradition as History.* Madison: University of Wisconsin Press.

Vaughan, M. (1991). *Curing Their Ills: Colonial Power and African Illness.* Stanford, CA: Stanford University Press.

Vincent, J. (1971). *African Elite: The Big Men of a Small Town.* New York: Columbia University Press.

————. (1991). Engaging historicism. In *Recapturing Anthropology: Working in the Present*, edited by R. G. Fox, 45–58. Santa Fe, NM: School for American Research Press.

Wakabi, W. (2008). New strategies sought in Uganda as HIV infections rise. *Lancet* 8 (5): 285.

————. (2009). Condoms still contentious in Uganda's struggle over AIDS. *Lancet* 367 (9520): 1387–88.

Wardlow, H. (2006). *Wayward Women: Sexuality and Agency in a New Guinea Society.* Berkeley: University of California Press.

————. (2007). Men's extramarital sexuality in rural Papua New Guinea. *American Journal of Public Health* 97 (6): 1006–14.

Wardlow, H., and J. S. Hirsch. (2006). Introduction. In *Modern Loves: The Anthropology of Romantic Courtship and Companionate Marriage*, edited by J. S. Hirsch and H. Wardlow, 1–34. Ann Arbor: University of Michigan Press.

Warner, M. (1999). *The Trouble with Normal: Sex, Politics, and the Ethics of Queer Life.* Cambridge, MA: Harvard University Press.

————. (2002). *Publics and Counterpublics.* Brooklyn, NY: Zone Books.

Washington, H. (2006). *Medical Apartheid: The Dark History of Medical Experimentation on Black Americans from Colonial Times to the Present.* New York: Doubleday.

Watney, S. (1989). Missionary positions: AIDS, "Africa," and race. *Critical Quarterly* 31 (3): 45–62.

Wawer, M. J., D. Serwadda, R. H. Gray, N. K. Sewankambo, C. Li, F. Nalugoda, T. Lutalo, and J. K. Konde-Lule. (1997). Trends in HIV-1 prevalence may not reflect trends in incidence in mature epidemics: Data from the Rakai population-based cohort, Uganda. *AIDS* 11 (8): 1023–30.

Wawer, M. J., N. K. Sewnakambo, S. Berkley, D. Serwadda, S. D. Musgrave, R. H. Gray, M. Musugara, R. Y. Stallings, and J. K. Konde-Lule. (1991). Incidence of HIV-1 infection in a rural region of Uganda. *British Medical Journal* 308 (6922):171–73.

Weeks, J. (1982). *Sex, Politics, and Society: The Regulation of Sexuality since 1800.* New York: Longman.

West, M. O. (2002). *The Rise of an African Middle Class: Colonial Zimbabwe, 1898–1965.* Bloomington: Indiana University Press.

White, L. (1990). *The Comforts of Home: Prostitution in Colonial Nairobi.* Chicago: University of Chicago Press.

White, L., S. F. Miescher, and D. W. Cohen, eds. (2001). *African Words, African Voices: Critical Practices in Oral History.* Bloomington: University of Indiana Press.

Whiting, B. B., and J. W. M. Whiting. (1975). *Children of Six Cultures: A Psychosocial Analysis.* Cambridge, MA: Harvard University Press.

WHO (World Health Organization). (2013). *Consolidated Guidelines on the Use of Antiretroviral Drugs for Treating and Preventing HIV Infection.* Geneva, Switzerland: World Health Organization. *www.who.int.*

Whyte, S. R. (1997). *Questioning Misfortune: The Pragmatics of Uncertainty in Eastern Uganda.* Cambridge: Cambridge University Press.

Whyte, S. R., M. A. Whyte, L. Meinert, and B. Kyaddondo. (2004). Treating AIDS: Dilemmas of unequal access in Uganda. *Journal of Social Aspects of HIV/AIDS Research Alliance* 1 (1):14–26.

Wilk, R. R., and L. C. Cliggett. (2007). *Economies and Cultures: Foundations of Economic Anthropology.* Boulder, CO: Westview Press.

Williams, R. (1991). The dream world of mass consumption. In *Rethinking Popular Culture,* edited by C. Mukerji and M. Schudson, 198–235. Berkeley: University of California Press.

Wolf, E. (1982). *Europe and the People without History.* Berkeley: University of California Press.

Worobey, M., M. Gemmel, D. E. Teuwen, T. Haselkorn, K. Kunstman, M. Bruce, J. J. Kabongo, R. M. Kalengayi. E. Van Marck, M. T. Gilbert, and S. M. Wolinsky. (2008). Direct evidence of extensive diversity of HIV-1 in Kinshasa by 1960. *Nature* 455 (7213): 661–64.

Yan, Y. (2005). The individual and transformation of bridewealth in rural north China. *Journal of the Royal Anthropological Institute* 11 (4): 637–58.

Index

Numbers in *italic* refer to figures; numbers in **bold** refer to tables.